Pediatric Pain Management

for Primary Care

2nd Edition

Editors

Joseph D. Tobias, MD, FAAP

Jayant K. Deshpande, MD, MPH, FAAP

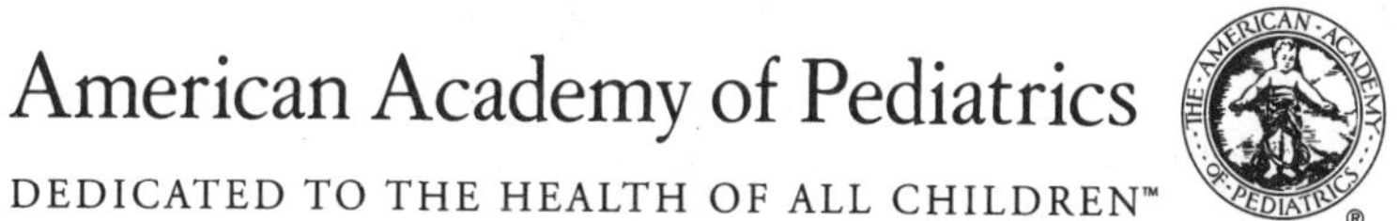

AAP Department of Marketing and Publications Staff

Maureen DeRosa
Director, Department of Marketing and Publications

Mark Grimes
Director, Division of Product Development

Diane E. Beausoleil
Senior Product Development Editor

Holly Kaminski
Coordinator, Product Development

Sandi King
Director, Division of Publishing and Production Services

Kate Larson
Manager, Editorial Services

Leesa Levin-Doroba
Manager, Print Production Services

Linda Diamond
Manager, Graphic Design

Jill Ferguson
Director, Division of Marketing and Sales

Linda Smessaert
Manager, Publication and Program Marketing

2nd edition
1st edition—©1996 Mosby-Yearbook, Inc.

Library of Congress Control Number: 2004101687
ISBN: 1-58110-133-3
MA0277

The recommendations in this publication do not indicate an exclusive course of treatment or serve as a standard of medical care. Variations, taking into account individual circumstances, may be appropriate.

Contributors

Chris L. Algren, RN, MSN, EdD
Vanderbilt University, Nashville, TN

John T. Algren, MD, FAAP
Professor of Anesthesiology and Pediatrics
Vice-Chair for Educational Affairs
Vanderbilt University Medical Center, Nashville, TN

Kanwaljeet J. S. Anand, MBBS, DPhil, FAAP, FCCM, FRCPCH
Morris and Hettie Oakley Endowed Chair of Critical Care Medicine
Professor of Pediatrics, Anesthesiology, Pharmacology, and Neurobiology
University of Arkansas College of Medicine, Little Rock
Director, Pain Neurobiology Laboratory
Arkansas Children's Hospital Research Institute, Little Rock

John W. Berkenbosch, MD, FAAP
Associate Professor
Department of Child Health, Division of Pediatric Critical Care
Director, Pediatric Procedural Sedation Service
University of Missouri, Columbia

Jayant K. Deshpande, MD, MPH, FAAP
Professor of Anesthesiology and Pediatrics
Departments of Anesthesiology and Pediatrics
Vanderbilt Children's Hospital, Nashville, TN

Stephen R. Hayes, MD, FAAP
Assistant Professor, Anesthesiology and Pediatrics
Vanderbilt University Medical Center, Nashville, TN
Director, Pediatric Pain Services
Vanderbilt Children's Hospital, Nashville, TN

Constance S. Houck, MD, FAAP
Senior Associate in Perioperative Anesthesia
Children's Hospital, Boston, MA
Assistant Professor of Anesthesia
Harvard Medical School, Boston, MA

Lynne Maxwell, MD, FAAP
Associate Professor of Anesthesiology
University of Pennsylvania
The Children's Hospital of Philadelphia

Allison Kinder Ross, MD
Associate Professor of Pediatric Anesthesia
Associate Chief, Division of Pediatric Anesthesia and Critical Care Medicine
Duke University Medical Center, Durham, NC

Santhanam Suresh, MD, FAAP
Codirector, Pain Management Services
Children's Memorial Hospital, Chicago, IL
Associate Professor of Anesthesiology and Pediatrics
Feinberg School of Medicine, Northwestern University

Sally E. Tarbell, PhD
Associate Professor of Psychiatry and Behavioral Sciences
The Feinberg School of Medicine, Northwestern University
Children's Memorial Hospital, Chicago, IL

Joseph D. Tobias, MD, FAAP
Vice-Chair, Department of Anesthesiology
Chief, Division of Pediatric Anesthesiology/Pediatric Critical Care
Russell and Mary Shelden Chair of Pediatric Intensive Care Medicine
Professor of Anesthesiology and Pediatrics
University of Missouri, Columbia

Dedication

To Julie, my wife and best friend, for her unconditional love and support.

Joseph D. Tobias

Foreword

Albert Camus once said words to the effect that "perhaps we can never create a world where there are no suffering children, but we can create a world where there are fewer suffering children." At the heart of safe patient centered care is the relief of pain especially for infants and children who put their trust in those who provide medical care. Pain management is a key measure of quality in children's healthcare and addressing this problem requires specialized knowledge, skill, and most importantly a commitment to provide care as pain-free as possible for each child.

In their second edition, Drs Tobias and Deshpande and their colleagues have improved on an already excellent effort to address this important issue. Their handbook provides knowledge that, translated into practice, will benefit children across a wide range of pediatric situations. As pain becomes considered the "fifth" vital sign, this book is essential reading for health professionals caring for children.

Paul V. Miles, MD
Vice President, Director of Quality Improvement
and Practice Assessment
The American Board of Pediatrics, Inc.
Chapel Hill, NC

Preface

The treatment of pain in neonates, infants, and children of all ages has seen dramatic improvements over the past 25 years; however, there is still much work to be done. So much has changed since 1996 when we first published our text. With the significant changes that have occurred during the past 8 years, there has been a considerable revision of the initial text with the addition of 4 new chapters. These chapters focus on areas that now rightfully receive significant attention in the field of pediatric pain management including pharmacology; the issues of tolerance, dependency, and withdrawal with prolonged administration of sedative and analgesic agents; treatment of chronic pain; and the use of non-pharmacologic means in the treatment and prevention of pain.

Another change is that this revised edition is being published by the American Academy of Pediatrics. We are honored and delighted that the leader in the care of children has agreed to partner with us. We are also honored to have a group of accomplished physicians with significant clinical expertise and experience in the field collaborate in the creation of this text. Drs Maxwell, Suresh, and Tobias discuss the pharmacology of analgesic and sedative medications in Chapter 2. Many new medications and new applications of medications familiar to the practitioner can be used to reduce or eliminate pain in children. The past decade has provided pediatric anesthesia practitioners with significant experience with neuraxial blockade in children. Nearly 300 articles have been published on the use of regional anesthesia in children during this time. The chapters by Drs Tobias and Hays on spinal and caudal anesthesia and Dr Kinder Ross on peripheral regional blockade provide the reader with concise reviews of these subjects with practical guidelines for the applications of these techniques in infants and children of all ages. In Chapter 5, Dr Berkenbosch provides a review of the topic of treatment of procedure-related pain. The pediatric care provider increasingly is called on to care for the child who requires a procedure that may be painful, stressful, or both. The chapter provides a guide through the entire process including the pre-sedation evaluation, intraoperative monitoring, suggestions for medications depending on the type and duration of procedure, and post-procedure recovery and discharge parameters. From the near complete absence of awareness of the pain and anxiety suffered by children in the intensive care unit, critical care has evolved to include significant consideration and discussion regarding the pain management and sedation of critically ill patients. The Joint Commission even has identified pain as the "fifth vital sign" in the hospitalized patient. Dr Tobias discusses the challenges of accurate assessment and treatment of infants and children needing intensive care and outlines techniques for the provision of sedation and analgesia during critical illnesses. Specific issues of postoperative pain management can be perplexing and challenging. Children are expected to have pain after surgery. Often the health care provider may consider a child in pain "normal" and attribute a child's crying or suffering as "whining" or parental anxiety. However, proper and timely treatment of pain in the perioperative setting can reduce hospital stays and improve patient outcomes. In Chapter 8, Dr Tobias describes techniques to treat acute pain of various etiologies. Neonatal pain management has also evolved substantially. In Chapter 9, Dr Houck presents a review of the evolving biology of pain in infants and methods for managing pain in this population. Acute medical conditions may be associated with significant pain that is acute, chronic, or recurrent. Children suffer short-term and potentially long-term morbidity because of undertreated pain associated with an underlying illness. Chapter 10 addresses some of the more common medical conditions in children that may cause acute pain. Options for the evaluation of pain associated with medical illnesses and its treatment are reviewed. Recent interest has focused on alternatives to the pharmacologic treatment of pain and anxiety in children. Techniques such as distraction, psychological preparation and awareness, and other "nontraditional" methods may be extremely effective in children and also infants. Drs Algren and Algren have summarized these approaches in Chapter 11. The authors present an informative examination of the topic and provide specific and useful means for the non-pharmacologic approaches to pain management. In the final chapter, Drs Suresh and Tarbell tackle the subject of chronic pain in children and, in particular, children with cancer. This population presents a unique challenge because the pain that children with oncologic diseases suffer includes both acute, severe episodes of pain that may be short-lived as well as unresolving chronic pain. Untreated or undertreated pain in these children can be associated with major emotional problems, physical dysfunction, and long-term disability. The goal of therapy often is to improve the functioning of the child to the point that he or she is able to carry on activities of daily living near normal for age.

This book is a not meant to be an exhaustive treatise on pediatric pain. Rather, we have attempted to review the literature and incorporate it with our clinical experience into a practical approach to the challenging issue of pain management in pediatric patients. We hope to provide practical information to assist health care providers in preventing and treating pain in infants and children on a daily basis.

Joseph D. Tobias, MD, FAAP
Jayant K. Deshpande, MD, MPH, FAAP

Contents

1 Neurobiology of the Pain System 1
Kanwaljeet J. S. Anand, MBBS, DPhil, FAAP, FCCM, FRCPCH
Jayant K. Deshpande, MD, MPH, FAAP
Joseph D. Tobias, MD, FAAP

2 Sedatives and Analgesics: General Principles and Pharmacology 39
Lynne Maxwell, MD, FAAP
Santhanam Suresh, MD, FAAP
Joseph D. Tobias, MD, FAAP

3 Neuraxial Blockade: Epidural and Spinal Anesthesia/Analgesia 93
Stephen R. Hays, MD, FAAP
Joseph D. Tobias, MD, FAAP

4 Peripheral Regional Blockade 141
Allison Kinder Ross, MD
Santhanam Suresh, MD, FAAP

5 Managing Procedure-Related Pain and Anxiety 183
John W. Berkenbosch, MD, FAAP

6 Sedation in the Pediatric Intensive Care Unit 229
Joseph D. Tobias, MD, FAAP

7 Tolerance, Physical Dependency, and Withdrawal 289
Joseph D. Tobias, MD, FAAP

8 Acute and Postoperative Pain Management 321
Joseph D. Tobias, MD, FAAP

9 Neonatal Pain Management 357
Constance S. Houck, MD, FAAP

10 Treatment of Acute Pain Associated With Medical Illnesses 379
Stephen R. Hays, MD, FAAP
Jayant K. Deshpande, MD, MPH, FAAP
Joseph D. Tobias, MD, FAAP

11 Non-pharmacologic Techniques for the Management of Pediatric Pain 417
John T. Algren, MD, FAAP
Chris L. Algren, RN, MSN, EdD

12 Chronic and Cancer Pain Management 435
Santhanam Suresh, MD, FAAP
Sally E. Tarbell, PhD

Index 461

Chapter 1

Neurobiology of the Pain System

Kanwaljeet J. S. Anand, MBBS, DPhil, FAAP, FCCM, FRCPCH
Jayant K. Deshpande, MD, MPH, FAAP
Joseph D. Tobias, MD, FAAP

The Anatomy of Pain
Development of the Pain System
- Peripheral Pain Mechanisms
  - Cutaneous Receptors and Nerve Terminals
  - Sensory Neurons and Peripheral Nerves
  - The Long-term Effects of Early Tissue Injury
- Spinal Pain Mechanisms
  - Central Afferent Terminals
  - Spinal Nerve Tracts
  - Development of Descending Inhibitory Controls
- Supraspinal Pain Mechanisms
  - Development of the Cortex
  - Development of the Thalamus
  - Development of the Hypothalamus
  - Endogenous Analgesic Symptoms
  - Long-term Effects of Visceral Pain
  - Long-term Effects of Somatic Pain

The Physiology of Pain
- Excitatory Neurotransmitters and Receptor Systems
  - Neurotrophins and Their Receptor Systems
  - Glutamate and Its Receptors
  - Substance P and Neurokinin Receptors
  - Excitatory Ion Channels and Receptors

- Inhibitory Neurotransmitters and Receptor Systems
  - Opioid Peptides and Their Receptors
  - GABA and Its Receptors
  - Nitric Oxide and Its Synthetases
- Regulation of the Pain Threshold

Pediatric and Neonatal Pain Management

The Anatomy of Pain

Pain was previously described as a process in which specific nociceptive receptors are stimulated, thereby producing standard responses within the dorsal horn neurons of the spinal cord, with well-defined patterns of conduction to the brainstem, thalamus, and other subcortical centers. Such concepts of the pain system and other simple explanations of pain mechanisms were abandoned because accumulating clinical and experimental evidence described the phenomenon of pain as a remarkable adaptive neuronal and neurochemical process, the elements of which may increase or decrease in number. Such adaptive processes were noted to be dependent on the characteristics of the noxious stimulus, the context in which it was applied, the behavioral state at the time of application, and various other factors, all of which produced significant alterations in the form or degree of pain experienced.

The nociceptive system develops during the second and third trimesters of human gestation, with additional maturation changes occurring during the first 2 years of postnatal life.[1-3] Thereafter, although the perception of pain changes very little, major changes occur in the emotional processing of painful experiences, interpretations of the importance and meaning of pain, repertoire of behavioral and cognitive expressions of pain, and pattern of responses and adaptations to continued pain. Traditionally, the pain system was thought to be underdeveloped in the neonate and older infant. Because neonates and nonverbal infants are incapable of reporting and describing the subjective phenomenon of pain, it was concluded that these age groups were also incapable of pain perception.[4,5] These widespread notions led to the clinical practices of providing either minimal or no anesthesia during major surgical procedures, following surgery, and for invasive procedures.[6,7] These practices were common in newborns, particularly preterm neonates, in whom there was also a significant fear regarding the potential adverse cardiorespiratory effects of opioids and other analgesic agents. Recommendations for analgesia or sedation during intensive care also were made without considering the developmental neurobiology of pain mechanisms or the physiologic and behavioral responses to pain and stress in neonates and small infants.[8-11]

The mature pain system may be traced from peripheral sensory receptors to the cerebral cortex (Figure 1-1). The developmental changes occurring at each of these levels of processing, from peripheral to spinal to supraspinal, provide a framework to study the development of the pain system. It is important to realize that the pain system develops as a "whole," rather than the sequential development of its separate parts, and is functional at each of these developmental stages such that developmental or detrimental changes occurring at each level of processing will affect the architecture and function of the entire pain system.[12-14]

The perception of pain begins with the activation of peripheral nociceptors and free nerve endings located in various layers of the skin, mucus membranes, ligaments and tendons, deep muscle fibers, and viscera. These first-order neurons carry the nociceptive input to the dorsal horn of the spinal cord, where the nociceptive input is modulated (amplified and inhibited) by descending fibers from the central nervous system (CNS) and interneurons within the dorsal horn. This modulation is mediated via various compounds (substance P, adrenergic agonists, serotonin, and endogenous opioids) that interact with either the first- or second-order neurons in the spinal or supraspinal areas. A complex circuitry in the dorsal horn of the spinal cord allows the input from first-order neurons to be processed via multiple opposing or convergent neuronal synapses, which are received by deep-seated projection neurons (in laminae V, VIII, and X of the spinal gray matter) (Figure 1-2). In the dorsal horn of the spinal cord, the first-order neurons synapse with second-order neurons, which then cross the midline and ascend in various pathways, including the spinothalamic, spinoreticular, and spinomesencephalic tracts. These projection neurons (axons of the second-order neurons) form synapses at multiple levels of the brainstem, midbrain, hypothalamus, and thalamus. Thalamic

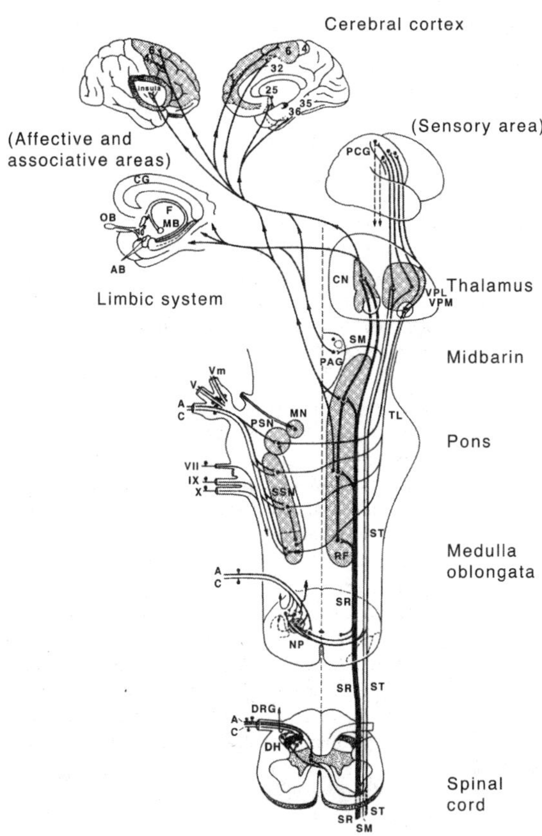

Figure 1-1
Graphical representation of the mature pain system. Numbers in the cerebral cortex indicate the cortical fields of Broadmann. A = A-δ fibers, C = C fibers, DRG = dorsal root ganglion, DH = dorsal horn of the spinal cord, SR = spinoreticular tract, SM = spinomesencephalic tract, ST = lateral spinothalamic tract, NP = nucleus proprius, RF = medullary and pontine reticular formation, PAG = periaqueductal gray matter, VPL = ventroposterolateral nucleus of the thalamus, VPM = ventroposteromedial nucleus of the thalamus, CN = central and intralaminary nuclei of the thalamus, OB = olfactory bulb, F = fornix, MB = mammiliary bodies, AB = amygdaloid body (central nucleus of the amygdala), H = hippocampus, CG = cingulate gyrus, PCG = postcentral gyrus, V & Vm = sensory and motor roots of the trigeminal nerve, MN = motor nucleus of the trigeminal nerve, PSN = principal sensory nucleus of the trigeminal nerve, SSN = spinal sensory nucleus of the trigeminal nerve, TL = trigeminal lemniscus, VII = facial nerve, IX = glossopharyngeal nerve, X = vagus nerve.

processing may be responsible for the first "perception" of the sensory-motivational aspects of pain,[15] through interactions with the hippocampus, amygdala, and other components of the limbic system; the hypothalamus; and multiple subcortical areas. Thalamic projection neurons also connect with multiple areas of the cortex, primarily the anterior insula, precentral gyrus, and anterior cingulate gyrus.[15-17] Neuroimaging studies using functional magnetic resonance imaging and positron emission tomography scans have begun to unravel the complex cortical processing of acute and prolonged pain, the effects of distraction, and placebo analgesia in humans.[18-21]

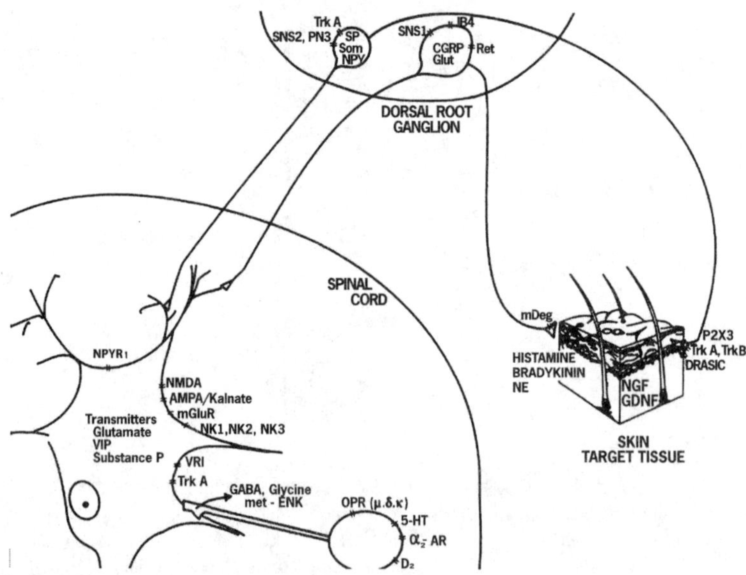

Figure 1-2
Schematic outline of the connections between the skin or other target tissue, the dorsal root ganglion, and neurons in the dorsal horn of the spinal cord. Trk= tyrosine kinase, NGF=nerve growth factor, GDNF=glial derived neurotrophic factor, SP = substance P, Glut=glutamate, CGRP=calcitonin gene related peptide, Som=somatostatin, NPY=neuropeptide Y, NMDA=N-methyl D-aspartate, GABA=gamma amino butyric acid, NK=neurokinin, OPR=opioid receptors (m, d, k), 5-HT=5-hydroxytryptamine or serotonin, VR=vanilloid receptor, D=dopamine, a2-AR=a2-adrenergic receptor, VIP=vasoactive intestinal polypeptide, met-ENK=met-enkephalin.

Development of the Pain System

Pain associated with or without tissue injury causes the activation of widely distributed and highly variable elements in the peripheral and central nervous systems, dependent on the features of the noxious stimulus, the context in which pain occurs, and characteristics of the subject (eg, age, species, gender, disease states, previous experiences of pain, etc). The 3 types of pain (namely physiologic or related to tissue injury, inflammatory, and neuropathic) are transmitted by distinct molecular mechanisms and alter pain sensitivity via the activation, modulation, or modification of different elements within the pain system.[22]

Peripheral Pain Mechanisms

Cutaneous Receptors and Nerve Terminals

Neurogenesis in the developing brain is completed by birth, but considerable growth and reorganization of peripheral nerve terminals occurs during infancy that progressively alters the reactions to noxious stimuli. At birth, the skin is fully innervated with a dense plexus of sensory fibers and nociceptors, which are located close to the surface[23] because the stratum corneum is rudimentary at this time. Polymodal nociceptors (PMNs) respond to mechanical, thermal, or chemical stimuli via transducer receptors or ion channels, which include the vanilloid receptor (VR1),[24] acid sensing ion channels (ASICs), nociceptor-specific sodium channels, and adenosine triphosphate (ATP) receptors (P2X3), producing depolarizing currents in unmyelinated C fibers[25] (Figure 1-2).

Neurotrophic factors play a crucial role in survival and maintenance of primary afferent neurons. The terminal density of cutaneous fibers is regulated by the release of nerve growth factor (NGF), brain-derived neurotrophic factor (BDNF), and others.[26] The onset of NGF synthesis is correlated with the onset of innervation. During normal development, skin NGF levels remain steady in fetal life and increase progressively around birth and early infancy before decreasing to adult levels.

High-threshold mechanoreceptors develop later than PMNs, with significant increases in their firing frequencies and stimulation thresholds, possibly transduced via the mDeg ion channel.[22,25,27] Tissue injury gives rise to sharp, well-localized "first pain" mediated by action potentials in thinly myelinated A-δ fibers that arise from high-threshold mechanoceptors,[27,28] whereas the dull aching pain that follows tissue injury or inflammation is transduced by PMNs, ASICs, P2X3, VR1, and SNa-2 receptors and transmitted by unmyelinated C fibers.[29] The immature properties of these receptors, with widespread activation of the dorsal horn neurons and bilateral activation of supraspinal areas following unilateral stimuli, may partially explain the poor localization of painful stimuli during infancy and early childhood.[27,29,30]

Sensory Neurons and Peripheral Nerves

In the developing dorsal root ganglia (DRG), cell death begins at embryonic day 15 (E15) in the rat, peaks at E17 to E19, and correlates with innervation of the cord by central sensory axons. Despite this, surviving cell numbers increase steadily until birth and then decrease by 16%, which correlates with the peripheral sensory axons that have found their distal peripheral targets, with axonal transport of NGF or other growth factors.[23, 31] Thus prenatal cell death in DRGs is controlled by local (ganglionic) or central (spinal) factors, whereas postnatal cell death depends on peripheral targets.

Nociceptive nerve fibers (A-δ and C) in immature animals have the same properties as those in the adult pain system, although faster nerve conduction occurs from the periphery to the DRG and spinal cord because of the shorter distances traveled. There is a loss of nearly 50% of afferent axons from birth to adulthood, which cannot be explained by neuronal cell death.[32]

The Long-term Effects of Early Tissue Injury

Skin injury at birth causes an increased expression of NGF and other neurotrophic factors,[26] leading to marked hyperinnervation with exuberant sprouting of cutaneous nerve fibers following neonatal skin wounds.[33] This nerve sprouting is 6-fold greater than that following adult skin injury, and withdrawal reflex thresholds in the areas of neonatally injured skin may be reduced (increased sensitivity) during childhood and adolescence.[34] Nerve sprouting is inhibited by anti-NGF antibody in adult rats, but not in neonatal rats, indicating a role for other neurotrophic factors[34] that are not altered by sciatic nerve blockade.[35] During maturation of these peripheral nociceptors, the central terminals of primary afferent neurons continue to express the mRNA of axonal growth cone proteins (eg, GAP-43) until well after birth, thus allowing peripheral nerve injury or inflammation to permanently alter spinal patterns of innervation.[36]

Spinal Pain Mechanisms

Central Afferent Terminals

During development, thickly myelinated A-β fibers are the first to penetrate the dorsal horn of the fetal spinal cord, whereas the central terminals of A-δ and C fibers penetrate the dorsal horn later during development.[37-40] Synaptogenesis of A-δ and C fibers with neurons in the substantia gelatinosa (laminae I and II of the dorsal horn of the spinal cord) occurs in a somatotopically precise manner. In the mature spinal cord, A-β fibers, subserving touch and proprioception, form connections with deep neurons in laminae III and IV of the dorsal horn, but in the developing cord their collateral terminals extend up to nociception-specific neurons in the substantia gelatinosa.[41] By the time synaptogenesis between C-fiber terminals and substantia gelatinosa neurons is completed, these unique superficial terminals from the A-β fibers disappear.[41] Thus in the newborn period it is fascinating that the same high-velocity A-β axons transmit both tactile and noxious impulses, with similar patterns of neuronal activation following noxious and innocuous stimuli.[42,43] Because of immature synapses with the dorsal horn, pure C–fiber stimulation may remain subthreshold until late in gestation.[44] Acute pain or inflammation produces robust and specific pain behaviors, neuronal *Fos* expression in the dorsal horn,[43] leading to A-δ fiber mediated sensitization and C-fiber mediated windup (the mechanisms underlying primary and secondary hyperalgesia).[22,44,45]

Spinal Nerve Tracts

This complex circuitry regulates the spinal modulation of noxious afferent impulses and terminates on projection neurons located mostly in layer V of the dorsal horn. Prenatal growth of axons from spinal projection neurons (second-order neurons) reach the thalamic nuclei by the early second trimester,[46-48] which is also the time when thalamocortical axons (third-order neurons) penetrate the subplate zone of the developing neocortex.[49-52] Spinal projection neurons (second-order neurons) primarily establish connections with the brainstem and thalamic nuclei associated with pain via the spinothalamic, spinohypothalamic, spinomesencephalic, spinopontoamygdaloid, and spinoreticular nerve tracts located mainly in the anterolateral and lateral white matter of the spinal cord.[53]

Lack of myelination in these nerve tracts was proposed as an index of immaturity in the neonatal CNS and was used to support the argument that neonates cannot feel pain. This argument was widely accepted despite the common knowledge that incomplete myelination does not imply lack of function, but merely imposes a slower conduction velocity in the central nerve tracts of neonates.[2,54] However, any slowing in the central conduction velocity would be completely offset by the shorter distances traveled by the impulse. Nociceptive nerve tracts to the brainstem and thalamus undergo myelination by 30 weeks of human gestation, and the thalamocortical pain fibers show some myelination in the term neonate.[55,56]

Development of Descending Inhibitory Controls

Descending axons from the brainstem grow caudad from the periaqueductal gray matter, pontine reticular nuclei, locus coeruleus, and other foci in the brainstem into the spinal cord in early fetal life and extend collateral branches into the dorsal horn later in gestation.[57] Boucher and colleagues[58] demonstrated that the development of diffuse noxious inhibitory controls (DNICs) was functionally mature in 21-day-old rats, but not effective in 12-day-old rats. The maturation of DNICs follows a rostrocaudal pattern as these fibers grow down the length of the spinal cord, thus explaining the higher pain thresholds in the upper limbs compared with the lower limbs in premature infants and rat pups.[57,59,60]

This delayed maturation of descending inhibition may be due to a deficiency of neurotransmitters (dopamine, serotonin, and norepinephrine) in the axon terminals or lack of specific receptors (α_2-adrenergic, $5HT_{1A}$) in their spinal targets.[57,61-66] Alternatively, a delayed maturation of inhibitory interneurons[48] or the excitatory role of neurotransmitters such as γ-aminobutyric acid (GABA) and glycine in the dorsal horn may contribute to the delayed maturation of inhibitory mechanisms in the spinal cord.[67-69] While GABA and glycine are inhibitory neurotransmitters in the adult, in the neonatal dorsal horn, they mediate increased calcium influx into immature neurons and enhance the action potential duration from these neurons.[68] Because of immature gating mechanisms, newborns are notoriously incapable of filtering out sensory stimulation from the periphery and their behavioral responses to all sensory inputs are exaggerated and generalized.[70-73] Given the plasticity of the supraspinal foci involved in sensory processing, repetitive pain during infancy may cause widespread changes in the developing brain.

Supraspinal Pain Mechanisms

The development of supraspinal pain mechanisms in the human fetus, neonate, infant, and young child has not been investigated, apart from the documentation of pain behaviors, pain thresholds, and the social and cultural correlates of pain processing. Yet multiple studies have shown that painful experiences in the neonatal period will have epochal and long-term, if not permanent, effects on the subsequent processing of pain, stress, and negative affect throughout the life of an individual.

Development of the Cortex

The time course of developmental gene expression in the brain critically depends on afferent inputs from the periphery. Thus "neurons that fire together wire together" or activity-dependent changes in gene expression lead to the establishment of cortical maps during development.[52,74] The roles of molecular factors regulating the growth and differentiation of the cerebral cortex include insulin-like growth factor (IGF-1) and its receptor,[75] other trophic factors (such as BDNF, neurotrophin [NT]-4/5 and NT-3, via specific ligand activity on tyrosine kinase [Trk] B receptors),[76] hepatic leukemia factor,[77] steroid neurohormones (DHEA and DHEAS),[78] calcium-binding proteins (eg, parvalbumin),[79] neurogranin (a substrate for protein kinase C),[80] and other factors altering cell-cycle kinetics.[81]

Changes in the expression of neurotransmitters in the developing cerebral cortex may be related to the functional maturation of distinct cortical areas. At birth, the α_1-subunit of the $GABA_A$ receptor selectively demarcates the boundaries of the primary somatosensory (S1) cortex in layers III and IV. Differences in the laminar distribution of α_1-$GABA_A$ receptors persists at least until late infancy.[82] The excitatory role of $GABA_A$ receptors occurs transiently during early postnatal development noted in cultured immature neurons, the neonatal spinal cord, and in supraspinal areas of the postnatal rat brain.[83] Presynaptic inhibition by $GABA_B$ receptors is already functional in early development, but postsynaptic inhibition in the hippocampal and cortical neurons does not develop until much later.[83] The density of *N*-methyl-D-aspartate (NMDA) receptors increases rapidly in the cortex, hippocampus, and other supraspinal areas.[83] Their composition is different between neonatal and adult brains, with significantly increased expression of the NR1 and NR2B subunits in the neonatal hippocampus and the cerebral cortex.[84,85]

Repetitive stimulation of thalamic neurons in newborn rats produces changes in the slope of the excitatory postsynaptic potential response recorded from the somatosensory cortex, indicating the presence of NMDA-mediated long-term potentiation, which was absent in the rats studied at P8 to P14.[86] NMDA-mediated afferent input from thalamic neurons is critically important for the formation of cortical columns and topographical maps in the cortex.[87-89] The formation and maturation of cortical barrels in the somatosensory cortex is critically dependent on serotonergic and $GABA_A$ activity during this period.[82,90] These findings correlate well with functional studies showing that evoked potentials from the forepaw in the rat somatosensory cortex reach maturity in infancy.[91]

Several forms of behavior imply cortical function during fetal life, including defined periods of quiet sleep, active sleep, and wakefulness; behavioral responses to pain; evidence for learning and memory; and cognitive and associative capabilities in response to external stimuli. Functional maturity of the cerebral cortex is further suggested by fetal and neonatal electroencephalographic (EEG) patterns and evoked responses. Intermittent EEG bursts in both cerebral hemispheres are first seen at 19 to 20 weeks of gestation, become sustained at 22 weeks, and are bilaterally synchronous at 26 to 27 weeks of gestation.[4] By 30 weeks, EEG patterns can distinguish between wakefulness and sleep and the effects of opioid analgesia.[92] Cortical components of somatosensory, auditory, and visually evoked potentials have been recorded in preterm infants before 26 weeks of gestation.[93]

The timing of the thalamocortical connection is of crucial importance for cortical perception, because most sensory pathways to the neocortex have synapses in the thalamus.[52] In the primate fetus, thalamic neurons produce axons that arrive in the cerebrum before midgestation. These fibers remain just below the neocortex until migration and dendritic arborization of cortical neurons are complete and finally establish synaptic connections at 20 to 22 weeks of gestation.

Development of the Thalamus

Areas of the thalamus associated with pain processing include the ventroposterior lateral, ventroposterior medial, and ventroposterior inferior nuclei in the lateral nociceptive system and the centrolateral nuclei, the ventrocaudal part of medial dorsal nucleus, parafascicular nuclei, and the posterior part of ventromedial nucleus in the medial nociceptive system.[15,16] A developmental sequence for the growth and synaptogenesis of thalamocortical fibers and their effects on the somatosensory cortex was described previously. Spinothalamic afferents relay in the ventroposterior lateral and ventroposterior inferior nuclei, and finally project to the primary and secondary somatosensory cortex, whereas the midline thalamic nuclei project into the anterior cingulate, insular cortex, and the limbic system.[15,16] The immature action potentials of neonatal thalamic neurons are primarily dependent on Na^+-currents, but gain significant Ca^{++}-components in the second postnatal week associated with supra-threshold oscillations of the membrane potential.[94]

Development of the Hypothalamus

Areas of the hypothalamus classically associated with responses to pain and stress include the periventricular and paraventricular nuclei, as well as sympathetic outflows from the posterior hypothalamus. More than 25 years ago it was observed that electrical stimulation of the periventricular hypothalamus and periaqueductal gray matter led to specific analgesic effects,[95,96] which were naloxone reversible.[97] Noxious inputs to the hypothalamus are derived from various sources.

- *Visceral and somatosensory input* is received from noradrenergic nuclei in the brainstem including the ventral tegmental area, nucleus of the solitary tract, and the locus coeruleus.
- *Emotional input* is transmitted to the corticolimbic system including the medial prefrontal cortex, the anterior cingulate, the bed nucleus of the stria terminalis, the ventral hippocampus, the amygdaloid complex, and the lateral septum.

- *Internal regulatory inputs* are received from the intrahypothalamic nuclei and circumventricular organs such as the subfornical organ.

All of these inputs, to varying degrees, activate neurons in the paraventricular nuclei and posterior hypothalamus, thus triggering the neuroendocrine and autonomic responses to pain and stress. Hypothalamic function in the newborn is characterized by increased vulnerability to permanent changes resulting from prolonged pain or stress, which may set the gain on future hypothalamic-pituitary-adrenal axis and autonomic responses.[98,99]

Endogenous Analgesic Systems

During fetal and early neonatal life, infants develop endogenous analgesic mechanisms that are mediated via 3 independent pathways, requiring orogustatory, orotactile, and generalized tactile inputs. Orogustatory inputs activate an opioid-mediated system that is activated by fat and milk proteins in the newborn rat, and by sweet taste in human newborns.[100,101] Nonnutritive sucking (or suckling at the breast) activates a second analgesic system, mediated via non-opioid mechanisms and independent of the taste-activated pathways, at least until it reaches the midbrain.[102] A third analgesic pathway is activated by whole body contact between mother and infant, which is not naloxone-reversible[102] and forms the basis for "kangaroo care" in critically ill preterm neonates.[103,104] The developmental maturation of descending inhibitory pathways and their supraspinal mechanisms await further investigation.

Long-term Effects of Visceral Pain

A recent epidemiologic study found that term, otherwise healthy, neonates exposed to gastric suctioning at birth had a 3-fold increase in the incidence of developing functional bowel disorders compared with sibling controls.[105] Why do noxious experiences in the neonatal period have such long-lasting effects? A mechanistic explanation for long-term changes in visceral pain may consider states of consciousness in the newborn.[106] At birth, neonates primarily exist in an interoceptive perceptual state with minimal attention to external stimuli.[107] Thus robust responses ensue from internal states such as hunger, thirst, or pain,[108] whereas external auditory, visual, or other stimuli may receive limited attention or brain processing. Maternal conditioning in early infancy entrains the cycles of feeding, sleep/arousal, and defecation, using external cues to regulate the visceral states experienced by the baby.[109] Newborn rats exposed to noxious (eg, visceral irritation) or disruptive (eg, maternal separation) conditions at birth developed abnormal neuronal processing related to their visceral function in adulthood.[110,111]

Emotions such as anxiety, fear, or anger may often lead to aversive visceral sensations ("gut feelings"), which is one aspect of our emotional intelligence.[112,113] In contrast to external signals, most interoceptive visceral stimuli remain subconscious and are mainly processed in the medial pain system, which regulates the autonomic, neuroendocrine, and affective responses to these stimuli via the medial prefrontal cortex, perigenual and anterior cingulate cortex, and anterior insula; areas that are closely interwoven with the emotional (limbic) system of the brain.[108,114,115] This may explain why 60% of patients with irritable bowel syndrome also show evidence of psychiatric or affective disorders.[116-118] It is possible that enhanced apoptosis or excitotoxic damage to immature neurons[119,120] or other mechanisms of brain plasticity may mediate these persistent behavioral patterns.[121,122]

Long-term effects of Somatic Pain

Different experimental paradigms have investigated the long-term effects of prolonged or repetitive pain occurring in the neonatal period. For example, neonatal rats exposed to repeated needle sticks from postnatal days 0 to 7 subsequently developed lower pain thresholds at 16 and 22 days of age,[123] perhaps associated with changes at several levels of the pain system. Localized inflammation for 5 to 7 days, caused by injecting complete Freund's adjuvant into the left hindpaw of neonatal rat pups, led to striking increases in the number of primary sensory fibers forming connections with superficial layers of the dorsal horn in adult rats.[124] These abnormal nerve fibers also extended into caudal segments of the spinal cord (L5, S1) that don't normally receive sensory input from the sciatic nerve. Hyperexcitability in the dorsal horn neurons noted by increased activity at rest and increased responses to tactile or noxious stimuli was correlated with increased pain behaviors in adult rats.[124] Localized inflammation for 48 hours, caused by injecting carrageenan into the hindpaws of 1-day-old rats, also led to marked reductions (33%) in the receptive field size of dorsal neurons to subsequent noxious stimulation (pinch).[125]

To summarize, neonatal interventions lead to permanent alterations in the structure and function of the pain system, with hyperinnervation in areas of wounded skin,[33] an increased sprouting of primary afferent fibers, and hyperexcitability of dorsal horn neurons,[124] leading to adaptive changes within the dorsal horn that decrease the receptive field size of these afferent neurons.[125] The long-term effects of peripheral nerve damage in the neonate have also been reviewed recently.[126]

The Physiology of Pain

Physiological regulation of the pain system mainly depends on the interaction of various excitatory and inhibitory influences mediated via specific neurotransmitters and receptor systems, voltage- or ligand-gated ion channels, membrane proteins, and small molecules at the cellular level of processing, as well as on the interaction of different populations of neuronal and glial elements at the architectural and anatomical level of processing. A brief description of the excitatory and inhibitory systems follows, although a comprehensive review of the areas is beyond the scope of this chapter.

Excitatory Neurotransmitters and Receptor Systems

Neurotrophins and Their Receptors

Sensory neurons are critically dependent on neurotrophins for survival during the period of embryonic neurogenesis,[126] with an upregulation of NT-3, BDNF, and NGF noted at days 11 and 12 of embryogenesis. Neurotrophin-3 synthesized by embryonic DRG cells is subsequently downregulated to undetectable levels by birth. At day 12 of embryogenesis, glial derived neurotrophic factor (GDNF) mRNA is present in the proximal limb bud and in Schwann cells, and in the dermis by day 14 to 16 of embryogenesis. Dorsal root ganglion cells also depend on neurturin, which is expressed at high levels in the skin during the late embryonic and early postnatal stages.[127] During days 11 and 12 of embryogenesis, the neurotrophin receptor p75 is upregulated and required to mediate neuronal survival with NGF in the spinal cord.[128] Tyrosine kinase receptor proteins are expressed in embryonic sensory neurons, with widely variable levels of expression from day 10 to 13 of embryogeneis. This period is characterized by striking cell death, temporally correlated with decreasing expression of TrkC, and increasing expression of TrkA. TrkB mRNA reaches maximal levels around birth in the spinal cord, gradually declining to adulthood, whereas trkA mRNA expression in the DRG similarly decreases 2-fold during postnatal days 0 to 14. Dorsal root ganglion neurons expressing the surface lectin IB4 lose their TrkA positivity after birth, associated with increased expression of tyrosine kinase Ret during this period.[129]

Glutamate and Its Receptors

Glutamate is the primary excitatory neurotransmitter in the spinal cord and brain and its receptors can be grouped into 3 classes: NMDA receptors, the AMPA/kainate receptors, and the metabotropic glutamate receptors, each of which have further subtypes. Progressively accumulating data have described the important and multiple roles played by NMDA and other glutamate receptors in the mechanisms underlying brain plasticity and pain transmission. The density of NMDA receptors increases postnatally, reaching a peak at postnatal day 7 to 10 in the rat neonatal brain.[130,131] The subtype of NMDA receptors expressed in the neonatal spinal cord has an increasing binding affinity to glutamate, which causes greater increases in intracellular calcium following neurotransmitter binding compared with adult subtypes.[132] Whole-cell patch clamp analysis has demonstrated NMDA-induced Ca^{++} currents developing at postnatal day 7, whereas AMPA/kainate-induced currents were larger and developed earlier.[133] Metabotropic glutamate receptors are coupled to the Gs protein and second messenger pathways and generate slow synaptic responses. Depending on the cellular context, Ca^{++} influx via the NMDA receptors may activate postnatal neurons or lead to excitotoxic cell death.[84,134,135] The peak susceptibility to NMDA-mediated excitotoxicity occurs between postnatal day 7 through 15 from an accentuation of its metabolic effects,[136,137] a reduction of the voltage-dependent Mg^{++} block,[138] coupled with the synergistic effects of GABAergic excitation.[139] These properties were correlated with the unique expression of NMDA subunits in immature neurons.[84,85] NMDA receptors play a central role in the activity-dependent changes of dendritic length or spine density, synaptic stability, long-term potentiation or depression, and other processes that mediate a heightened plasticity in the neonatal brain.[49,140,141] NMDA-dependent mechanisms were not only implicated in the spinal transmission of pain, but also in the long-term effects of pain (such as hyperalgesia, allodynia, windup, and central sensitization).[142]

Substance P and Neurokinin Receptors

The NK receptors (NK-1, NK-2, and NK-3) are members of the 7 transmembrane domains, G-protein bound superfamily of receptors, with signal transduction from NK-1 and NK-2 receptors mediated via the inositol triphosphate pathway. Substance P is colocalized with glutamate in the central terminals of C fibers forming connections in the substantia gelatinosa of the dorsal horn of the spinal cord. Substance P and other tachykinins (NK-A, NK-B) bind to neurokinin receptors distributed evenly throughout the gray matter in the neonatal spinal cord and play a major role in nociceptive transmission.[27] As a neurotransmitter, substance P is released from primary afferent terminals, intrinsic spinal cord neurons, and brainstem axons terminating in the dorsal horn.[22] The density of neurokinin receptors decreases 6-fold during the postnatal period, to reach an adult distribution pattern primarily localized to the substantia gelatinosa.[40,48]

Substance P-containing neurons first appear at embryonic day 14 in the primordium of the epithalamus and extend around the posterior commissure.[143] Soon thereafter, substance P immunoreactivity develops rapidly in the parafascicular and interpeduncular nuclei, the bed nucleus of the stria terminalis, the amygdaloid complex, around the third ventricle, and in the frontal cortex. Substance P neurons and nerve terminals appear in multiple hypothalamic nuclei and the hippocampus by embryonic day 19, increasing markedly in number and density during the perinatal period. Maximum substance P expression occurs from postnatal days 5 to 15, with dense representations in the frontal and piriform cortex, the limbic system, and thalamic and hypothalamic nuclei.[143,144]

Excitatory Ion Channels and Receptors

These include the ATP-gated inotropic channels (P2X, P2Y purinoceptors), noxious heat-activated ion channels (VR1), proton-gated channels (ASIC, DRASIC), and tetrodotoxin-resistant sodium channels (PN3/SNS, NaN/SNS-2). Although the activities of these ion channels play important roles in the molecular regulation of inflammatory or neuropathic pain, a detailed description is omitted from this review because very little is known of their developmental expression (during embryonic or postnatal development) or their specific roles in the transmission of pain in immature animals.

In general, the development of excitatory processes precedes that of inhibitory processes in the developing pain system (Figure 1-3). In the immature spinal cord, synaptic connections between the C fibers and dorsal horn neurons cause prolonged excitation following a single stimulus, and repetitive stimulation leads to temporal summation or windup, associated with considerable background activity and lowered thresholds to subsequent stimuli. In addition, the receptive fields of adjacent dorsal horn neurons are large and overlapping, allowing for spatial summation, whereby weak peripheral stimuli produce exaggerated withdrawal reflexes in the newborn rats, associated with reflex radiation and facilitated transmission to supraspinal centers.[27, 28]

Inhibitory Neurotransmitters and Receptor Systems

Opioid Peptides and Their Receptors

The molecular diversity and widespread distribution of endogenous opioid peptides and their receptors in the developing nervous system highlights their involvement in various physiologic functions other

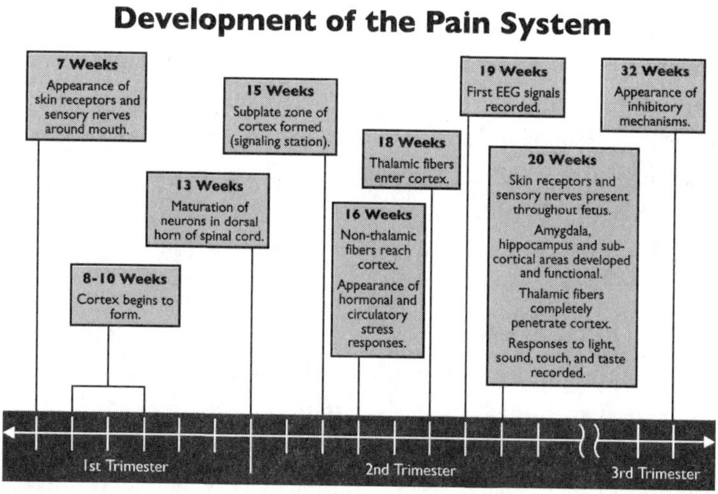

Figure 1-3

Salient events occurring in the ontogeny of the pain system during fetal life. If cortical function is necessary for pain perception, these developmental changes suggest that the fetus starts experiencing pain between 20 and 24 weeks of gestation. According to a new view of supraspinal pain processing, however, if pain perception occurs at the level of the thalamus, then the fetus may experience pain as early as 16 to 18 weeks of development.

than pain modulation. There is definite evidence that endogenous opioid systems contribute to functional analgesic mechanisms in the early postnatal period.[145] Endorphins are potent agonists for μ-opioid receptors located in the neocortex, thalamus, hippocampus, amygdala, periaqueductal gray matter, and the spinal gray matter. Functional opioid receptors were demonstrated as early as embryonic day 17, with robust receptor binding observed at postnatal day 1.[146,147] The mature pattern of opioid receptor binding shows high densities of opioid receptors in laminae I and II of the dorsal horn and moderate densities in laminae III through V, IX, and X. The dynorphin binding δ-opioid receptors appear widely distributed throughout forebrain, midbrain, and brainstem, although comprising only 10% of total opioid receptors. Functional δ-opioid receptors are observed on embryonic day 17, with progressive increases in density until postnatal day 10.[146,147] Comparative data from mature and immature spinal cords demonstrate that a 5-fold density of δ-opioid binding sites in postnatal day 9 through 16 infant rats compared with adult rats.[148] In contrast, binding sites for κ-opioid receptors are not detected until postnatal day 10, and peak levels of expression developed by day 25.[147] Opioid receptor activity mediates much of the inhibitory mechanisms in the dorsal horn, although other physiologic roles have been illustrated, such as the regulation of dendritic growth and spine formation in developing neurons.[149]

GABA and Its Receptors

GABA is an inhibitory neurotransmitter that hyperpolarizes neuronal membranes through the activation of postsynaptic $GABA_A$ and $GABA_B$ receptors, thus inhibiting neurotransmitter release or the development of excitatory postsynaptic potentials. As noted previously, $GABA_A$ receptors mediate an excitatory drive during early development.[150] It is overexpressed transiently in the developing spinal cord during the first 2 postnatal weeks, with gradual downregulation after this age.[151]

Nitric Oxide and Its Synthetases

Early expression of neuronal nitric oxide synthase (NOS) suggests its developmental role in the thalamic and hypothalamic pain system of fetal and neonatal rats. Weak NOS-like immunoreactivity is present in the anterior hypothalamus at embryonic day 15, with strong NOS expression in the developing neurons of the hypothalamic paraventricular nucleus at embryonic day 17. In the thalamic paramedial nucleus, a strong NOS occurs during the embryonic and perinatal periods with progressively weaker intensity during infancy, whereas NOS-positive neurons are not detected in the adolescent or adult rats.[152]

Regulation of the Pain Threshold

The cutaneous flexor reflex, a well-accepted measure of the pain thresholds, has a lower threshold in preterm neonates than in term neonates or adults.[153] Thresholds for the flexor withdrawal reflex are further decreased (sensitized) after previous stimulation or local tissue injury in preterm neonates, which can be abolished by topical analgesia.[45,71,154] Sensitization of this reflex may result from immature segmental or descending inhibition in the spinal cord; the immaturity of other spinal or supraspinal mechanisms; or factors associated with intensive care,[155] the environment (eg, noise[156]), and critical illness.[157,158]

A further decrease in the pain threshold, also known as the windup phenomenon, occurs in preterm neonates after exposure to a painful stimulus or experience. The windup phenomenon results from exaggerated responses of neurons in the dorsal horn of the spinal cord.[159] The temporal summation of these responses produces a condition of prolonged or recurrent hypersensitivity that is far out of proportion to the extent of the original injury.[72,73] During these prolonged periods of hypersensitivity, even non-noxious stimuli (such as those produced by handling, physical examination, and checking vital signs) are perceived as noxious stimuli, producing stress and stimulating the systemic physiologic stress responses.[4] Increased responses to acute pain are related to prior tissue injury, but also occur after physical handling,[160] while decreased responses occur following maternal contact,[103] demonstrating the supraspinal control of stimulus responsiveness in preterm and term neonates. Recent data suggest that following acute pain, an uncoupling of opioid receptors occurs in the forebrain, leading to decreased inhibitory tone along the pain system, which is manifested as hyperalgesia and decreased pain thresholds.[161] These data suggest a novel set of mechanisms regulating pain responsiveness via changes in the forebrain.

Pediatric and Neonatal Pain Management

The management of pain and its effective treatment in infants and children has evolved over the past generation from the mere hope and mission of patient advocates to a patient right and an expectation by the family. Many factors have led to this transformation. Clinical studies have shown that pain in children, regardless of its etiology, is frequently undertreated.[162-164] Evidence has emerged that preterm infants continue to experience pain from a variety of causes, including medical procedures and interventions.[164] The most recent information regarding the development of the pain system has demonstrated that term and preterm infants are placed at a disadvantage in the perception of pain. Premature infants who undergo repeated painful procedures, such as heel stick, have subsequently demonstrated increased agitation and irritability to non-threatening touch. The landmark research by Anand and Hickey[54] demonstrated significantly improved survival in infants after surgery for congenital heart disease if they received adequate treatment of postoperative pain as part of their intensive care support. Treatment of pain and stress not only results in improved short-term outcomes, but also has long-term effects. Infants and children who have received inadequate treatment or prevention of their procedural pain or stress may have significant behavioral or school-related problems long after the actual procedure or hospitalization.[165] The clinician's awareness of the needs of children with terminal illnesses, such as cancer, has also evolved. Palliative care and hospice care long have been available for adults. However, a lack of understanding of the patients' needs, combined with a lack of familiarity with analgesic medications, has resulted in many children with terminal illnesses not being offered adequate treatment.[166,167]

A means of assessing pain is paramount in determining the severity of pain and evaluating the patient's response to therapy. Early tools to assess pain in adult patients, which relied on self-reporting, were difficult to apply to younger children. Although tools have been developed to assess pain in infants and children,[168] the clinical practice of routine and standardized assessment of pain in infants and children remains inconsistent at best. A key in our ability to better manage pain in infants and children will be the routine assessment of pain scores as the fifth vital sign. New pain scales or tools also will be instrumental for future clinical research in the development of novel techniques and the assessment of new pharmacologic agents to control pain in infants and children.

Concurrent with the evolving clinical movement to appropriately treat pain in infants and children is the growing body of evidence on the mechanisms of pain, even in the smallest of infants. It has been demonstrated that the neonate's nervous system is more hypersensitive to painful stimuli than that of the adult and demonstrates a reduced threshold to certain stimuli. The myth that the infant's brain is immature and, therefore, unable to sense pain has been thoroughly refuted. The immaturity of the nervous system involves key descending, inhibitory pathways, thereby making the neonatal nervous system hypersensitive to nociceptive input. The nervous system continues to mature from birth until early childhood. Brain maturation involves changes in synaptic receptor type and density, which can affect both sensory input and the brain's response. Sensory neuronal function, ascending and descending transmission of neuronal impulses, and the nervous system's processing of painful stimuli evolve throughout early childhood. All of these changes affect the way infants and children respond to pain.

This growing body of clinical knowledge has coincided with the growing awareness of the public of the importance of pain management to the well-being of infants and children. The American Academy of Pediatrics has published position statements advocating the proper assessment and treatment of pain in infants and children.[169,170] Governing entities and other professional organizations have become vocal advocates for the adequate treatment of pain and stress in children. The Joint Commission on Accreditation of Healthcare Organizations (JCAHO) has focused on the issue of pain assessment and treatment in its guidelines and surveys. These guidelines require all hospitals to establish system-wide methods to deal with pain management and procedural-sedation in patients, including infants and children. Compliance with these guidelines has been a major area of focus of the annual site visits performed by the JCAHO.

Summary

The treatment of pain in children of all ages has seen dramatic improvements over the past 25 years; however, there is still much work to be done. Elegant developmental neuroanatomical studies have refuted the myth that preterm and term infants do not feel pain because of the immaturity of their nervous systems. These studies have demonstrated that these patients are at a disadvantage, given the immaturity of the inhibitory pathways that normally regulate the nociceptive input and modulate its transmission. Clinical studies have demonstrated an exaggerated stress response in neonates and infants with catecholamine and other stress hormone levels that are 3 to 5 times those of adults undergoing similar surgical procedures. Following major surgical procedures for repair of congenital heart disease, the quality of postoperative analgesia has been shown to influence morbidity and even mortality. Additionally, the undertreatment of pain may have consequences that persist for many years. Given these issues and our obvious humanitarian concerns, we continue to strive to improve the quality of pain control in pediatric patients. This text is designed to provide health care practitioners with a basic understanding of the issues surrounding the management of pain in infants and children. It is our hope that this book will provide practical information to assist health care providers in preventing and treating pain in infants and children on a daily basis.

References

1. Smith RP, Gitau R, Glover V, Fisk NM. Pain and stress in the human fetus. *Eur J Obstet Gynecol Reprod Biol.* 2000;92:161-165
2. Anand KJS, Hickey PR. Pain and its effects in the human neonate and fetus. *N Engl J Med.* 1987;317:1321-1329
3. Anand KJS, Maze M. Fetuses, fentanyl, and the stress response: signals from the beginnings of pain? *Anesthesiology.* 2001;95:823-825
4. Anand KJS. Clinical importance of pain and stress in preterm neonates. *Biol Neonate.* 1998;73:1-9
5. Hadjistavropoulos HD, Craig KD, Grunau RE, Whitfield MF. Judging pain in infants: behavioural, contextual, and developmental determinants. *Pain.* 1997;73:319-324
6. Betts EK, Downes JJ. Anesthetic considerations in newborn surgery. *Semin Anesth.* 1984;3:59-74
7. Purcell-Jones G, Dormon F, Sumner E. Paediatric anaesthetists' perceptions of neonatal and infant pain. *Pain.* 1988;33:181-187
8. Franck LS. A national survey of the assessment and treatment of pain and agitation in the neonatal intensive care unit. *J Obstet Gynecol Neonatal Nurs.* 1987;16:387-393
9. Fitzgerald M. Pain and analgesia in neonates. *Trends Neurosci.* 1987;10:344-346
10. Anand KJ, Carr DB. The neuroanatomy, neurophysiology, and neurochemistry of pain, stress, and analgesia in newborns and children. *Pediatr Clin North Am.* 1989;36:795-822
11. Dixon S, Snyder J, Holve R, Bromberger P. Behavioral effects of circumcision with and without anesthesia. *J Dev Behav Pediatr.* 1984;5:246-250
12. Johnston CC, Stevens B, Craig KD, Grunau RV. Developmental changes in pain expression in premature, full-term, two- and four-month-old infants. *Pain.* 1993;52:201-208
13. Fitzgerald M, Beggs S. The neurobiology of pain: developmental aspects. *Neuroscientist.* 2001;7:246-257
14. Anand KJS, Grunau RE, Oberlander T. Developmental character and long-term consequences of pain in infants and children. *Child Adolesc Psychiatr Clin North Am.* 1997;6:703-724

15. Craig AD. A new view of pain as a homeostatic emotion. *Trends Neurosci.* 2003;26:303-307
16. Price DD. Psychological and neural mechanisms of the affective dimension of pain. *Science.* 2000;288:1769-1772
17. Rainville P, Duncan GH, Price DD, Carrier B, Bushnell MC. Pain affect encoded in human anterior cingulate but not somatosensory cortex. *Science.* 1997;277:968-971
18. Zubieta JK, Smith YR, Bueller JA, et al. Regional mu opioid receptor regulation of sensory and affective dimensions of pain. *Science.* 2001;293:311-315
19. Wager TD, Rilling JK, Smith EE, et al. Placebo-induced changes in FMRI in the anticipation and experience of pain. *Science.* 2004;303:1162-1167
20. Fitzek S, Fitzek C, Huonker R, et al. Event-related fMRI with painful electrical stimulation of the trigeminal nerve. *Magn Reson Imaging.* 2004;22:205-209
21. Valet M, Sprenger T, Boecker H, et al. Distraction modulates connectivity of the cingulo-frontal cortex and the midbrain during pain—an fMRI analysis. *Pain.* 2004;109:399-408
22. Woolf CJ, Salter MW. Neuronal plasticity: increasing the gain in pain. *Science.* 2000;288:1765-1769
23. Fitzgerald M. Spontaneous and evoked activity of fetal primary afferents in vivo. *Nature.* 1987;326:603-605
24. Caterina MJ, Leffler A, Malmberg AB, et al. Impaired nociception and pain sensation in mice lacking the capsaicin receptor. *Science.* 2000;288:306-313
25. McCleskey EW, Gold MS. Ion channels of nociception. *Ann Rev Physiol.* 1999;61:835-856
26. Constantinou J, Reynolds ML, Woolf CJ, Safieh-Garabedian B, Fitzgerald M. Nerve growth factor levels in developing rat skin: upregulation following skin wounding. *Neuroreport.* 1994;5:2281-2284
27. Fitzgerald M, Anand KJS. The developmental neuroanatomy and neurophysiology of pain. In: Schechter N, Berde C, Yaster M, eds. *Pain Management in Infants, Children and Adolescents.* Baltimore, MD: Williams & Wilkins, 1993:11-32
28. Anand KJS. Physiology of pain in infants and children. *Annales Nestle.* 1999;57:7-18
29. Narsinghani U, Anand KJS. Developmental neurobiology of pain in neonatal rats. *Lab Anim.* 2000;29:27-39
30. Bartocci M, Bergqvist L, Ihre E, et al. Changes in cerebral haemodynamics during pain in newborn infants: a near infrared spectroscopy study. *Pediatr Res.* 2001;49:643A

31. Coggeshall RE, Pover CM, Fitzgerald M. Dorsal root ganglion cell death and surviving cell numbers in relation to the development of sensory innervation in the rat hindlimb. *Brain Res Dev Brain Res.* 1994;82:193-212
32. Jenq CB, Chung K, Coggeshall RE. Postnatal loss of axons in normal rat sciatic nerve. *J Comp Neurol.* 1986;244:445-450
33. Reynolds ML, Fitzgerald M. Long-term sensory hyperinnervation following neonatal skin wounds. *J Comp Neurol.* 1995;358:487-498
34. Reynolds M, Alvares D, Middleton J, Fitzgerald M. Neonatally wounded skin induces NGF-independent sensory neurite outgrowth in vitro. *Brain Res Dev Brain Res.* 1997;102:275-283
35. De Lima J, Alvares D, Hatch DJ, Fitzgerald M. Sensory hyperinnervation after neonatal skin wounding: effect of bupivacaine sciatic nerve block. *Br J Anaesth.* 1999;83:662-664
36. Fitzgerald M, Reynolds ML, Benowitz LI. GAP-43 expression in the developing rat lumbar spinal cord. *Neurosciences.* 1991;41:187-199
37. Tohyama l, Lee VM, Roche LB, Trojanowski JQ. Molecular milestones that signal axonal maturation and the commitment of human spinal cord precursor cells to the neuronal or glial phenotype in development. *J Comp Neurol.* 1991;310:285-299
38. Konstantinidou AD, Silos-Santiago I, Flaris N, Snider WD. Development of primary afferent projection in human spinal cord. *J Comp Neurol.* 1995;354:1-12
39. Fitzgerald M. Cutaneous primary afferent properties in the hind limb of the neonatal rat. *J Physiol.* 1987;383:79-92
40. Pignatelli D, Ribeiro-da-Silva A, Coimbra A. Postnatal maturation of primary afferent termintions in the substantia gelatinosa of the rat spinal cord. An electron microscope study. *Brain Res.* 1989;491:33-44
41. Fitzgerald M, Butcher T, Shortland P. Developmental changes in the laminar termination of A fibre cutaneous sensory afferents in the rat spinal cord dorsal horn. *J Comp Neurol.* 1994;348:225-233
42. Jennings E, Fitzgerald M. C-fos can be induced in the neonatal rat spinal cord by both noxious and innocuous peripheral stimulation. *Pain.* 1996;68:301-306
43. Yi DK, Barr GA. The induction of Fos-like immunoreactivity by noxious thermal, mechanical and chemical stimuli in the lumbar spinal cord of infant rats. *Pain.* 1995;60:257-265
44. Jennings E, Fitzgerald M. Postnatal changes in responses of rat dorsal horn cells to afferent stimulation: a fibre-induced sensitization. *J Physiol.* 1998;509:859-868

45. Fitzgerald M, Millard C, McIntosh N. Cutaneous hypersensitivity following peripheral tissue damage in newborn infants and its reversal with topical anaesthesia. *Pain.* 1989;39:31-36
46. Kostovic I, Goldman-Rakic PS. Transient cholinesterase staining in the mediodorsal nucleus of the thalamus and its connections in the developing human and monkey brain. *J Comp Neurol.* 1983;219:431-447
47. Ulfig N, Nickel J, Bohl J. Transient features of the thalamic reticular nucleus in the human foetal brain. *Eur J Neurosci.* 1998;10:3773-3784
48. Bicknell HR Jr, Beal JA. Axonal and dendritic development of substantia gelatinosa neurons in the lumbosacral spinal cord of the rat. *J Comp Neurol.* 1984;226:508-522
49. Kostovic I, Rakic P. Developmental history of the transient subplate zone in the visual and somatosensory cortex of the macaque monkey and human brain. *J Comp Neurol.* 1990;297:441-470
50. Molliver ME, Kostovic I, van der Loos H. The development of synapses in cerebral cortex of the human fetus. *Brain Res.* 1973;50:403-407
51. Mrzljak L, Uylings HB, Kostovic I, Van Eden CG. Prenatal development of neurons in the human prefrontal cortex: I. A qualitative Golgi study. *J Comp Neurol.* 1988;271:355-386
52. Erzurumlu RS, Jhaveri S. Thalamic axons confer a blueprint of the sensory periphery onto the developing rat somatosensory cortex. *Brain Res Dev Brain Res.* 1990;56:229-234
53. Millan MJ. The induction of pain: an integrative review. *Prog Neurobiol.* 1999;57:1-164
54. Anand KJS, Hickey PR. Halothane-morphine compared with high-dose sufentanil for anesthesia and postoperative analgesia in neonatal cardiac surgery. *N Engl J Med.* 1992;326:1-9
55. Childs AM, Ramenghi LA, Cornette L, et al. Cerebral maturation in premature infants: quantitative assessment using MR imaging. *AJNR Am J Neuroradiol.* 2001;22:1577-1582
56. Huppi PS, Warfield S, Kikinis R, et al. Quantitative magnetic resonance imaging of brain development in premature and mature newborns. *Ann Neurol.* 1998;43:224-235
57. Fitzgerald M, Koltzenburg M. The functional development of descending inhibitory pathways in the dorsolateral funiculus of the newborn rat spinal cord. *Brain Res.* 1986;389:261-270
58. Boucher T, Jennings E, Fitzgerald M. The onset of diffuse noxious inhibitory controls in postnatal rat pups: a C-Fos study. *Neurosci Lett.* 1998;257:9-12

59. Kinney HC, Ottoson CK, White WF. Three-dimensional distribution of 3H-naloxone binding to opiate receptors in the human fetal and infant brainstem. *J Comp Neurol.* 1990;291:55-78
60. Ren K, Blass EM, Zhou Q, Dubner R. Suckling and sucrose ingestion suppress persistent hyperalgesia and spinal Fos expression after forepaw inflammation in infant rats. *Proc Natl Acad Sci U S A.* 1997;94:1471-1475
61. Omote K, Kawamata T, Kawamata M, Namiki A. Formalin-induced nociception activates a monoaminergic descending inhibitory system. *Brain Res.* 1998;814:194-198
62. Aimone LD, Gebhart GF. Spinal monoamine mediation of stimulation-produced antinociception from the lateral hypothalamus. *Brain Res.* 1987;403:290-300
63. Zhuo M, Gebhart GF. Spinal cholinergic and monoaminergic receptors mediate descending inhibition from the nuclei reticularis gigantocellularis and gigantocellularis pars alpha in the rat. *Brain Res.* 1990;535:67-78
64. Ossipov MH, Gebhart GF. Opioid, cholinergic and alpha-adrenergic influences on the modulation of nociception from the lateral reticular nucleus of the rat. *Brain Res.* 1986;384:282-293
65. Budai D, Harasawa I, Fields HL. Midbrain periaqueductal gray (PAG) inhibits nociceptive inputs to sacral dorsal horn nociceptive neurons through $alpha_2$-adrenergic receptors. *J Neurophysiol.* 1998;80:2244-2254
66. Calejesan AA, Kim SJ, Zhuo M. Descending facilitatory modulation of a behavioral nociceptive response by stimulation in the adult rat anterior cingulate cortex. *Eur J Pain.* 2000;4:83-96
67. Obrietan K, van den Pol AN. GABA neurotransmission in the hypothalamus: developmental reversal from Ca^{2+} elevating to depressing. *J Neurosci.* 1995;15:5065-5077
68. Wang J, Reichling DB, Kyrozis A, MacDermott AB. Developmental loss of GABA- and glycine-induced depolarization and Ca^{2+} transients in embryonic rat dorsal horn neurons in culture. *Eur J Neurosci.* 1994;6:1275-1280
69. Reichling DB, Kyrozis A, Wang J, MacDermott AB. Mechanisms of GABA and glycine depolarization-induced calcium transients in rat dorsal horn neurons. *J Physiol.* 1994;476:411-421
70. Andrews K, Fitzgerald M. The cutaneous withdrawal reflex in human neonates: sensitisation, receptive fields and the effects of contralateral stimulation. *Pain.* 1994;56:95-101
71. Andrews K, Fitzgerald M. Cutaneous flexion reflex in human neonates: a quantitative study of threshold and stimulus-response characteristics after single and repeated stimuli. *Dev Med Child Neurol.* 1999;41:696-703

72. Andrews KA, Desai D, Dhillon HK, Wilcox DT, Fitzgerald M. Abdominal sensitivity in the first year of life: comparison of infants with and without prenatally diagnosed unilateral hydronephrosis. *Pain.* 2002;100:35-46
73. Andrews K, Fitzgerald M. Wound sensitivity as a measure of analgesic effects following surgery in human neonates and infants. *Pain.* 2002;99:185-195
74. Jones EG. The role of afferent activity in the maintenance of primate neocortical function. *J Exp Biol.* 1990;153:155-176
75. Bondy CA, Lee WH. Patterns of insulin-like growth factor and IGF receptor gene expression in the brain. Functional implications. *Ann N Y Acad Sci.* 1993;692:33-43
76. Behar TN, Dugich-Djordjevic MM, Li YX, et al. Neurotrophins stimulate chemotaxis of embryonic cortical neurons. *Eur J Neurosci.* 1997;9:2561-2570
77. Hitzler JK, Soares HD, Drolet DW, et al. Expression patterns of the hepatic leukemia factor gene in the nervous system of developing and adult mice. *Brain Res.* 1999;820:1-11
78. Compagnone NA, Mellon SH. Dehydroepiandrosterone: a potential signalling molecule for neocortical organization during development. *Proc Natl Acad Sci U S A.* 1998;95:4678-4683
79. Solbach S, Celio MR. Ontogeny of the calcium binding protein parvalbumin in the rat nervous system. *Anat Embryol.* 1991;184:103-124
80. Alvarez-Bolado G, Rodriguez-Sanchez P, Tejero-Diez P, Fairen A, Diez-Guerra FJ. Neurogranin in the development of the rat telencephalon. *Neuroscience.* 1996;73:565-580
81. Kornack DR, Rakic P. Changes in cell-cycle kinetics during the develop ment and evolution of primate neocortex. *Proc Natl Acad Sci U S A.* 1998;95:1242-1246
82. Paysan J, Bolz J, Mohler H, Fritschy JM. GABAA receptor alpha-1 subunit, an early marker for area specification in developing rat cerebral cortex. *J Comp Neurol.* 1994;350:133-149
83. Ben-Ari Y, Khazipov R, Leinekugel X, Caillard O, Gaiarsa JL. GABAA, NMDA and AMPA receptors: a developmentally regulated 'menage a trois'. *Trends Neurosci.* 1997;20:523-529
84. Lipton SA, Nakanishi N. Shakespeare in love—with NMDA receptors? *Nat Med.* 1999; 5:270-271
85. Kim WT, Kuo MF, Mishra OP, Delivoria-Papadopoulos M. Distribution and expression of the subunits of N-methyl-D-aspartate (NMDA) receptors; NR1, NR2A and NR2B in hypoxic newborn piglet brains. *Brain Res.* 1998;799:49-54

86. Isaac JT, Crair MC, Nicoll RA, Malenka RC. Silent synapses during development of thalamocortical inputs. *Neuron.* 1997;18:269-280
87. Feldman DE, Nicoll RA, Malenka RC, Isaac JT. Long-term depression at thalamocortical synapses in developing rat somatosensory cortex. *Neuron.* 1998;21:347-357
88. Feldman DE, Nicoll RA, Malenka RC. Synaptic plasticity at thalamocortical synapses in developing rat somatosensory cortex: LTP, LTD, and silent synapses. *J Neurobiol.* 1999;41:92-101
89. Benedetti F. Differential formation of topographic maps on the cerebral cortex and superior colliculus of the mouse by temporally correlated tactile-tactile and tactile-visual inputs. *Eur J Neurosci.* 1995;7:1942-1951
90. Osterheld-Haas MC, van der Loos H, Hornung JP. Monoaminergic afferents to cortex modulate structural plasticity in the barrelfield of the mouse. *Brain Res Dev Brain Res.* 1994;77:189-202
91. Thairu BK. Post-natal changes in the somaesthetic evoked potentials in the albino rat. *Nat New Biol.* 1971;231:30-31
92. Eaton DG, Wertheim D, Oozeer R, Royston P, Dubowitz L, Dubowitz V. The effect of pethidine on the neonatal EEG. *Dev Med Child Neurol.* 1992;34:155-163
93. Klimach VJ, Cooke RW. Maturation of the neonatal somatosensory evoked response in preterm infants. *Dev Med Child Neurol.* 1988;30:208-214
94. MacLeod N, Turner C, Edgar J. Properties of developing lateral geniculate neurones in the mouse. *Int J Dev Neurosci.* 1997;15:205-224
95. Richardson DE, Akil H. Pain reduction by electrical brain stimulation in man. Part 1: acute administration in periaqueductal and periventricular sites. *J Neurosurg.* 1977;47:178-183
96. Richardson DE, Akil H. Pain reduction by electrical brain stimulation in man. Part 2: chronic self-administration in the periventricular gray matter. *J Neurosurg.* 1977;47:184-194
97. Hosobuchi Y, Adams JE, Linchitz R. Pain relief by electrical stimulation of the central gray matter in humans and its reversal by naloxone. *Science.* 1977;197:183-186
98. Liu D, Diorio J, Tannenbaum B, et al. Maternal care, hippocampal glucocorticoid receptors, and hypothalamic-pituitary-adrenal responses to stress. *Science.* 1997;277:1659-1662
99. Grunau RE, Weinberg J, Whitfield MF. Neonatal procedural pain and preterm infant cortisol response to novelty at 8 months. *Pediatrics.* 2004;114:e77-84

100. Blass EM, Watt LB. Suckling- and sucrose-induced analgesia in human newborns. *Pain.* 1999;83:611-623
101. Barr GA. Antinociceptive effects of locally administered morphine in infant rats. *Pain.* 1999;81:155-161
102. Blass EM, Shide DJ, Zaw-Mon C, Sorrentino J. Mother as shield: differential effects of contact and nursing on pain responsivity in infant rats—evidence for nonopioid mediation. *Behav Neurosci.* 1995;109:342-353
103. Gray L, Watt L, Blass EM. Skin-to-skin contact is analgesic in healthy newborns. *Pediatrics.* 2000;105:e14
104. Ludington-Hoe SM, Swinth JY. Developmental aspects of kangaroo care. *J Obstet, Gynecol Neonat Nurs.* 1996;25:691-703
105. Anand KJS, Runeson B, Jacobson B. Gastric suction at birth associated with long-term risk for functional intestinal disorders in later life. *J Pediatr.* 2004;144:449-454
106. Anand KJS, Rovnaghi C, Walden M, Churchill J. Consciousness, behavior, and clinical impact of the definition of pain. *Pain Forum.* 1999;8:64-73
107. Jouen F, Gapenne O. Interactions between the vestibular and visual systems in the neonate. In: Rochat P, ed. *The Self in Infancy: Theory and Research.* Vol 112. Amsterdam, Netherlands: North-Holland/Elsevier Science Publishers; 1995:277-301
108. Saper CB. Pain as a visceral sensation. *Prog Brain Res.* 2000;122:237-243
109. Read NW. Bridging the gap between mind and body: do cultural and psychoanalytic concepts of visceral disease have an explanation in contemporary neuroscience? *Prog Brain Res.* 2000;122:425-443
110. Al-Chaer ED, Kawasaki M, Pasricha PJ. A new model of chronic visceral hypersensitivity in adult rats induced by colon irritation during postnatal development. *Gastroenterology.* 2000;119:1276-1285
111. Coutinho SV, Plotsky PM, Sablad M, et al. Neonatal maternal separation alters stress-induced responses to viscerosomatic nociceptive stimuli in rat. *Am J Physiol Gastrointest Liver Physiol.* 2002;282:G307-G316
112. Goleman D. *Emotional Intelligence: Why It Can Matter More Than IQ.* New York, NY: Bantam Books; 1995
113. Damasio AR. *Descartes' Error.* New York, NY: G.P. Putnam's Sons; 1994
114. Naliboff BD, Chang L, Munakata J, Mayer EA. Towards an integrative model of irritable bowel syndrome. *Prog Brain Res.* 2000;122:413-423
115. Mayer EA, Naliboff BD, Munakata J. The evolving neurobiology of gut feelings. *Prog Brain Res.* 2000;122:195-206
116. Lydiard RB. Irritable bowel syndrome, anxiety, and depression: what are the links? *J Clin Psychiatry.* 2001;62:38-45

117. Mayer EA, Craske M, Naliboff BD. Depression, anxiety, and the gastrointestinal system. *J Clin Psychiatry.* 2001;62:28-36
118. Poitras MR, Verrier P, So C, Paquet S, Bouin M, Poitras P. Group counseling psychotherapy for patients with functional gastrointestinal disorders: development of new measures for symptom severity and quality of life. *Dig Dis Sci.* 2002;47:1297-1307
119. Bhutta AT, Anand KJS. Abnormal cognition and behavior in preterm neonates linked to smaller brain volumes. *Trends Neurosci.* 2001;24:129-130
120. Anand KJS. Pain, plasticity, and premature birth: a prescription for permanent suffering? *Nat Med.* 2000;6:971-973
121. Anand KJS. Effects of perinatal pain. In: Mayer EA, Saper CB, eds. *The Biological Basis for Mind-Body Interactions.* Vol 122. New York NY: Elsevier Science; 2000:117-129
122. Ladd CO, Huot RL, Thrivikraman KV, Nemeroff CB, Meaney MJ, Plotsky PM. Long-term behavioral and neuroendocrine adaptations to adverse early experience. *Prog Brain Res.* 2000;122:81-103
123. Anand KJS, Coskun V, Thrivikraman KV, Nemeroff CB, Plotsky PM. Long-term behavioral effects of repetitive pain in neonatal rat pups. *Physiol Behav.* 1999;66:627-637
124. Ruda MA, Ling QD, Hohmann AG, Peng YB, Tachibana T. Altered nociceptive neuronal circuits after neonatal peripheral inflammation. *Science.* 2000;289:628-631
125. Rahman W, Fitzgerald M, Aynsley-Green A, Dickenson AH. The effects of neonatal exposure to inflammation and/or morphine on neuronal responses and morphine analgesia in adult rats. In: Jensen TS, Turner JA, Wiesenfeld-Hallin Z, eds. *Proceedings of the 8th World Congress on Pain.* Vol 8. Seattle, WA: IASP Press; 1997:783-794
126. Alvares D, Fitzgerald M. Building blocks of pain: the regulation of key molecules in spinal sensory neurones during development and following peripheral axotomy. *Pain.* 1999;Suppl 6:S71-S85
127. Kotzbauer PT, Lampe PA, Heuckeroth RO, et al. Neurturin, a relative of glial-cell-line-derived neurotrophic factor. *Nature.* 1996;384:467-470
128. Barrett GL, Bartlett PF. The p75 nerve growth factor receptor mediates survival or death depending on the stage of sensory neuron development. *Proc Natl Acad Sci U S A.* 1994;91:6501-6505
129. Molliver DC, Wright DE, Leitner ML, et al. IB4-binding DRG neurons switch from NGF to GDNF dependence in early postnatal life. *Neuron.* 1997;19:849-61

130. Rao H, Jean A, Kessler JP. Postnatal ontogeny of glutamate receptors in the rat nucleus tractus solitarii and ventrolateral medulla. *J Auton Nerv Syst.* 1997;65:25-32
131. Chahal H, D'Souza SW, Barson AJ, Slater P. Modulation by magnesium of N-methyl-D-aspartate receptors in developing human brain. *Arch Dis Child Fetal Neonatal.* 1998;78:F116-F120
132. Hori Y, Kanda K. Developmental alterations in NMDA receptor-mediated [Ca2+]i elevation in substantia gelatinosa neurons of neonatal rat spinal cord. *Brain Res Dev Brain Res.* 1994;80:141-148
133. Colwell CS, Cepeda C, Crawford C, Levine MS. Postnatal development of glutamate receptor-mediated responses in the neostriatum. *Dev Neurosci.* 1998;20:154-163
134. Ghosh A, Greenberg ME. Calcium signaling in neurons: molecular mechanisms and cellular consequences. *Science.* 1995;268:239-247
135. McDonald JW, Johnston MV. Physiological and pathophysiological role of excitatory amino acids during central nervous system development. *Brain Res Brain Res Rev.* 1990;15:41-70
136. Lipartiti M, Lazzaro A, Zanoni R, Mazzari S, Toffano G, Leon A. Monosialoganglioside GM1 reduces NMDA neurotoxicity in neonatal rat brain. *Exp Neurol.* 1991;113:301-305
137. Jacquin T, Gillet B, Fortin G, Pasquier C, Beloeil JC, Champagnat J. Metabolic action of N-methyl-D-aspartate in newborn rat brain ex vivo: 31p magnetic resonance spectroscopy. *Brain Res.* 1989;497:296-304
138. Mitani A, Watanabe M, Kataoka K. Functional change of NMDA receptors related to enhancement of susceptibility to neurotoxicity in the developing pontine nucleus. *J Neurosci.* 1998;18:7941-7952
139. Serafini R, Valeyev AY, Barker JL, Poulter MO. Depolarizing GABA-activated Cl- channels in embryonic rat spinal and olfactory bulb cells. *J Physiol.* 1995;488:371-386
140. Kim JJ, Foy MR, Thompson RF. Behavioral stress modifies hippocampal plasticity through N-methyl-D-aspartate receptor activation. *Proc Natl Acad Sci U S A.* 1996;93:4750-4753
141. Vicario-Abejon C, Collin C, McKay RD, Segal M. Neurotrophins induce formation of functional excitatory and inhibitory synapses between cultured hippocampal neurons. *J Neurosci.* 1998;18:7256-7271
142. Kim YI, Na HS, Yoon YW, Han HC, Ko KH, Hong SK. NMDA receptors are important for both mechanical and thermal allodynia from peripheral nerve injury in rats. *Neuroreport.* 1997;8:2149-2153

143. Inagaki S, Sakanaka M, Shiosaka S, et al. Ontogeny of substance P-containing neuron system of the rat: immunohistochemical analysis—I. Forebrain and upper brain stem. *Neuroscience.* 1982;7:251-277
144. McGregor GP, Woodhams PL, O'Shaughnessy DJ, Ghatei MA, Polak JM, Bloom SR. Developmental changes in bombesin, substance P, somatostatin and vasoactive intestinal polypeptide in the rat brain. *Neurosci Lett.* 1982;28:21-27
145. Marsh DF, Hatch DJ, Fitzgerald M. Opioid systems and the newborn. *Br J Anaesth.* 1997;79:787-795
146. Spain JW, Roth BL, Coscia CJ. Differential ontogeny of multiple opioid receptors (mu, delta, and kappa). *J Neurosci.* 1985;5:584-588
147. Rahman W, Dashwood MR, Fitzgerald M, Aynsley-Green A, Dickenson AH. Postnatal development of multiple opioid receptors in the spinal cord and development of spinal morphine analgesia. *Brain Res Dev Brain Res.* 1998;108:239-254
148. Allerton CA, Smith JA, Hunter JC, Hill RG, Hughes J. Correlation of ontogeny with function of [3H]U69593 labelled kappa opioid binding sites in the rat spinal cord. *Brain Res.* 1989;502:149-157
149. Hauser KF, McLaughlin PJ, Zagon IS. Endogenous opioid systems and the regulation of dendritic growth and spine formation. *J Comp Neurol.* 1989;281:13-22
150. Strata F, Cherubini E. Transient expression of a novel type of GABA response in rat CA3 hippocampal neurones during development. *J Physiol.* 1994;480:493-503
151. Schaffner AE, Behar T, Nadi S, Smallwood V, Barker JL. Quantitative analysis of transient GABA expression in embryonic and early postnatal rat spinal cord neurons. *Brain Res Dev Brain Res.* 1993;72:265-276
152. Gorbatyuk O, Landry M, Emson P, Akmayev I, Hokfelt T. Developmental expression of nitric oxide synthase in the rat diencephalon with special reference to the thalamic parataenial nucleus. *Int J Dev Neurosci.* 1997;15:931-938
153. Fitzgerald M, Shaw A, MacIntosh N. Postnatal development of the cutaneous flexor reflex: a comparative study in premature infants and newborn rat pups. *Dev Med Child Neurol.* 1988;30:520-526
154. Fitzgerald M, Millard C, MacIntosh N. Hyperalgesia in premature infants. *Lancet.* 1988;1:292
155. Ward-Larson C, Horn RA, Gosnell F. The efficacy of facilitated tucking for relieving procedural pain of endotracheal suctioning in very low birthweight infants. *MCN Am J Maternal Child Nurs.* 2004;29:151-156

156. Philbin MK, Ballweg DD, Gray L. The effect of an intensive care unit sound environment on the development of habituation in healthy avian neonates. *Dev Psychobiol.* 1994;27:11-21
157. Stevens BJ, Johnston CC, Horton L. Factors that influence the behavioral pain responses of premature infants. *Pain.* 1994;59:101-109
158. Johnston CC, Stevens BJ, Franck LS, Jack A, Stremler R, Platt R. Factors explaining lack of response to heel stick in preterm newborns. *J Obstet Gynecol Neonatal Nurs.* 1999;28:587-594
159. Arendt-Nielsen L, Petersen-Felix S. Wind-up and neuroplasticicty: is there a correlation to clinical pain? *Eur J Anesthesiol.* 1995;10:1-7
160. Porter FL, Wolf CM, Miller JP. The effect of handling and immobilization on the response to acute pain in newborn infants. *Pediatrics.* 1998;102:1383-1389
161. Liu JG, Rovnaghi CR, Garg S, Anand KJS. Hyperalgesia in young rats associated with opioid receptor desensitization in the forebrain. *Eur J Pharmacol.* 2004;491:127-136
162. Walco GA, Cassidy RC, Schechter NL. Pain, hurt, and harm. The ethics of pain control in infants and children. *N Engl J Med.* 1994;331:541-544
163. Johnston CC, Collinge JM, Henderson SJ, Anand KJS. A cross-sectional survey of pain and pharmacological analgesia in Canadian neonatal intensive care units. *Clin J Pain.* 1997;13:308-312
164. Simons SHP, van Dijk M, Anand KJS, Roofthooft D, van Lingen RA, Tibboel D. Do we still hurt newborn babies? A prospective study of procedural pain and analgesia in neonates. *Arch Pediatr Adolesc Med.* 2003;157:1058-1064
165. Porter FL, Grunau RVE, Anand KJS. Long-term effects of neonatal pain. *J Behav Dev Pediatr.* 1999;20:253-261
166. Kane JR, Primomo M. Alleviating the suffering of seriously ill children. *Am J Hospice Palliat Care.* 2001;18:161-169
167. Gauthier JC, Finley GA, McGrath PJ. Children's self-report of postoperative pain intensity and treatment threshold: determining the adequacy of medication. *Clin J Pain.* 1998;14:116-120
168. Bird J. Selection of pain measurement tools. *Nurs Stand.* 2003;18:33-39
169. American Academy of Pediatrics Committee on Fetus and Newborn. The prevention and management of pain and stress in the neonate. *Pediatrics.* 2000;105:454-461
170. American Academy of Pediatrics Committee on Psychosocial Aspects of Child and Family Health. The assessment and management of acute pain in infants, children, and adolescents. *Pediatrics.* 2001;108:793-797

Chapter 2

Sedatives and Analgesics: General Principles and Pharmacology

Lynne Maxwell, MD, FAAP
Santhanam Suresh, MD, FAAP
Joseph D. Tobias, MD, FAAP

- Specific Agents
  - Opioids
    - Opioid Receptors
    - Opioid Chemistry and Metabolism
    - Opioid Antagonists
    - Adverse Effects of Opioids
    - Adverse Effects of Opioid Antagonists
  - Propofol
  - Ketamine
  - Etomidate
  - Barbiturates
  - Nitrous Oxide
  - Chloral Hydrate
  - Benzodiazepines
  - Dexmedetomidine
- Local Anesthetic Agents
  - Local Anesthetics—Amides
    - Lidocaine
    - Bupivacaine
    - Ropivacaine
    - Levobupivacaine
  - Local Anesthetics—Esters
- Topical Anesthesia

Introduction

Several agents are now available that provide analgesia, amnesia, and anxiolysis. Some of these medications also have been used as therapeutic agents (eg, barbiturates for the treatment of intracranial hypertension or propofol for the treatment of refractory status epilepticus). In most clinical scenarios, these drugs are incrementally titrated until the desired effect (sedation or analgesia) is achieved. Basic knowledge about the pharmacologic profile, metabolism, and adverse effects of these agents will help the clinician to select the appropriate agent for a specific clinical scenario. This may be especially critical for patients who have altered renal or hepatic function, which may affect the pharmacologic profile of these medications. This chapter reviews the basic principles and pharmacology of the analgesic and sedative agents that are discussed throughout this handbook.

Specific Agents

Opioids

Opioid Receptors

Opioid receptors and endogenous endorphins are classified as agonists, antagonists, and mixed agonist-antagonists, based on their receptor affinity.[1] The interaction between opioid medications and receptors is responsible for their desired analgesic and sedative effects, as well as their less desirable adverse effects.[2]

As outlined in Table 2-1, there are 4 primary opioid receptor types: μ, κ, δ, and σ. Sites of binding of agonists and antagonists range from the peripheral nervous system to the spinal cord to the brain. The μ receptor has 2 subtypes: μ_1 and μ_2. The μ_1 receptor is responsible for supraspinal analgesia and the development of dependence. The μ_2 receptor is associated with most opioid adverse effects, including respiratory depression, slowing of gastrointestinal (GI) motility, nausea/vomiting, pruritus, and sedation. The κ receptor is responsible for spinal analgesia and also contributes to opioid-induced sedation.[2]

The κ and δ receptors have been subtyped as well, although specific differentiation of physiologic effects has not been fully determined. It is likely that other receptors and subtypes remain to be discovered.

As is true for other classes of receptors, drugs exist that are pure agonists at one or more opioid receptors. Other drugs are antagonists at some or all of these same receptors, and a third group of drugs may be agonists at one receptor and antagonists at another receptor. These are the so-called mixed agonist/antagonists. Agonists interact with the receptor and trigger a series of subcellular or intracellular processes, which serve to translate the binding into the definitive end-organ effect. The analgesic effect is modulated through the activation of signaling proteins (such as G proteins). The end effect is modulation of nociceptive neurotransmission (signal transduction) either through a direct effect on the nociceptive neuron or through inhibitory neurons that secondarily affect the primary nociceptive pathway.[3] Antagonists

Table 2-1. Opioid Receptors and Their Effects

Receptor	Agonists	Antagonists	Effects	Adverse Effects
μ	Morphine Fentanyl(s) Meperidine Remifentanil	Naloxone Nalmefene Butorphanol	μ_1 Supraspinal analgesia μ_2 Sedation	μ_1 Dependence μ_2 Respiratory depression, inhibition of gastrointestinal motility, urinary retention, bradycardia, pruritus
κ	Butorphanol Nalbuphine	Naloxone Nalmefene	Spinal analgesia, sedation	Miosis, inhibition of antidiuretic hormone release
δ	Enkephalins	Analgesia		
σ	Ketamine* Butorphanol	Naloxone Nalmefene		Dysphoria, hallucinations, psychomotor stimulation

*Ketamine, although not an opioid, does affect the σ receptor.

bind to the same receptor(s), but do not result in transduction. They may displace the agonist agent and, therefore, reverse its effect (or side effect). Antagonists commonly used in the context of sedation include naloxone and, more recently, nalmefene. A third class of drugs has actions both as agonists at one or more receptors and antagonists at other receptors. These drugs, butorphanol (Stadol, Bristol-Meyers-Squibb, Princeton, NJ) and nalbuphine (Nubain, Endo Pharmaceuticals, Chadds Ford, PA), are rarely used for procedural sedation/analgesia, but sometimes are used to provide analgesia when there is an increased risk of respiratory depression (central nervous system [CNS] or pulmonary disease) or to treat opioid side effects. Table 2-1 lists the medications that interact with the various opioid receptors and are commonly used to implement or reverse sedation/analgesia in children. Although δ receptors are known to bind enkephalins and some experimental drugs resulting in spinal and supraspinal analgesic effects, none of the opioids commonly used in clinical medicine bind to these receptors.[2]

Opioid Chemistry and Metabolism

Morphine is a phenanthrene alkaloid, which is derived from the poppy plant because it is difficult to synthesize in the laboratory. The major route of morphine metabolism is hepatic glucuronidation with a major metabolite being the active moiety, morphine-6-glucuronide (M6G), which is several times as potent as morphine systemically; however, given its water solubility, it has limited penetration through the blood-brain barrier. It is excreted by the kidneys and may accumulate in patients with renal failure. The 3-glucuronide by-product does not bind to opioid receptors. The half-life of morphine is approximately 2 to 3 hours, but may be longer in infants younger than 3 months due to decreased glucuronidation and/or renal excretion, especially of the active M6G metabolite.[1] The age at which adult-like morphine metabolism and excretion develops varies, but it has been shown to occur between the ages of 1 and 3 months in term infants.[1,4] The significance of the developmental aspects of morphine metabolism is much greater in long-term neonatal intensive care unit or pediatric intensive care unit (PICU) sedation by infusion than in the acute sedation/analgesia setting. Another of the opioid agonists, hydromorphone, shares a similar half-life with morphine (2 to 3 hours in adults), but lacks active hepatic metabolites.

Metabolism of synthetic opioids such as fentanyl is dependent on the hepatic enzyme system. Unlike morphine, synthetic opioids have no active metabolites and their half-life is less dependent on renal function. The pharmacokinetics of fentanyl and its congeners (sufentanil, alfentanil) have been less well studied in healthy, term infants, but clearance is reduced and half-life increased in preterm infants.[5] The metabolism of fentanyl and sufentanil is relatively unaffected in patients with liver disease. Another of the synthetic opioids, remifentanil, is different from all other opioids in that it undergoes non-hepatic metabolism and is rapidly metabolized (cleaved) by plasma esterases. Therefore, its half-life is independent of liver and kidney function and does not vary among neonates, infants, and older children. Its ultra-short half-life requires administration by continuous infusion for prolonged analgesia.

Opioid Antagonists

Naloxone (Narcan, Endo Pharmaceuticals, Chadds Ford, PA) and its longer-acting cousin, nalmefene, are μ-receptor antagonists and, therefore, can be used to reverse both the analgesic/sedative effects and side effects of opioids acting at the μ receptor.[1] Naloxone is rapidly distributed, metabolized by glucuronide conjugation, and excreted in the urine, with a half-life of approximately 1 hour in children and adults and 90 minutes to 3 hours in neonates.[6] Naloxone has been used safely to treat opioid overdose in children of all ages including neonates, although there is risk of precipitating an abstinence syndrome (irritability, sweating, diarrhea, tachycardia) in neonates of opioid-addicted mothers or any patient with a history of long-term opioid use. The long half-life of some opioids compared with the short half-life of naloxone may require repeated doses or an infusion to avoid recurrence of opioid-induced adverse effects. In addition to a shorter half-life, naloxone has lower affinity for μ receptors than most opioids; therefore, it leaves the site of action more rapidly than even the shorter half-life would predict. In the treatment of respiratory depression during sedation/analgesia, the use of naloxone (or nalmefene) is preferable to the use of mixed agonists/antagonists such as nalbuphine or butorphanol, which may have less predictable antagonistic effects. While opioid antagonists commonly are regarded as antagonists only at the μ receptor, they have been found to be effective in reversing the κ-receptor mediated respiratory depression and sedation caused by mixed agonist-antagonist agents. Nalmefene (Revex, Ivax Corporation, Miami, FL) is a naltrexone derivative that is a pure opioid antagonist without agonist effects. It has a longer duration of effect than naloxone and is a more potent antagonist than naloxone at all types of opioid receptors. Nalmefene is 4 times as potent as naloxone in antagonizing effects at the μ receptor and more potent than naloxone in antagonizing effects at the κ receptor.[1]

Adverse Effects of Opioids

Common adverse effects of opioids include respiratory depression and effects on the cardiovascular and nervous systems (Table 2-2). Opioid agonists depress ventilatory drive by reducing sensitivity of the respiratory center to hypercarbia and hypoxia as well as breathing rhythm, which results first in a decrease in the respiratory rate followed by a decrease in tidal volume with increasing doses. This is reflected in a decrease in the slope and a rightward shift of the carbon dioxide response curve. What is even more concerning in the setting of procedural sedation/analgesia is the routine coadministration of opioids with a range of sedative drugs, such as benzodiazepines, phenothiazines, barbiturates, and propofol, which causes the carbon dioxide response curve to shift and flatten even further, greatly increasing the

Table 2-2. Serious Adverse Effects of Opioids

Adverse Effect	Mechanism	Causative Agents	Reversal Agent
Respiratory depression: Central*	CNS: brainstem, μ mediated Brainstem: medullary, pontine centers	All opioids	Naloxone/nalmefene
Other CNS effects: Seizures	Inhibition of inhibitory interneurons μ receptor mediated	Opioids (especially meperidine); morphine in neonates	Naloxone; lower dose
Myoclonic movements	Unknown	Meperidine (normeperidine)	None known
Sedation, dysphoria	μ receptor effects (dysphoria μ_2)	All opioids	Naloxone/nalmefene
	κ receptor effects	Morphine, butorphanol	
	σ receptor effects (dysphoria)	Butorphanol, nalbuphine	
Other respiratory: Chest wall rigidity	μ_1 and κ mediated GABA modulation	Fentanyl, sufentanil, alfentanil, remifentanil (large bolus; lower doses in neonates)	Naloxone/nalmefene, neuromuscular blocking agent with endotracheal intubation
Cardiovascular: Hypotension†	Histamine release and decreased sympathetic outflow from μ agonism in brainstem and periphery	Morphine and all opioids except meperidine	Naloxone/nalmefene
Bradycardia	Decreased sympathetic outflow from μ agonism	Fentanyl, sufentanil, alfentanil, remifentanil	Anticholinergic agents (atropine); opioid antagonists (naloxone or nalmefene)
Tachycardia and arrhythmia	Anticholinergic effects and catecholamine release	Meperidine‡	None known

*Respiratory depression exacerbated with combinations of medications.
†Hypotension potentiated with combinations of medications or in patients with compromised cardiovascular function or hypovolemia.
‡Arrhythmia seen primarily in overdose.

risk of hypoventilation, desaturation, and even apnea despite hypercarbia and hypoxemia.[6] This effect has been seen in healthy adult volunteers and in children.[6,7] In preterm infants and neonates, the rate of metabolism and excretion of opioid agonists is extremely variable (because of immaturity of hepatic enzyme systems and decreased renal clearance) and is inversely related to postconceptional age.[8] Although respiratory depression occurs more frequently in this age group, a direct correlation between respiratory depression and plasma drug levels generally has not been found. However, Quinn and Vokes[9] found lower respiratory rates in preterm infants and higher levels of M6G after a continuous infusion of morphine.

In addition to the centrally mediated adverse effects on ventilation, another respiratory effect of opioids is chest wall rigidity, which has been reported with the synthetic opioids including fentanyl, sufentanil and, more recently, remifentanil.[10] The mechanism of this effect is thought to be mediated in part by the modulation of γ-aminobutyric acid (GABA) pathways at the spinal cord and basal ganglia levels through synthetic opioid binding to μ_1 and κ receptors. Other opioids (morphine, meperidine) also bind to these receptors, but have not been reported to cause chest wall rigidity. Rigidity caused by fentanyl and its congeners may be related to faster onset, increased lipophilicity and, therefore, increased CNS penetration, and differences in binding and intracellular transduction. Although chest wall rigidity has been noted in adult patients after bolus administration of large doses during anesthetic induction, it has been reported in neonates, both term and preterm, at lower doses (1-2 μg/kg).[11,12] In a study by Fahnenstich et al,[11] 3 to 5 μg/kg of fentanyl was administered to 97 preterm and term infants (25-40 weeks' gestational age). Chest wall rigidity was observed in 8 patients. All 8 had respiratory distress, hypercarbia, and hypoxemia, followed by bradycardia. Laryngospasm was noted in 2 patients, which prevented endotracheal intubation. Chest wall rigidity was quickly and easily reversed in less than 1 minute by the administration of naloxone in a dose of 20 to 40 μg/kg. One of the patients in this study and one reported by Muller and Vogtmann[12] received only 2 μg/kg. In addition, chest wall rigidity has been reported in a 2-month-old patient after 35 minutes of receiving a continuous infusion of fentanyl at 4.3 μg/kg/h with no bolus administration.[11] These cases emphasize the necessity of administering boluses of these drugs slowly in small increments, especially in neonates, and having naloxone available at the bedside. Because it may take as long as 1 minute for naloxone to reverse rigidity, neuromuscular blocking agents also should be immediately available in the event that severe hypoxemia with inability to ventilate is not immediately reversed by naloxone administration.

Meperidine (Demerol, Sanofi-Synthelabo, Paris, France) has a high incidence of CNS side effects, which is unique among the opioids. This is due primarily to meperidine's principle metabolite, normeperidine, which can cause tremors, muscle twitches, hyperactivity of reflexes, and seizures.[1] These effects are more likely after prolonged administration. After 3 days (or more quickly in patients with renal failure), normeperidine may accumulate.[1] Anticonvulsants (eg, phenytoin, phenobarbital, and phenothiazines) increase the conversion of meperidine to normeperidine.[13] Therefore, the frequency of seizures may increase in patients with epilepsy who are treated with anticonvulsants and also receive meperidine.

Although CNS effects are much more common with meperidine, they have been reported with all other opioids, including morphine,[14,15] fentanyl, alfentanil, and remifentanil,[16,17] with an increased incidence in neonates, perhaps because of their more permeable blood-brain barrier. There have been reports of "seizures" including tonic-clonic movements with all of these drugs, but studies in which an electroencephalogram (EEG) was recorded during administration of large doses of opioids showed no cortical epileptiform activity during periods of muscle rigidity and myoclonic limb movements in older patients.[15] However, in neonates, EEG abnormalities have been reported after morphine and fentanyl administration[15] and, in one case, the abnormalities were terminated by a naloxone infusion. As is the case with chest wall rigidity, CNS effects are thought to be related to excitation of pyramidal neurons of the hippocampus due to inhibition of nearby interneurons of the GABA class.[1]

Sedation is an intrinsic effect of opioid binding to the μ receptor and usually desirable. Opioids that bind to the κ receptor, such as morphine and the agonist-antagonist butorphanol, have an even more exaggerated sedative effect than those opioids that bind only to the μ receptor (fentanyl, meperidine). Although tolerance to the sedative effects develops rapidly when compared with other adverse effects of opioids, with long-term infusions (eg, the terminal cancer patient), stimulant medications occasionally are needed to prevent excessive sedation. The dysphoric effects of opioids are due in part to the μ_2-related CNS excitatory phenomena discussed previously but, in the mixed agonist-antagonist drugs, are also due to σ receptor binding (Table 2-1).

Opioids exhibit variable hemodynamic effects. Morphine can cause vasodilation (especially venodilation), which is due to histamine release and not a μ receptor effect.[18] Venodilation is a primary reason why morphine historically was used in adults with heart failure and pulmonary edema as a means of reducing venous return (preload) and "unloading" the heart. Despite these effects, morphine usually is not accompanied by a significant change in cardiac output except in patients who are hypovolemic or in an upright posture. Although other opioids alone rarely cause hypotension, all other opioids may cause hypotension when used with other sedative drugs, especially propofol or benzodiazepines, with a more exaggerated effect in hypovolemic patients.

Many of the cardiovascular side effects of opioid administration are neurologically mediated. Opioid receptors are widely distributed throughout the central and peripheral nervous system and the hemodynamic effects of exogenous and endogenous opioids are related to binding at receptors in multiple areas, including the brainstem (nucleus solitarius and nucleus ambiguus), periaqueductal grey matter, and in the periphery of the sympathetic nervous system.[19] Opioids, especially the synthetic agents, also modulate the stress response through receptor-mediated actions on the hypothalamic-pituitary-adrenal axis, thereby decreasing endogenous catecholamine release during surgical procedures. Most opioids reduce sympathetic and enhance vagal and parasympathetic tone. If not countered by indirect effects (eg, catecholamine release) or the coadministration of drugs with anticholinergic or sympathomimetic activity (eg, atropine, ephedrine), opioids can cause bradycardia and hypotension. Patients who are volume depleted, or individuals dependent on high sympathetic tone or exogenous catecholamines to maintain cardiovascular function (such as those with heart failure) are predisposed to hypotension after opioid administration. Meperidine, alone among opioids, may cause tachycardia and arrhythmias. These may be due to both vagolytic and central stimulant actions. Tachycardia after meperidine administration may be related to its structural similarity to atropine, normeperidine (its principal metabolite), or its CNS stimulatory effects.

Adverse Effects of Opioid Antagonists

It is commonly thought that naloxone and nalmefene have no pharmacologic or physiologic effects in patients who have no opioids in their system. Doses as high as 4 mg/kg have been administered intravenously to healthy adult volunteers without adverse physiologic effects.[20] However, use of opioid antagonists to reverse opioid sedation and respiratory depression has been associated with significant complications, including pulmonary edema, tachycardia, hypertension, and even death. These adverse effects may be particularly prominent in children and young adults in whom pain is still present.[21] Seizures have been reported after naloxone administration, but only in patients with CNS pathology who receive relatively large doses.

In some pediatric studies, routine reversal of opioid effect has been used at the end of a procedure for which sedation/analgesia is administered.[22] Previous reports of life-threatening complications after opioid reversal would dictate caution in advocating "universal reversal." Reversal should be used only in situations in which respiratory depression or obstruction cannot be relieved with stimulation and airway positioning. Even in such situations, naloxone or nalmefene administration should be titrated in small increments to mitigate the respiratory depression and/or sedation without reversing analgesia. Commonly recommended doses of naloxone as high as 0.1 mg/kg with a maximum of 2 mg per dose are appropriate only for patients presenting with acute opioid ingestions or intoxications. During sedation, doses as low as 0.001 mg/kg should be used to achieve reversal of side effects only. Repeat doses can be administered at 1-minute intervals until there is reversal of respiratory depression. By doing this, it is possible to reverse respiratory depression without reversing analgesia. Larger, yet still relatively small (0.08-0.8 mg), doses in the immediate postoperative setting have been associated with the onset of acute pulmonary edema in healthy children and young adults.[21] Naloxone has been reported to induce an acute rise in blood pressure in adults receiving clonidine chronically. It is unknown whether this may occur in children receiving clonidine for either blood pressure or pain control, but caution should be taken when administering opioid antagonists in this setting. Another situation in which opioid reversal by naloxone might be ill-advised is in patients with, or at risk for, glaucoma, because intraocular opioid receptors are involved in regulation of intraocular pressure. Opioids reduce intraocular pressure and antagonist administration reverses the effect.[23]

Overdoses of nalmefene have not been reported, but the possibility of naloxone-like catecholamine stimulation should be considered because it may induce arrhythmias and hypertension, especially in patients receiving clonidine. Because of its prolonged duration of action, nalmefene has potential advantages over naloxone. As with naloxone, pulmonary edema has been reported in a young healthy patient after opioid reversal with nalmefene.[24] However, there is less risk of recurrent respiratory depression given the longer half-life (Table 2-3).

Gastrointestinal effects of all opioids include nausea and/or vomiting, which may be mitigated by coadministration of propofol or prophylactic use of an anti-emetic such as ondansetron. Nausea and/or vomiting and biliary spasm may occur after a single short-term use of opioids for sedation, whereas other GI effects, such as decreased bowel motility (constipation, ileus), occur with long-term administration of opioids. Even with long-term administration, tolerance to the GI effects of opioids occurs slowly if at all. Therefore, appropriate attention to bowel habits is mandatory in any patient receiving opioids.

The main genitourinary effect of opioids is a decrease in tone of the urinary tract, resulting in the potential for urinary retention. This is compounded by an increase in antidiuretic hormone release. This effect is more common with morphine and meperidine than with the fentanyl class of opioids.[1] Opioids also decrease intravesical pressure and increase bladder compliance by partially inhibiting discharge of parasympathetic nerves that innervate the bladder and control bladder tone and contraction. This has been reported more frequently in the setting of long-term sedation in preterm infants.[25]

Short-term use of opioids, such as for relatively brief sedation/analgesia, may result in mild pruritus. With more prolonged opioid use, as in a patient in the intensive care unit (ICU) or during the postoperative period, pruritus may cause great discomfort. Opioid-induced itching is caused by μ receptor binding.[26] When morphine is used,

Table 2-3. Pharmacokinetic Characteristics of Opioid Antagonists

Drug	Onset	Duration of Action	$T_{1/2}$ (Serum)	Dose*
Naloxone (Narcan)	1-2 minutes	20-30 minutes	63 minutes	1-2 μg/kg q. 1-2 minutes
Nalmefene (Revex)	1-2 minutes	4 hours	10-12 hours	0.25 μg/kg q. 2 minutes

*Dose cited refers to sedation situation, not acute opioid overdose.

the effect may be exacerbated by histamine release, resulting in wheal formation where the intravenous morphine is injected. With short-term opioid use, itching will subside as opioid levels recede, but in longer-term use, or if pruritus is severe, treatment may be necessary. Antihistamines such as diphenhydramine or hydroxyzine are usually effective, but may increase sedation and respiratory depression. Likewise, a small dose of a mixed agonist-antagonist, such as nalbuphine (0.01 mg/kg as opposed to the analgesic dose of 0.05 mg/kg) or butorphanol, is effective in treating itching but may result in increased sedation because of the κ binding of these agents. In situations in which increased sedation is undesirable, a low-dose infusion of an opioid antagonist such as naloxone, or bolus administration of the longer-acting nalmefene, will decrease itching without reversing analgesia or causing sedation. Alternatively, switching from morphine to hydromorphone is another option because hydromorphone may cause less histamine release.

Opioid receptor binding modulates immune function by incompletely understood mechanisms. Newly discovered opioid receptors outside the CNS through which opioid binding modulates pain also are present on immune cells, which participate in inflammatory processes. The presence of immune cells with opioid receptors at the site of inflammation may enhance the efficacy of opioids to mitigate the pain in inflammatory processes. Opioids may, in some cases, interfere with positive aspects of the inflammatory response, as has been shown in the case of increased viral loads in patients with HIV who are taking methadone.[27] In addition, morphine has been shown to cause some degree of macrophage injury in a mouse model, which is mitigated by naloxone pretreatment. Opioids also can modulate cytokine production.[28] Whether any of these effects on immune function occur or are clinically significant in the short-term sedation setting is unknown, but may be of more concern in immunosuppressed patients (eg, transplant or oncology) who require long-term analgesia.

Propofol

Propofol (2,6-di-isoprophylphenol) is commonly classified as an intravenous anesthetic agent. Because of its insolubility in water, it is commercially available in a soy-egg lecithin emulsion as a 1% (10 mg/mL) solution. Its chemical structure is distinct from that of the barbiturates and other commonly used anesthetic induction agents. Propofol is a sedative/amnestic agent, possesses no analgesic properties, and should be combined with an opioid when analgesia is required. Like the barbiturates (discussed later), its effects are mediated through the GABA receptor system resulting in an increase in the duration of time that the GABA molecule occupies the receptor. This interaction increases chloride conductance across the cell membrane.

The anesthetic induction dose of propofol in healthy adults ranges from 1.5 to 3 mg/kg with recommended maintenance infusion rates of 50 to 200 µg/kg/min; the exact dose depends on the depth of sedation required. Following intravenous administration, propofol is rapidly cleared from the central compartment and undergoes hepatic metabolism to inactive water-soluble metabolites, which are then renally cleared. Propofol's clearance rate exceeds hepatic blood flow, suggesting an extrahepatic route of elimination. Propofol's rapid clearance and metabolism provide rapid awakening when the infusion is discontinued. Clearance in patients with hepatic or renal dysfunction is not altered.

Although initially introduced for anesthetic induction and maintenance, propofol's pharmacodynamic profile, including a rapid onset, rapid recovery time, and lack of active metabolites, led to its evaluation as an agent for ICU and procedural sedation.[29,30] In addition to its favorable properties with regard to sedation and recovery times, propofol has beneficial effects on CNS dynamics, including a decreased cerebral metabolic rate for oxygen ($CMRO_2$), cerebral vasoconstriction, and lowering of intracranial pressure (ICP).[31] These effects are clinically similar to those seen with the barbiturates and etomidate and suggest that propofol may be an effective and beneficial agent for sedation in patients with altered intracranial compliance, provided that ventilation is controlled to prevent increases in $PaCO_2$ related to the respiratory depressant properties of propofol.

Despite encouraging animal studies demonstrating a decreased $CMRO_2$, cerebral vasoconstriction, and lowering of ICP,[32,33] a review of the literature concerning propofol use in humans provides somewhat contradictory results. Although several studies demonstrate a decrease in ICP, there also is a lowering of the mean arterial pressure (MAP). This decrease in cerebral perfusion pressure may lead to reflex cerebral vasodilation to maintain cerebral blood flow (CBF), which may result in an increase in ICP and negate the decrease in ICP induced by the direct effects of propofol on $CMRO_2$.[34-38] Further study is necessary to fully evaluate the role of propofol in controlling ICP. With control of MAP, the initial clinical and laboratory evidence suggests that propofol can be used to decrease $CMRO_2$, CBF, and ICP. Additionally, propofol maintains CBF autoregulation in response to changes in MAP and $PaCO_2$. Preliminary evidence suggests a CNS protective effect, similar to that reported with the barbiturates, during periods of cerebral hypoperfusion and ischemia.[39-41]

Depending on the clinical scenario, the beneficial physiologic effects of propofol may be offset by adverse effects. Propofol decreases MAP related to peripheral vasodilation and negative inotropic properties.[42] Propofol alters the baroreflex responses, resulting in a smaller increase in heart rate for a given decrease in blood pressure. These cardiovascular effects are especially pronounced following bolus administration. Although well-tolerated by patients with adequate cardiovascular function, these effects may result in detrimental physiologic effects in patients with compromised cardiovascular function. Tritapepe et al[43] demonstrated that the administration of calcium chloride (10 mg/kg) may prevent the deleterious cardiovascular effects of propofol during anesthetic induction in patients undergoing coronary artery bypass grafting. Additional cardiovascular effects relate to propofol's augmentation of central vagal tone leading to bradycardia or even asystole when combined with other medications that decrease cardiac chronotropic function (fentanyl, succinylcholine).[44,45]

Reported neurologic manifestations and movement disorders with intravenous administration of propofol include opisthotonic posturing, myoclonic movements (especially in children), and even seizure-like activity.[46-49] Although actual clinical seizure activity has been reported, these concerns have most likely been overemphasized, because no electroencephalographic evidence of seizure activity has been documented during the abnormal movements seen with propofol administration. Additionally, propofol has been used as a therapeutic agent for refractory status epilepticus.[50]

Like many of the sedative/analgesic agents discussed in this chapter, propofol has significant respiratory-depressant effects, which may be increased when combined with other agents (eg, opioids). Studies of its use for procedural sedation in spontaneously breathing patients report a high incidence of respiratory effects including hypoventilation, upper airway obstruction, and apnea.[51] Despite its respiratory depressant effects, laboratory and clinical studies have suggested that propofol may be beneficial for endotracheal intubation of patients with asthma. In an animal model, Chih-Chung et al[52] demonstrated attenuation of carbachol-induced airway constriction by propofol via a decrease in intracellular inositol phosphate and limitation of intracellular calcium availability.

A major concern with prolonged (>48 hours) administration of propofol for sedation in the PICU setting are reports of unexplained metabolic acidosis, bradydysrhythmias, and fatal cardiac failure.[53-55] In 1992, Parke et al[53] reported a series of 5 children with respiratory infections and respiratory failure who received prolonged propofol infusions in doses up to 13.6 mg/kg/h who developed metabolic acidosis and eventually died from bradydysrhythmias and cardiac failure. Bray[55] reported 18 children with suspected propofol infusion syndrome and identified risk factors for the syndrome, including administration for more than 48 hours or doses greater than 4 mg/kg/h. Another associated factor was age; 13 of the 18 patients were 4 years old or younger and only 1 of 18 was more than 10 years old. Since the review of Bray,[55] the syndrome has been reported in a 17-year-old patient and in a cohort of adults with closed head injury.[56] In addition to the cardiovascular manifestations, signs and symptoms include metabolic acidosis, lipemic serum, hepatomegaly, and muscle involvement with rhabdomyolysis. Interruption of mitochondrial oxidative phosphorylation by propofol or a metabolite has been suggested as a possible mechanism for the syndrome. Recommended treatment includes immediate discontinuation of the propofol followed by symptomatic treatment of the cardiovascular dysfunction. In patients with rhabdomyolysis and renal failure, hemodialysis has been used. Although effective in the management of patients with associated renal insufficiency/failure, it has not been determined whether the role of hemodialysis is to manage renal dysfunction or whether it also may have a therapeutic effect through the removal of a toxic metabolite. Caution is suggested with the administration of propofol by continuous infusion in the ICU setting for more than 48 hours.

Additional problems with propofol relate to its delivery in a lipid emulsion, similar to that used for parenteral hyperalimentation. There are reports of anaphylactoid reactions, which may be more likely in patients with a history of egg allergy.[57] Pain occurs with propofol administration through a peripheral infusion site. Preadministration of lidocaine, pretreatment with thiopental, mixing the lidocaine and propofol in a single solution, diluting the concentration of the propofol, cooling the solution prior to bolus administration, or the administration of ketamine (0.5 mg/kg) may decrease the incidence of pain.[58-60] Given the limited analgesic properties of propofol, concomitant administration of ketamine and propofol can take advantage of the analgesia of ketamine and the rapid recovery of propofol. The high lipid content of the solution also can result in hypertriglyceridemia and potentially hypercarbia with high infusion rates over prolonged periods.[61,62] The lipid content of propofol should be considered when calculating the patient's daily caloric intake. A propofol infusion of 2 mg/kg/h provides 0.5 g/kg/d of fat. To limit the total lipid administration, especially with higher infusion rates such as those used in the ICU setting, a 2% solution containing 20 mg/mL of propofol is being investigated as opposed to 10 mg/mL in a 1% solution.

The initial formulation of propofol did not contain preservatives. Laboratory investigation has demonstrated that the lipid emulsion of propofol is a suitable culture medium for bacteria, and reports have linked systemic bacteremia and postoperative wound infections to extrinsically contaminated propofol.[63,64] Current preparations of propofol include either ethylenediaminetetraacetic acid (EDTA) or sodium metabisulfite as preservatives. Despite the recent improvements, meticulous aseptic technique is required when using propofol, and opened but unused vials should be disposed of immediately.

Ketamine

Ketamine was introduced in the 1960s and generally is classified as an intravenous anesthetic agent that is structurally related to phencyclidine. Ketamine provides amnesia and analgesia, which makes it particularly attractive for sedation during procedures. Its molecular structure contains a chiral center at the C2 carbon of the cyclohexanone ring, resulting in both an S (+) and R (–) enantiomer. Preliminary data suggest that the S (+) isomer may possess clinical advantages including a more potent anesthetic/analgesic effect, a more limited duration of action with a more rapid awakening, and fewer psychomimetic effects (hallucinations and emergence delirium).[65]

Ketamine's anesthetic and analgesic properties result from poorly defined mechanisms within the limbic and thalamic systems, providing what has been termed "dissociative anesthesia." Additional sites of action include the *N*-methyl-D-aspartate (NMDA) receptor as well as the σ-opioid receptor. Commercially available ketamine is a racemic mixture of 2 optical isomers in a concentration of 10 mg/mL (1%), 50 mg/mL (5%), or 100 mg/mL (10%). Metabolism occurs primarily by hepatic N-methylation. One metabolite, norketamine, is further metabolized via hydroxylation pathways with subsequent urinary excretion. Norketamine retains one third of the analgesic and sedative properties of the parent compound. Ketamine's bioavailability is 100% following intravenous or intramuscular administration, but is markedly decreased with oral or rectal administration because of limited absorption and a high degree of first-pass hepatic metabolism. Metabolism of ketamine to norketamine during first pass metabolism may account for most of its anesthetic effect following oral or rectal administration. Infusion doses should be reduced in patients with hepatic dysfunction.

Ketamine maintains cardiovascular function and has limited effects on respiratory mechanics. In most clinical scenarios, ketamine causes a dose-related increase in heart rate and blood pressure, which is mediated through the sympathetic nervous system response with the release of endogenous catecholamines.[66,67] Increased heart rate and blood pressure can increase myocardial oxygen consumption, which can alter the balance between myocardial oxygen demand and delivery, inducing ischemia in patients with ischemic heart disease. Hypertension and tachycardia following ketamine administration can be decreased by the administration of ketamine with a benzodiazepine, a barbiturate, propofol, or synthetic opioid. Although ketamine's indirect sympathomimetic effects generally overshadow its direct negative inotropic properties, hypotension may occur in patients with diminished myocardial contractility.[68,69] In patients with compromised myocardial function, ketamine's direct negative inotropic properties predominate because the endogenous catecholamine stores have been depleted.

Ketamine's effects on pulmonary vascular resistance (PVR) remain controversial. Initial studies involved patients with spontaneous ventilation and the reported alterations in PVR may have been related to increases in $PaCO_2$ and not a direct effect of ketamine on the pulmonary vasculature. Morray et al[70] noted a mean pulmonary artery pressure increase from 20.6 to 22.8 mmHg and increases in PVR following ketamine administration to infants with congenital heart disease during spontaneous ventilation. In contrast, Hickey et al[71] reported no change in PVR in intubated infants (7 with normal and 7 with elevated baseline PVR) receiving minimal ventilatory support. Despite the controversy about its effects on PVR, the available literature on infants and children with cyanotic and non-cyanotic congenital heart disease shows beneficial effects of ketamine on overall cardiovascular performance with maintenance or improvement of oxygen saturation.[72]

Functional residual capacity, minute ventilation, and tidal volume remain unchanged following ketamine administration.[73] In an animal model of reactive airway disease, Hirshman et al[74] demonstrated improved pulmonary compliance, decreased resistance, and prevention of bronchospasm. The effects on respiratory mechanisms have been attributed partially to effects from the release of endogenous catecholamines.[75] Although minute ventilation is generally maintained, hypercarbia and a depressed ventilatory response to carbon dioxide may occur.[75,76]

Additional issues surround ketamine's effect on protective airway reflexes. Although clinical use and experimental studies suggest that airway reflexes are maintained, aspiration and laryngospasm have been reported following ketamine administration in patients who are spontaneously breathing without a protected airway.[77] Ketamine can cause apnea, especially in higher doses, when combined with other sedative/analgesic agents, or in critically ill patients. An additional effect that may influence airway patency and compromise respiratory function is increased oral secretions, which is mediated via stimulation of central cholinergic receptors. To lessen such problems, an antisialagogue such as atropine or glycopyrrolate can be administered before ketamine.

Another controversial issue about ketamine is its effect on CBF and ICP, with some studies demonstrating increased ICP and others decreased ICP.[78-81] The risk-benefit ratio must be considered when using ketamine in patients with altered intracranial compliance. As with any sedative/analgesic agent administered to patients with altered intracranial compliance who are spontaneously ventilating, a secondary effect may be seen if the agent depresses ventilatory function resulting in hypercarbia, which secondarily leads to cerebral vasodilation and increased ICP.

Ketamine may cause emergence phenomena or hallucinations. Emergence phenomena are dose-related, and clinical practice suggests that they occur more commonly in adolescents and adults. Their incidence can be decreased by the pre- or concomitant administration of a barbiturate, propofol, or benzodiazepine.[82] Emergence phenomena may result from the alteration of auditory and visual relays in the inferior colliculus and the medical geniculate nucleus with a misinterpretation of visual and auditory stimuli.

Etomidate

Etomidate is a carboxylated, imidazole-containing intravenous anesthetic agent. It was initially synthesized in 1964 and introduced into clinical anesthesia practice in 1972. Because the aqueous solution of etomidate is unstable at physiologic pH, it is available in a 0.2% (2 mg/mL) solution with 35% propylene glycol. The pH of 6.9 of this solution and the carrier vehicle, propylene glycol, account for the high incidence of pain and the potential for thrombophlebitis with administration through peripheral intravenous cannulae. As with other medications that contain propylene glycol as a diluent (eg, lorazepam), one-time administration is not a problem, but propylene glycol toxicity has been reported following long-term infusions.[83] Etomidate provides its anesthetic effects through the GABA system with alterations of chloride conductance across the cell membrane.[84] When compared with the barbiturates and propofol, etomidate has little effect on cardiovascular performance, even in patients with altered myocardial contractility, making it a popular anesthetic induction agent in this population.[85, 86] Anesthetic induction doses range from 0.2 to 0.4 mg/kg and provide a rapid onset of amnesia and sedation with a rapid emergence time following a one-time bolus dose. Etomidate undergoes hepatic ester hydrolysis with the formation of inactive water-soluble metabolites. The elimination half-life is prolonged in patients with hepatic dysfunction. Because etomidate possesses limited analgesic properties, it may not effectively blunt the hemodynamic response to endotracheal intubation in patients with normal cardiovascular function, and coadministration of a synthetic opioid is frequently used in anesthetic practice to provide a more stable hemodynamic profile.

Etomidate decreases the $CMRO_2$, resulting in cerebral vasoconstriction and a decrease in CBF and ICP. Cerebral perfusion pressure is maintained, making it a suitable induction agent for patients with altered myocardial contractility and increased ICP. In most patients, etomidate produces EEG changes similar to that of the barbiturates; however, it also can produce epileptic-like EEG potentials without accompanying motor activity in patients with seizure disorders.[87] Etomidate also frequently produces myoclonic movements following bolus administration. This is not associated with EEG changes suggestive of epileptic activity.

Most clinical experience with etomidate involves using a single dose for the induction of anesthesia in adults. Kay[88] noted a rapid onset of anesthesia with etomidate and limited effects on cardiovascular function in 198 infants and children ranging in age from 1 day to 15 years. Tobias[89] reported anecdotal experience with the use of etomidate for anesthetic induction in 3 children in various clinical scenarios where cardiovascular function was compromised, including a 33-month-old with a dilated cardiomyopathy, a 9-year-old trauma victim with hypovolemia and increased ICP, and a 10-year-old with aortic stenosis and respiratory failure. Canessa et al[90] evaluated 4 anesthetic agents (thiopental 3 mg/kg, etomidate 0.15 mg/kg, midazolam 0.15 mg/kg, and propofol 1.5 mg/kg) during cardioversion in adults. Etomidate caused mild pain on injection and myoclonus, but was the only agent that did not affect blood pressure.

The most significant concern about etomidate is its effect on the endogenous production of corticosteroids. These effects limit its use for prolonged sedation in the ICU setting.[91] Etomidate inhibits the function of an enzyme , 11-β hydroxylase, which is necessary for the production of cortisol, aldosterone, and corticosterone. Although temporary inhibition is present after a single dose of etomidate,[92] this effect is not believed to be of clinical significance. Given this effect, etomidate is no longer used for prolonged sedation in the ICU setting.

Barbiturates

The barbiturates are among the medications most used in the practice of anesthesia. They can be classified according to their duration of activity or their chemical structure. Short-acting agents include methohexital, thiopental, and thiamylal. Pentobarbital is considered an intermediate-acting agent, and phenobarbital is considered a long-acting agent. Due to their rapid redistribution, the short-acting agents have a duration of action of 5 to 10 minutes following a single bolus dose. Their clinical use generally includes a single intravenous bolus dose for brief procedures such as the induction of anesthesia and endotracheal intubation. If a more prolonged effect is needed, a continuous infusion is required to maintain plasma concentrations. Accumulation throughout the body may occur resulting in a prolonged duration of action when the infusion is discontinued.

Thiopental and thiamylal are thiobarbiturates containing a sulfur molecule in its ring structure, while methohexital is an oxybarbiturate (oxygen molecule in the ring structure). Thiopental and thiamylal are commercially provided as racemic mixtures of the 2 optical isomers. The L-isomer of either drug is twice as potent as the D-isomer. These drugs are reconstituted with sterile saline to provide solutions of 1% to 2.5% for clinical use. Induction doses vary based on the potency of the agent. Methohexital is the most potent (2.5-3 times that of thiopental), while thiopental is the least potent. Induction doses also are higher in neonates and infants. Anesthetic induction doses for thiopental vary from 3 to 5 mg/kg in healthy adults, 5 to 6 mg/kg in children, and up to 6 to 8 mg/kg in neonates and infants. Barbiturates undergo predominantly hepatic metabolism, except for phenobarbital, which also undergoes renal elimination. The rapid dissipation of clinical effect is not related to hepatic metabolism, but rather redistribution from the central compartment.

Barbiturates decrease $CMRO_2$ with a reduction in CBF, cerebral vasoconstriction, and a decrease in ICP. They produce dose-dependent degrees of EEG suppression and, in sufficient doses, produce electrical silence. The barbiturates are potent anticonvulsants and may provide cerebral protective effects in that they may decrease CNS damage during periods of cerebral hypoxia or hypoperfusion.

Barbiturates' effects on cardiorespiratory function are dose dependent. In healthy patients, sedative doses have minimal effects on respiratory drive and airway protective reflexes, yet respiratory depression, apnea, or hypotension may occur with larger doses or with administration to patients with cardiorespiratory compromise. The cardiorespiratory effects are additive when the barbiturates are used with other agents such as opioids. Hypotension results from peripheral vasodilation with a decrease in preload/afterload and a direct negative inotropic effect.

Barbiturate solutions are alkaline, thereby making them incompatible with other medications and parenteral alimentation solutions. Therefore, they should be administered separately from other medications. When used for anesthetic induction with various neuromuscular blocking agents such as rocuronium, a precipitate may form, leading to obstruction of the intravenous infusion site. Local erythema and thrombophlebitis can occur with subcutaneous infiltration.

Nitrous Oxide

Nitrous oxide (N_2O), not to be confused with nitric oxide (NO) or nitrogen dioxide (NO_2), was synthesized in 1776 by Priestly. Humphrey Davy subsequently demonstrated its anesthetic properties in 1799. Despite Davy's opinion about the potential of nitrous oxide for the management of pain, it was not until 1844 that Gardner Colton used nitrous oxide as an anesthetic agent during a tooth extraction. Today, nitrous oxide remains one of the most widely used agents for intraoperative anesthetic care.

Nitrous oxide has a rapid onset of action; it is relatively easy and inexpensive to use; its effects dissipate rapidly once discontinued; and it provides amnesia, sedation, and analgesia. Because of its low blood-gas partition coefficient (relative insolubility in blood), its alveolar concentration rises rapidly, resulting in a rapid onset of activity. In addition to its intraoperative use, nitrous oxide is used in some centers for the prevention of procedure-related pain such as tooth extraction, burn dressing changes, and reduction of orthopedic fractures.[93, 94]

Nitrous oxide's minimum alveolar concentration, or MAC (a measure of anesthetic potency that describes the anesthetic concentration at which 50% of patients will not move in response to surgical incision), is 105%. Because this is impossible to achieve at normal barometric pressure, additional agents may be necessary. In clinical practice, nitrous oxide is administered in concentrations varying from 50% to 80% by a face or nasal mask. Alternatively, a weighted mouthpiece that is held in place by the patient during administration can be used. If the patient becomes excessively sedated, the device falls from the patient, thereby interrupting the administration of nitrous oxide.

Nitrous oxide should be administrated only with standard procedural-sedation monitoring plus a monitor of the inspired oxygen concentration, a device that limits the ratio of the flow rates of oxygen to nitrous oxide (a proportioning system so that less than 20% to 30% oxygen cannot be administered), and a system that cuts off the nitrous oxide flow if the oxygen supply fails. This eliminates the potential administration of 100% nitrous oxide if the oxygen supply is interrupted.

In the operating room, nitrous oxide and oxygen are administered from wall outlets connected to the hospital's central supply. In other areas when such a supply is not available, nitrous oxide can be administered from E cylinders and mixed with oxygen to provide the desired concentration. Alternatively, commercially available tanks are manufactured that contain a 50/50 oxygen and nitrous oxide mixture, thereby limiting the risk of a hypoxic mixture and the need for specialized equipment to mix oxygen and nitrous oxide from separate tanks. A scavenger device attached to the delivery system is also required to remove waste gases and prevent environmental pollution. Repeated exposure of the patient or health care workers to nitrous oxide can lead to teratogenic effects, increased risk of spontaneous abortion, bone marrow suppression or megaloblastic anemia, and peripheral neuropathy as a result of its effects on B_{12} metabolism and protein synthesis. Because of the potential for abuse and/or illicit use, nitrous oxide tanks should be kept under close surveillance.

Nitrous oxide exerts a dose-dependent negative depressant effect on myocardial contractility and increases pulmonary artery pressure. It also causes dose-dependent respiratory depression, resulting in an elevation of the resting $PaCO_2$ level and blunting of the central respiratory response to hypercarbia and hypoxemia.[95] Nitrous oxide increases the incidence of postoperative nausea and vomiting. It diffuses into air-filled spaces, increasing the volume and pressure of the space. This can be an issue with any collection of air (bowel obstruction, pneumothorax, air in the middle ear, lung cysts, or pneumocephalus). Nitrous oxide increases CBF/ICP and is relatively contraindicated in patients with closed head injury and altered intracranial compliance.

Despite its relative insolubility in blood, during the administration of nitrous oxide, a large amount is taken up into the blood. This latter effect, known as the second gas effect of anesthesia, increases the alveolar partial pressure of oxygen resulting in an added margin of safety during induction even if high concentrations of nitrous oxide (80%-90%) are administered. Once the administration of nitrous oxide is discontinued, this effect occurs in the opposite direction, resulting in a lowering of the alveolar partial pressure of oxygen, which can result in hypoxemia unless supplemental oxygen is administered until the nitrous oxide is eliminated from the body.

Chloral Hydrate

Chloral hydrate was originally synthesized in 1832 and introduced into clinical practice in 1869 by Liebreich. For street and recreational use, chloral hydrate is the ingredient combined with alcohol in mixtures known as "knockout drops" and "Mickey Finns." Chloral hydrate is available in several different preparations and concentrations including capsules (250 mg, 500 mg), syrup (250 mg/5 mL and 500 mg/5 mL), and suppositories (325 mg, 500 mg, and 650 mg). Chloral hydrate can be a GI irritant, especially when administered to patients who have been *nil per os,* resulting in nausea and vomiting. In younger children, these problems can be avoided with the use of suppositories. Chloral hydrate should be combined with an analgesic agent such as an opioid if analgesia is required.

Chloral hydrate is rapidly absorbed from the GI tract with a bioavailability that approaches 100%. Its onset of action is within 20 minutes, with a peak effect at 30 to 60 minutes. It undergoes hepatic metabolism by alcohol dehydrogenase to the active ingredient trichloroethanol (TCE). Trichloroethanol is then further metabolized by either glucuronidation or oxidation to inactive metabolites. Less than 10% of chloral hydrate undergoes renal excretion. The plasma half-life of TCE is 8 to 12 hours in children, but may be up to 24 to 36 hours in neonates and infants.[96] Additive and prolonged effects are commonly seen after repeated administration over a period of days.

Chloral hydrate and TCE are CNS depressants. In therapeutic doses, there are minimal effects on cardiorespiratory function and airway control. Apnea and hypotension can occur with excessive dosing or in patients with compromised cardiorespiratory or CNS function. Cardiovascular effects include decreased myocardial contractility, a shortened refractory period, and an altered sensitivity of the myocardium to endogenous catecholamines.[97] The latter 2 effects account for its pro-arrhythmogenic effects. Chloral hydrate should not be administered to patients who have ingested toxic amounts of drugs that may cause arrhythmias, such as tricyclic antidepressants.[98]

Benzodiazepines

Benzodiazepines bind to specific receptor sites that are part of the GABA receptor system, increasing the efficacy of the interaction between the GABA receptor and the chloride channel. Benzodiazepines provide sedation, anxiolysis, amnesia, anticonvulsant properties, and spinally mediated muscle relaxation. Increasing the rate of occupancy of the benzodiazepine receptor may result in an escalation of the benzodiazepine effect from anxiolysis to sedation to unconsciousness when 60% or more of the receptor sites are occupied.

Diazepam and lorazepam are insoluble in water. They are commercially available in a solution containing propylene glycol, which may result in tissue irritation, pain on injection, local thrombophlebitis, and even systemic toxicity, depending on the duration and dose of the infusion. These problems are not seen with midazolam, which is water-soluble. Diazepam also is available in a lipid emulsion, which may limit local tissue irritation and pain on injection. Metabolism of the benzodiazepines occurs via hepatic oxidation and glucuronidation.

Oxidative processes are primarily responsible for the metabolism of diazepam and midazolam, and glucuronidation pathways for lorazepam metabolism. Hepatic oxidative processes occurring via the P_{450} system decrease with hepatic dysfunction and are altered by the coadministration of several other medications, including cimetidine and anticonvulsants. Glucuronidation pathways are less influenced by hepatic dysfunction and are not altered by the coadministration of other mediations. As such, lorazepam pharmacokinetics are not significantly altered, even in patients with hepatic dysfunction. Hepatic oxidative metabolism of diazepam results in the active metabolites desmethyl-diazepam and 3-hydroxy-diazepam, both of which have significantly prolonged half-lives when compared with the parent compound. Oxidation of midazolam results in a hydroxy-metabolite, which also can result in a prolonged effect following a continuous infusion.

Benzodiazepines decrease $CMRO_2$, CBF, and ICP. They are effective anticonvulsants. However, even in high doses, they do not produce electrical silence on the EEG. When used alone, especially in patients without underlying systemic illness, they have limited effects on cardiorespiratory function. However, when combined with opioids or other sedative agents or administered to patients with cardiorespiratory compromise, they may produce respiratory depression, apnea, and hypotension by a direct negative inotropic effect and decrease in vascular resistance.

In contrast to other sedative agents, there is a specific reversal agent for benzodiazepines: flumazenil. Flumazenil's chemical structure resembles that of the benzodiazepines, except that it has a carbonyl group instead of a phenyl group. It undergoes rapid hepatic metabolism with an elimination half-life of 1 hour. When used to reverse the effects of longer-acting benzodiazepines, flumazenil may be metabolized more rapidly, resulting in a reappearance of the benzodiazepine's actions. There are reports of seizure activity following administration to patients chronically treated with benzodiazepines or patients who have ingested other medications that lower the seizure threshold, such as tricyclic antidepressants or phenothiazines. As such, it is intended only for the reversal of adverse clinical effects following the acute administration of benzodiazepines.

Dexmedetomidine

Dexmedetomidine (Precedex, Abbott Laboratories, Abbott Park, IL) is a novel α_2 adrenergic agonist. It is the pharmacologically active dextroisomer of medetomidine.[99] In general, the α_2 adrenergic agonist class of drugs can be divided into 3 groups: imidazolines, phenylethylamines, and oxalozepines. Both dexmedetomidine and clonidine are imidazole compounds that exhibit a high ratio of specificity for the α_2 versus the α_1 receptor. Clonidine exhibits an α_2:α_1 specificity ratio of 200:1 compared with 1600:1 for dexmedetomidine. Therefore, dexmedetomidine is considered a full agonist at the α_2 adrenoreceptor. The half-life is 12 to 24 hours for clonidine and 2 to 3 hours for dexmedetomidine. By activation of specific transmembrane α_2 adrenergic receptors at various locations throughout the central nervous system, dexmedetomidine provides sedation, anxiolysis, and analgesia. It has been used for intraoperative anesthetic care and as a sedative agent for adult patients during mechanical ventilation. United States Food and Drug Administration-approved labeling indicates that dexmedetomidine can be used for sedation for up to 24 hours in adults during mechanical ventilation in an intensive care unit setting.

The physiologic effects of dexmedetomidine are mediated via stimulation of postsynaptic α_2 adrenoceptors that activate a pertussis toxin-sensitive guanine nucleotide regulatory protein (G protein),[100] resulting in inhibitory feedback and decreased activity of adenylate cyclase.[101] The subsequent reduction in cyclic adenosine monophosphate (cAMP) and cAMP-dependent protein kinase activity causes a predominant dephosphorylation of various species of ion channels.[102] This modifies ion translocation and membrane conductance, resulting in decreased neuronal activation, causing sedation and anxiolysis.[103] The centrally acting α_2 agonists, including dexmedetomidine, activate receptors in the medullary vasomotor center, thereby reducing norepinephrine turnover and decreasing central sympathetic outflow resulting in alterations in sympathetic function and decreased heart rate and blood pressure. Additional effects result from the central stimulation of parasympathetic outflow and inhibition of sympathetic outflow from the locus ceruleus in the brainstem. The latter effect plays a prominent role in sedation and anxiolysis because decreased noradrenergic output from the locus ceruleus allows for increased firing of inhibitory neurons including the GABA system.[104-106] Dexmedetomidine also regulates the release of substance P, a powerful nociceptive mediator, resulting in primary analgesic effects as well as potentiation of opioid-induced analgesia. The activation of α_2 adrenoceptors in dorsal horn neurons of the spinal cord results in inhibition of the release of substance P, and several clinical trials have demonstrated opioid-sparing and analgesic/anesthetic effects of dexmedetomidine in acute pain syndromes and during intraoperative anesthetic care. However, animal data suggest limited efficacy in neuropathic pain.[107]

Based on data from healthy volunteers, the pharmacokinetic profile of dexmedetomidine includes a rapid distribution phase with a distribution half-life of approximately 6 minutes, an elimination half-life of approximately 2 hours, and a steady-state volume of distribution of approximately 118 L. Dexmedetomidine exhibits linear kinetics in the dosage range of 0.2 to 0.7 μ/kg/h when delivered via intravenous infusion for up to 24 hours. Dexmedetomidine is 94% protein bound to serum albumin and α_1-glycoprotein. It undergoes extensive hepatic metabolism with very little unchanged drug excreted in urine and feces. Renal excretion accounts for 95% of drug elimination, predominantly in the form of methyl and glucuronide conjugates. Other investigators have evaluated the pharmacokinetic profile of dexmedetomidine following intravenous administration in additional patient populations. Cunningham et al[108] evaluated dexmedetomidine pharmacokinetics following the administration of 0.6 μg/kg infused over 10 minutes in 5 individuals with severe hepatic failure and compared the results to 5 age-matched controls with normal hepatic function. Patients with hepatic dysfunction had a significantly increased volume of distribution at steady state (3.2 vs 2.2 L/kg, $P<.05$), an increased elimination half-life (7.5 vs 2.6 hours, $P<.05$), and a decreased clearance (0.32 vs 0.64 L/h/kg; $P<.05$) when compared with age-matched controls.

De Wolf et al[109] evaluated the pharmacokinetics of a single 0.6 μg/kg bolus dose of dexmedetomidine in 6 volunteers with severe renal disease compared with 6 volunteers with normal renal function. The subjects with severe renal disease had a prestudy 24-hour creatinine clearance of less than 30 mL/min, but were considered to have stable renal disease with no prior history of dialysis. They noted no statistically significant differences between the renal disease and control groups in the volume of distribution at steady state (1.81 ± 0.55 vs 1.54 ± 0.08 L/kg) or the elimination clearance (12.5 ± 4.6 vs 8.9 ± 0.7 mL/min/kg). However, the elimination half-life was decreased in the renal disease group (113.4 ± 11.3 vs 136.5 ± 13.0 minutes, $P<.05$). Despite the shorter elimination half-life, they also noted prolonged sedation in patients with renal failure. Those patients with renal failure had a 1-hour post-infusion visual analogue score of sedation (0 to 100) of 49.2 ± 25.4 vs 26.2 ± 18.3, $P<.05$. The authors postulated that the increased level of sedation was related to decreased protein binding in patients with renal impairment, resulting in an increased free fraction of the drug.

Dexmedetomidine can have deleterious effects on cardiorespiratory function. The latter may be particularly worrisome in the patient with underlying respiratory insufficiency or during the immediate postoperative period. In a study of adult patients undergoing vascular surgery, Venn et al[110] reported that 18 of the 66 patients who received dexmedetomidine experienced adverse hemodynamic effects, including hypotension (mean arterial pressure ≤60 mmHg or a greater than 30% decrease from baseline) or bradycardia (heart rate ≤50 beats per minute). In 11 of these 18 patients, the hemodynamic effects were noted during the bolus infusion. Hypertension also has been reported with the loading dose. This is thought to be mediated via peripheral α_1 adrenergic agonism (leading to vasoconstriction) before the onset of the central α_2 effects.

Talke et al[111] evaluated the efficacy of a dexmedetomidine infusion during vascular surgery in 41 adults. In the 22 patients who received the dexmedetomidine infusion, there was a lower heart rate, less tachycardia, and decreased norepinephrine levels during emergence from anesthesia. Adverse effects related to dexmedetomidine included one episode of postoperative hypotension and one patient who had a 5- to 10-second sinus pause after anesthetic induction with thiopental and fentanyl followed by endotracheal intubation. Two other patients who had received dexmedetomidine experienced a brief episode of sinus arrest following laryngoscopy and propofol administration, thereby suggesting the possibility of potentiation of the vagotonic effects by procedures (laryngoscopy) or medications (propofol, fentanyl). Bradycardia also has been reported with the concomitant administration of dexmedetomidine and digoxin in an infant.[112]

Initial clinical trials suggested that the potential for respiratory depression with dexmedetomidine seemed to be limited. Hall et al[113] demonstrated sedation, impairment of memory, and decreased psychomotor performance during dexmedetomidine infusions (0.6 μg/kg followed by either 0.2 or 0.6 μg/kg/h) in healthy adult volunteers. No changes were noted in hemodynamic variables or respiratory function (end-tidal carbon dioxide, oxygen saturation, respiratory rate). However, other studies have noted a modest increase in $PaCO_2$ values during dexme-detomidine infusions as well as a depression of the slope of the carbon dioxide response curve and blunting of the ventilatory response at a $PaCO_2$ level of 55 mmHg in healthy adult volunteers.[114]

No significant CNS effects from dexmedetomidine have been reported. In laboratory animals and humans, dexmedetomidine has been shown to have no clinically significant effect on ICP.[115,116] Animal studies have suggested a potential beneficial effect on neurologic outcome following global and focal ischemia with the administration of dexmedetomidine.[117,118] Future clinical trials are needed to fully determine the potential clinical applications of dexmedetomidine in this setting.

Local Anesthetic Agents

The use of local anesthetics in children has become widespread because of the increasing awareness of the need for providing both short-term and long-term analgesia for painful procedures. As the demands for regional anesthetic techniques expand, there is a need for a better understanding of the pharmacology, pharmacodynamics, and potential toxicities of local anesthetic solutions. The incidence of adverse effects can be reduced by calculating the total dose on a mg/kg basis prior to injection, being aware of the differential absorption depending on injection site, using a vasoconstrictor to reduce vascular absorption, understanding that specific medications may alter the toxic threshold in specific organ systems (eg, benzodiazepines reduce the CNS seizure threshold, but do not alter the cardiac toxicity of local anesthetics), and using careful injection techniques, including the use of repeated aspiration and small volume injections to identify inadvertent intravascular injection. Continuous observation of the shape of the electrocardiogram waveform during the slow incremental injection of local anesthetics is vital. With local anesthetics containing epinephrine (usually 1:200,000), intravascular injection may be heralded by a sudden increase in heart rate and/or blood pressure. There may also be a doubling or tripling in size of the T wave.[119] Vasoconstrictors should never be used where there is an end artery circulation (eg, fingers, toes, and penis).

Local Anesthetics—Amides

Lidocaine

Due to its rapid onset and short duration of action, lidocaine is commonly used in the perioperative setting. In the procedural setting, a longer-acting local anesthetic may be desired. Lidocaine can be combined with bupivacaine, a longer-acting amide, to provide early onset and prolonged analgesia.[120] Alkalinization of the solution enhances the onset of action of lidocaine and decreases the pain on injection.[121] All local anesthetic solutions will exist in solution in a combination of the unionized and ionized forms. Although the ionized form attaches to the ion channel and exerts the local anesthetic effect, it is the unionized form that penetrates the cell membrane and, as such, the onset of action is dependent on the quantity of the unionized form. Because these agents are weak bases with a pKa greater than 7.0, as the pH of the solution decreases, the unionized fraction decreases. Commercially prepared buffered lidocaine solution is available and is commonly used for infiltration anesthesia for suturing lacerations in the emergency department. Alternatively, a small amount of sodium bicarbonate (1 mL per 10 mL of local anesthetic solution) can be added to increase the pH of the solution.

Lidocaine toxicity usually can be avoided by carefully calculating the dose on a mg/kg basis and graded drug injection. Because of the rapid vascular absorption, seizures may be seen with lower mg/kg doses when lidocaine is used for intercostal nerve blocks compared with other blocks. Central nervous system toxicity is seen in doses greater than 5 mg/kg with plain lidocaine and 7 mg/kg when epinephrine is added to the solution. Central nervous system toxicity may be manifest as lightheadedness, tunnel vision, and tinnitus followed by seizures and coma. Various concentrations of lidocaine are available commercially including 0.5%, 1%, 1.5%, and 2.0% solutions with or without epinephrine.

Bupivacaine

This is the most commonly used local anesthetic solution for prolonged nerve blockade analgesia or for single-dose or continuous caudal/epidural analgesia in infants and children in North America. The pharmacokinetics and pharmacodynamics have been well studied. The average duration of analgesia is 5 to 6 hours after a single bolus injection in the epidural space.[122] The concentration of the local anesthetic used depends on the site of administration, the desired density of blockade, and the potential for toxicity. The concomitant use of other local anesthetics, including infiltration anesthesia, must be taken into consideration before a total volume of local anesthetic solution is selected. The preferred concentration for peripheral nerve blockade is 0.25% or 0.5%, with or without epinephrine depending on the site of injection. The preferred concentration for single-dose epidural/caudal blockade is 0.125% or 0.25% (usually with epinephrine 1:200,000 to provide a marker for intravascular injection and to prolong the duration of blockade). When a continuous infusion is desired, a 0.1% or 0.125% solution of bupivacaine is preferred to reduce the potential for motor block while also minimizing the potential for drug accumulation and toxicity. Care should be taken to decrease the infusion rates for neonates when compared with older children. The maximum rate of administration should be 0.2 mg/kg/h for neonates and infants up to 6 months of age and 0.4 mg/kg/h for older children.[123]

Bupivacaine is a racemic mixture of the levo-enantiomers and dextro-enantiomers. Although the levo-enantiomer is the active form that provides the clinical effect of the local anesthetic solution, the dextro-enantiomer causes the adverse effects related to local anesthesia, including cardiac and CNS toxicity. Recent development has led to the availability of the isolated isomer (levobupivacaine) for clinical use. The major adverse effect of bupivacaine is toxicity related to the cardiovascular system and the CNS. Local anesthetics have the ability to rapidly cross the blood-brain barrier and cause serious alterations in CNS function (CNS excitation manifests as ringing in the ears, tingling around the mouth, garrulous behavior, and generalized seizures). As the systemic concentration of the local anesthetic increases, the risk of complications from toxicity increases exponentially.[124] In pediatric patients, cardiac toxicity occurs sooner than neurotoxicity. This may be partly due to the fact that children may be anesthetized, thus masking the clinical manifestations of neurotoxicity until significant cardiac toxicity (dysrhythmias, vasodilation and hypotension, cardiac arrest) is observed.[125,126] This also may be affected by the concomitant use of volatile anesthetic agents and/or premedication with benzodiazepine.[127] With cardiac toxicity, resuscitation may be impossible and, therefore, inadvertent intravascular injection must be avoided.

Bupivacaine can be used for most peripheral nerve blocks as well as for epidural and caudal infusions in infants and children. The maximum dose suggested for bolus injections for older children is 3 mg/kg and for neonates and infants is 2 mg/kg. Dosage recommendations for continuous infusions include 0.3 to 0.4 mg/kg/h in older children and 0.2 mg/kg/h in neonates and infants.[123]

Ropivacaine

Ropivacaine is a newer amide local anesthetic. It is a levo-enantiomer, not a racemic mixture like bupivacaine, with fewer cardiovascular and CNS side effects compared with bupivacaine. The lethal dose in rats is higher than that of bupivacaine.[128,129] Its potency is approximately 60% to 70% that of an equivalent concentration of bupivacaine. Ropivacaine also produces less motor blockade when compared with bupivacaine, especially when a concentration of 0.375% is used. This may offer some advantages in an outpatient setting when the return of motor function for ambulation is required.[130] Several pediatric trials have demonstrated a longer duration of action of ropivacaine when compared with mepivacaine for peripheral nerve blocks in a clinical setting.[131]

However, there seems to be no difference in duration when compared with bupivacaine.

Caudal block with ropivacaine (2 mg/kg) in a study of children aged 1 to 8 years resulted in plasma concentrations of ropivacaine well below toxic levels in adults.[132] This dose also produced less motor block and yet provided adequate analgesia. The mean maximum plasma concentration of ropivacaine was 0.47 mg/L. A threshold of CNS toxicity was noted at a plasma concentration of 0.6 mg/L. Body weight adjusted clearance was the same as in adults (5 mL/ min/ kg). Ropivacaine clearance depends on the unbound fraction of ropivacaine rather than liver blood flow. Hence, toxicity is directly related to the amount of unbound drug that is present.

Although the safety of ropivacaine has been demonstrated in animal experiments, there have been reports of CNS toxicity with its use for epidural anesthesia.[133,134] Hence, it is imperative that doses remain within the recommended limits. Our recommended dose in the epidural space is a bolus dose of 2 mg/kg and an infusion rate of 0.2 to 0.4 mg/kg/h, depending on the age of the patient.

Levobupivacaine

Levobupivacaine is the levo-enantiomer of bupivacaine. Initial clinical trials in adults suggest that it has fewer adverse effects than bupivacaine.[135,136] To date, there are limited pediatric data available. Despite the advantage of the reduced potential for toxicity, there is still limited use of levobupivacaine in the United States.[137,138] In animal models, levobupivacaine has been shown to have less cardiotoxicity, decreased myocardial depression, and a lower incidence of fatal dysrhythmias than bupivacaine.[139] Pharmacokinetic studies have been performed in children and the data should be available soon.

Local Anesthetics—Esters

Commonly used ester local anesthetic agents include procaine, tetracaine, and 2-chloroprocaine. Tetracaine is used most commonly for spinal anesthesia, while chloroprocaine is used for epidural anesthesia.

Ester local anesthetics are metabolized by plasma cholinesterases.[140] In populations with decreased pseudocholinesterase concentrations (congenital or drug-induced deficiency of pseudocholinesterase), there may be an increased duration of activity and the potential for toxicity from drug accumulation. Given the increased body water and, therefore, the increased amount of pseudocholinesterase on a per kilogram basis in neonates and infants, the metabolism of the ester anesthetics is rapid. For prolonged procedures, when redosing with bupivacaine is not feasible due to the risks of toxicity, chloroprocaine has been used to provide 4 to 5 hours of intraoperative surgical anesthesia.[141] For this purpose, administration by continuous infusion for caudal/epidural blockade is needed due to its short duration of action.[141] One area of concern with the neuraxial use of chloroprocaine is evidence suggesting the potential for neurotoxicity with inadvertent intrathecal administration. Although controversial, this effect is thought to result from the preservative sodium metabisulfite, which was used in the original solution, not the chloroprocaine itself. A newer preparation contains the preservative EDTA, which, although thought to cause back pain following epidural administration, has not been associated with neurotoxicity. There is also a preservative-free solution available.

Topical Anesthesia

The most commonly used topical local anesthetic preparations include lidocaine, tetracaine, benzocaine, and prilocaine. When applied to skin they produce an effective, but relatively short duration of, analgesia. The topical anesthetic formulation eutectic mixture of local anesthetics (EMLA, AstraZeneca Pharmaceuticals) is a mixture of lidocaine 2.5% and prilocaine 2.5%.[142] There is extensive clinical experience with this agent for topical anesthesia in neonates, particularly for circumcision, as well as for venipunctures and lumbar punctures.[143-145] Although EMLA can provide effective analgesia for a circumcision, the analgesia is less than that provided by a dorsal nerve block with local anesthetic solution.[146]

The eutectic mixture of local anesthetics is applied under an occlusive dressing for 45 to 60 minutes to obtain effective cutaneous analgesia. Caution should be exercised to limit the surface area application and to apply EMLA to intact skin only while avoiding mucus membranes. A concern, especially in neonates, is the reduced activity of methemoglobin reductase. Metabolism of prilocaine results in the production of *o*-toluidine, which can cause methemoglobinemia. The combination of the increased susceptibility of fetal hemoglobin to oxidation and the reduced methemoglobin reductase make the neonate particularly susceptible to methemoglobinemia with prilocaine. Despite extensive clinical experience with EMLA, there have been no reports of methemoglobinemia in neonates with its appropriate use (correct dose and application only to intact normal skin).

Newer topical anesthetics are now available that may offer a faster rate of onset. ELA-Max, a 4% liposomal lidocaine solution, is used for topical anesthesia. There is no need for an occlusive dressing when ELA-Max is used, and it has the same efficacy as EMLA.[147] Liposome-encapsulated lidocaine and tetracaine have been shown to remain in the epidermis after topical application, affording a fast and lasting anesthetic effect.[148,149]

Summary

Pharmaceutical research continues to provide the health care professional with new and potentially better agents for the control of pain in infants and children. Despite extensive premarketing work in the adult population, it is feasible that there will be limited information about the pharmacokinetics of many of these agents in infants and children. Because there are differences in the metabolism of medications between adults and pediatric patients, toxicity may occur when these agents are used at similar doses in infants and children. Despite these concerns, these new agents may provide us with more effective alternatives. Therefore, we are in need of appropriate clinical trials with these agents in infants and children. Knowledge of the pharmacologic profiles, metabolism, and adverse effect profiles of these agents will guide the clinician in the selection of the appropriate agent for the specific scenario as well as the safe clinical use of these medications.

References

1. Reisine T, Pasternak G. Opioid analgesics and antagonists. In: Hardman JG, Limbird LE, eds. *Goodman and Gilman's The Pharmacologic Basis of Therapeutics.* New York, NY: McGraw-Hill; 1996:521-555
2. Satoh M, Minami M. Molecular pharmacology of the opioid receptors. *Pharmacol Ther.* 1995;68:343-364
3. Standifer KM, Pasternak GW. G proteins and opioid receptor-mediated signaling. *Cell Signal.* 1997;9:237-248
4. Lynn AM, Slattery JT. Morphine pharmacokinetics in early infancy. *Anesthesiology.* 1987;66:136-139
5. Greeley WJ, De Bruijn NP. Changes in sufentanil pharmacokinetics within the neonatal period. *Anesth Analg.* 1988;67:86-90
6. Yaster M, Maxwell LG. Opioid agonists and antagonists. In: Schecter NL, Berde CB, Yaster M, eds. *Pain in Infants, Children, and Adolescents.* Baltimore, MD: Williams and Wilkins; 1993:145-171
7. Bailey PL, Pace NL, Ashburn MA, et al. Frequent hypoxemia and apnea after sedation with midazolam and fentanyl. *Anesthesiology.* 1990;73:826-830
8. Saarenmaa E, Neuvonen PJ, Rosenberg P, Fellman V. Morphine clearance and effects in newborn infants in relation to gestational age. *Clin Pharmacol Ther.* 2000;68:160-166
9. Quinn MW, Vokes A. Effect of morphine on respiratory drive in trigger ventilated pre-term infants. *Early Hum Dev.* 2000;59:27-35
10. Breslin DS, Reid JE, Mirakhur RK, et al. Sevoflurane-nitrous oxide anaesthesia supplemented with remifentanil: effect on recovery and cognitive function. *Anaesthesia.* 2001;56:114-119
11. Fahnenstich H, Steffan J, Kau N, Bartmann P. Fentanyl-induced chest wall rigidity and laryngospasm in preterm and term infants. *Crit Care Med.* 2000;28:836-839
12. Muller P, Vogtmann C. Three cases with different presentation of fentanyl-induced muscle rigidity—a rare problem in intensive care of neonates. *Am J Perinatol.* 2000;17:23-26

13. Hershey LA. Meperidine and central neurotoxicity. *Ann Intern Med.* 1983;98:548-549
14. Da Silva O, Alexandrou D, Knoppert D, Young GB. Seizure and electroencephalographic changes in the newborn period induced by opiates and corrected by naloxone infusion. *J Perinatol.* 1999;19:120-123
15. De Armendi AJ, Fahey M, Ryan JF. Morphine-induced myoclonic movements in a pediatric pain patient. *Anesth Analg.* 1993;77:191-192
16. Scott JC, Sarnquist FH. Seizure-like movements during a fentanyl infusion with absence of seizure activity in a simultaneous EEG recording. *Anesthesiology.* 1985;62:812-814
17. Blair JM, Hill DA. Probable seizure after remifentanil in a 4-year-old boy. *Anaesthesia.* 2000;55:501
18. Grossmann M, Abiose A, Tangphao O, et al. Morphine-induced venodilation in humans. *Clin Pharmacol Ther.* 1996;60:554-560
19. Sato A, Sato Y, Schmidt RF. Modulation of somatocardiac sympathetic reflexes mediated by opioid receptors at the spinal and brainstem level. *Exp Brain Res.* 1995;105:1-6
20. Cohen MR, Cohen RM, Pickar D, et al. Behavioural effects after high dose naloxone administration to normal volunteers. *Lancet.* 1981;255:1110
21. Johnson C, Mayer P, Grosz D. Pulmonary edema following naloxone administration in a healthy orthopedic patient. *J Clin Anesth.* 1995;7:356-357
22. Chumpa A, Kaplan RL, Burns MM, Shannon MW. Nalmefene for elective reversal of procedural sedation in children. *Am J Emerg Med.* 2001;19:545-548
23. Drago F, Panissidi G, Bellomio F, et al. Effects of opiates and opioids on intraocular pressure of rabbits and humans. *Clin Exp Pharmacol Physiol.* 1985;12:107-113
24. Henderson CA, Reynolds JE. Acute pulmonary edema in a young male after intravenous nalmefene. *Anesth Analg.* 1997;84:218-219
25. Das UG, Sasidharan P. Bladder retention of urine as a result of continuous intravenous infusion of fentanyl: 2 case reports. *Pediatrics.* 2001;108:1012-1015
26. Kuraishi Y, Yamaguchi T, Miyamoto T. Itch-scratch responses induced by opioids through central mu opioid receptors in mice. *J Biomed Sci.* 2000;7:248-252
27. Suzuki S, Carlos MP, Chuang LF, et al. Methadone induces CCR5 and promotes AIDS virus infection. *FEBS Lett.* 2002;519:173-177

28. Carr DJ, Rogers TJ, Weber RJ. The relevance of opioids and opioid receptors on immunocompetence and immune homeostasis. *Proc Soc Exp Biol Med.* 1996;213:248-257
29. Harris CE, Grounds RM, Murray AM, et al. Propofol for long-term sedation in the intensive care unit. A comparison with papaveretum and midazolam. *Anaesthesia.* 1990;45:366-372
30. Beller JP, Pottecher T, Lugnier A, et al. Prolonged sedation with propofol in ICU patients: recovery and blood concentration changes during periodic interruption in infusion. *Br J Anaesth.* 1988;61:583-588
31. Van Hemelrijck JV, Fitch W, Mattheussen M, Van Aken H, Plets C, Lauwers T. Effect of propofol on cerebral circulation and autoregulation in the baboon. *Anesth Analg.* 1990;71:49-54
32. Nimkoff L, Quinn C, Silver P, Sagy M. The effects of intravenous anesthetics on intracranial pressure and cerebral perfusion pressure in two feline models of brain edema. *J Crit Care.* 1997;12:132-136
33. Watts AD, Eliasziw M, Gelb AW. Propofol and hyperventilation for the treatment of increased intracranial pressure in rabbits. *Anesth Analg.* 1998;87:564-568
34. Herregods L, Verbeke J, Rolly G, Colardyn F. Effect of propofol on elevated intracranial pressure. Preliminary results. *Anaesthesia.* 1988;43(suppl): 107-109
35. Pinaud M, Lelausque J, Chetanneau A, Fauchoux N, Menegalli D, Souron R. Effects of propofol on cerebral hemodynamics and metabolism in patients with brain trauma. *Anesthesiology.* 1990;73:404-409
36. Ravussin P, Guinard JP, Ralley F, Thorin D. Effect of propofol on cerebrospinal fluid pressure and cerebral perfusion pressure in patients undergoing craniotomy. *Anaesthesia* 1988;43(suppl):37-41
37. Farling PA, Johnston JR, Coppel DL. Propofol infusion for sedation of patients with head injury in intensive care. *Anaesthesia.* 1989;44:222-226
38. Spitzfaden AC, Jimenez DF, Tobias JD. Propofol for sedation and control of intracranial pressure in children. *Pediatr Neurosurg.* 1999;31:194-200
39. Yamaguchi S, Midorikawa Y, Okuda Y, Kitajima T. Propofol prevents delayed neuronal death following transient forebrain ischemia in gerbils. *Can J Anaesth.* 1999;46:593-598
40. Young Y, Menon DK, Tisavipat N, et al. Propofol neuroprotection in a rat model of ischaemia reperfusion injury. *Eur J Anesth.* 1997;14:320-326
41. Pittman JE, Sheng H, Pearlstein R, Brinkhous A, Dexter F, Warner DS. Comparison of the effects of propofol and pentobarbital on neurologic outcome and cerebral infarct size after temporary focal ischemia in the rat. *Anesthesiology.* 1997;87:1139-1144

42. Brussel T, Theissen JL, Vigfusson G, Lunkenheimer PP, Van Aken H, Lawin P. Hemodynamic and cardiodynamic effects of propofol and etomidate: negative inotropic properties of propofol. *Anesth Analg.* 1989;69:35-40
43. Tritapepe L, Voci P, Marino P, et al. Calcium chloride minimizes the hemodynamic effects of propofol in patients undergoing coronary artery bypass grafting. *J Cardiothorac Vasc Anaesth.* 1999;13:150-153
44. Scholal C, Van Deenen D, De Ville A, Goveart MJM. Heart block following propofol in a child. *Paediatr Anaes.* 1999;9:349-351
45. Egan TD, Brock-Utne JG. Asystole and anesthesia induction with a fentanyl, propofol and succinylcholine sequence. *Anesth Analg.* 1991;73:818-820
46. Trotter C, Serpell MG. Neurological sequelae in children after prolonged propofol infusions. *Anaesthesia.* 1992;47:340-342
47. Saunders PRI, Harris MNE. Opisthotonic posturing and other unusual neurological sequelae after outpatient anaesthesia. *Anaesthesia.* 1992;47:552-557
48. Collier C, Kelly K. Propofol and convulsions—the evidence mounts. *Anaesth Intensive Care.* 1991;19:573-575
49. Finley GA, MacManus B, Sampson SE, Fernandez CV, Retallick I. Delayed seizure following sedation with propofol. *Can J Anaesth.* 1993;40:863-865
50. Lowenstein DH, Alldredge BK. Status epilepticus. *N Engl J Med.* 1998;338:970-976
51. Hertzog JH, Campbell HJ, Dalton HJ, Hauser GJ. Propofol anesthesia for invasive procedures in ambulatory and hospitalized children: experience in the pediatric intensive care unit. *Pediatrics.* 1999;103:e30
52. Chih-Chung L, Ming-Hwang S, Tan PPC, et al. Mechanisms underlying the inhibitory effect of propofol on the contraction of canine airway smooth muscle. *Anesthesiology.* 1999:91:750-759
53. Parke TJ, Stevens JE, Rice AS, et al. Metabolic acidosis and fatal myocardial failure after propofol infusion in children: five case reports. *Br Med J.* 1992;305:613-616
54. Strickland RA, Murray MJ. Fatal metabolic acidosis in a pediatric patient receiving an infusion of propofol in the intensive care unit: is there a relationship? *Crit Care Med.* 1995;23:405-409
55. Bray RJ. Propofol infusion syndrome in children. *Paediatr Anaesth.* 1998;8:491-499
56. Hanna JP, Ramundo ML. Rhabdomyolysis and hypoxia associated with prolonged propofol infusion in children. *Neurology.* 1998;50:301-303

57. Laxenaire MC, Mata-Bermejo E, Moneret-Vautrin DA, Gueant JL. Life-threatening anaphylactoid reactions to propofol. *Anesthesiology.* 1992;77:275-280
58. Haugen RD, Vaghadia H, Waters T, Merrick PM. Thiopentone pretreatment for propofol injection pain in ambulatory patients. *Can J Anaesth.* 1995;42:1108-1112
59. Mangar D, Holak EJ. Tourniquet at 50 mmHg followed by intravenous lidocaine diminishes hand pain associated with propofol injection. *Anesth Analg.* 1992;74:250-252
60. Tobias JD. Prevention of pain associated with the administration of propofol in children: lidocaine versus ketamine. *Am J Anesthesiol.* 1996;23:231-232
61. Sosis MB, Braverman B. Growth of *Staphylococcus aureus* in four intravenous anesthetics. *Anesth Analg.* 1993;77:766-768
62. Centers for Disease Control and Prevention. Postsurgical infections associated with extrinsically contaminated intravenous anesthetic agent—California, Illinois, Maine, and Michigan, 1990. *MMWR Morb Mortal Wkly Rep.* 1990;39:426-427
63. Gottardis M, Khunl-Brady KS, Koller W, Sigl G, Hackl JM. Effect of prolonged sedation with propofol on serum triglyceride and cholesterol concentrations. *Br J Anaesth.* 1989;62:393-396
64. Valente JF, Anderson GL, Branson RD, Johnson DJ, Davis K Jr, Porembka DT. Disadvantages of propofol sedation in the critical care unit. *Crit Care Med.* 1994;22:710-712
65. White PF, Ham J, Way WL, Trevor AJ. Pharmacology of ketamine isomers in surgical patients. *Anesthesiology.* 1980;52:231-239
66. Chernow B, Laker CR, Creuss D, et al. Plasma, urine, and CSF catecholamine concentration during and after ketamine sedation. *Crit Care Med.* 1982;10:600-603
67. Waxman K, Shoemaker WC, Lippmann M. Cardiovascular effects of anesthetic induction with ketamine. *Anesth Analg.* 1980;59:355-358
68. Spotoft H, Korshin JD, Sorensen MB, Skovsted P. The cardiovascular effects of ketamine used for induction of anesthesia in patients with valvular heart disease. *Can Anaesth Soc J.* 1979;26:463-467
69. Gooding JM, Dimick AR, Travakoli M, Corssen G. A physiologic analysis of cardiopulmonary responses to ketamine anesthesia in noncardiac patients. *Anesth Analg.* 1977;56;813-816
70. Morray JP, Lynn AM, Stamm SJ, Herndon PS, Kawabori I, Stevenson JG. Hemodynamic effects of ketamine in children with congenital heart disease. *Anesth Analg.* 1984;63:895-899

71. Hickey PR, Hansen DD, Cramolini GM, Vincent RN, Lang P. Pulmonary and systemic hemodynamic responses to ketamine in infants with normal and elevated pulmonary vascular resistance. *Anesthesiology.* 1985;62:287-293
72. Fleischer F, Polarz H, Lang J, Bohrer H. Changes in oxygen saturation following low-dose intramuscular ketamine in pediatric cardiac surgical patients. *Paediatr Anaesth.* 1991;1:33-36
73. Mankikin B, Cantineau JP, Sartene R, Clergue F, Viars P. Ventilatory and chest wall mechanics during ketamine anesthesia in humans. *Anesthesiology.* 1986;65:492-499
74. Hirshman CA, Downes H, Farbood A, Bergman NA. Ketamine block of bronchospasm in experimental canine asthma. *Br J Anaesth.* 1979;51:713-718
75. Bourke DL, Malit LA, Smith TC. Respiratory interactions of ketamine and morphine. *Anesthesiology.* 1987;66:153-156
76. Lanning CF, Harmel MH. Ketamine anesthesia. *Annu Rev Med.* 1975;26:137-141
77. Taylor PA, Towey RM. Depression of laryngeal reflexes during ketamine administration. *Br Med J.* 1971;2:688-689
78. Shapiro HM, Wyte SR, Harris AB. Ketamine anesthesia in patients with intracranial pathology. *Br J Anaesth.* 1972;44:1200-1204
79. Gardner AE, Dannemiller FJ, Dean D. Intracranial cerebrospinal fluid pressure in man during ketamine anesthesia. *Anesth Analg.* 1972;51: 741-745
80. Reicher D, Bhalla P, Rubenstein EH. Cholinergic cerebral vasodilator effect of ketamine in rabbits. *Stroke.* 1987;18:445-449
81. Oren RE, Rasool NA, Rubinstein EH. Effect of ketamine on cerebral cortical blood flow and metabolism in rabbits. *Stroke.* 1987;18:441-444
82. White PF, Way WL, Trevor AJ. Ketamine—its pharmacology and therapeutic uses. *Anesthesiology.* 1982;56:119-136
83. Van de Wiele B, Rubinstein E, Peacock W, Martin N. Propylene glycol toxicity caused by prolonged infusion of etomidate. *J Neurosurg Anesth.* 1995;7:259-262
84. Belelli D, Pistis M, Peters JA, Lambert JJ. The interaction of general anesthetics and neurosteroids with GABA(A) and glycine receptors. *Neurochem Int.* 1999;34:447-452
85. Giese JL, Stockham RJ, Stanley TH, Pace NL, Nellison RH. Etomidate versus thiopental for induction of anesthesia. *Anesth Analg.* 1985;64:871-876

86. Brussel T, Theissen JL, Vigfusson G, Lunkenheimer PP, Van Aken H, Lawin P. Hemodynamic and cardiodynamic effects of propofol and etomidate: negative inotropic properties of propofol. *Anesth Analg.* 1989;69:35-40
87. Modica PA, Tempelhoff R, White PF. Pro- and anticonvulsant effects of anesthetics (part 2). *Anesth Analg.* 1990;70:433-439
88. Kay B. A clinical assessment of the use of etomidate in children. *Br J Anaesth.* 1976;48:207-210
89. Tobias JD. Etomidate: applications in pediatric anesthesia and critical care. *J Intensive Care Med.* 1997;12:324-326
90. Canessa R, Lema G, Urzua J, Dagnino J, Concha M. Anesthesia for elective cardioversion: a comparison of four anesthetic agents. *J Cardiothorac Vasc Anesth.* 1991;5:566-568
91. Wagner RL, White PF, Kan PB, Rosenthal MH, Feldman D. Inhibition of adrenal steroidogenesis by the anesthetic etomidate. *N Engl J Med.* 1984;310:1415-1421
92. Absalom A, Pledger D, Konig A. Adrenocortical function in critically ill patients 24 hours after a single dose of etomidate. *Anaesthesia.* 1999;54:861-867
93. Holst JJ. Use of nitrous oxide-oxygen analgesia in dentistry. *Int Dent J.* 1962;12:47-51
94. Griffin GC, Campbell VD, Jones R. Nitrous oxide-oxygen sedation for minor surgery: experience in a pediatric setting. *JAMA.* 1981;245: 2411-2413
95. Litman RS, Berkowitz RJ, Ward DS. Levels of consciousness and ventilatory parameters in young children during sedation with oral midazolam and nitrous oxide. *Arch Pediatr Adolesc Med.* 1996;150: 671-675
96. Mayers DJ, Hindmarsh KW, Sankaran K, Gorecki DK, Kasian GF. Chloral hydrate disposition following single-dose administration to critically ill neonates and children. *Dev Pharmacol Ther.* 1991;16:71-77
97. Graham SR, Day RO, Lee R, et al. Overdose with chloral hydrate: a pharmacological and therapeutic review. *Med J Aust.* 1988;149:686-688
98. Seger D, Schwartz G. Chloral hydrate: a dangerous sedative for overdose patients? *Pediatr Emerg Care.* 1994;10:349-350
99. Virtanen R, Savola JM, Saano V, Nyman L. Characterization of selectivity, specificity, and potency of medetomidine as an alpha$_2$-adrenoceptor agonist. *Eur J Pharmacol.* 1998;150:9-14
100. Correa-Sales C, Reid K, Maze M. Pertussis toxin mediated ribosylation of G proteins blocks the hypnotic response to an alpha$_2$ agonist in the locus cereleus of the rat. *Pharmacol Biochem Behav.* 1992;43:723-727

101. Correa-Sales C, Nacif-Coelho C, Reid K, Maze M. Inhibition of adenylate cyclase in the locus cereleus mediates the hypnotic response to an alpha$_2$ agonist in the rat. *J Pharmacol Exp Ther.* 1992;263:1046-1050
102. Nacif-Coelho C, Correa-Sales C, Chang LL, Maze M. Perturbation of ion channel conductance alters the hypnotic response to the alpha$_2$ adrenergic agonist dexmedetomidine in the locus cereleus of the rat. *Anesthesiology.* 1994;81:1527-1534
103. Sculptoreanu A, Scheuer T, Catterall WA. Voltage-dependent potentiation of L-type Ca^{2+} channels due to phosphorylation by cAMP-dependent protein kinase. *Nature.* 1993;364:240-243
104. Correa-Sales C, Rabin BC, Maze M. A hypnotic response to dexmedetomidine, an alpha$_2$ agonist, is mediated in the locus ceruleus in rats. *Anesthesiology.* 1992;76:948-952
105. Doze VA, Chen BX, Maze M. Dexmedetomidine produces a hypnotic-anesthetic action in rats via activation of central alpha-2 adrenoceptors. *Anesthesiology.* 1989;71:75-79
106. Nelson LE, Lu J, Guo T, Saper CB, Franks NP, Maze M. The alpha$_2$-adrenoceptor agonist dexmedetomidine converges on an endogenous sleep-promoting pathway to exert its sedative effects. *Anesthesiology.* 2003;98:428-436
107. Kontinen VK, Paananen S, Kalso E. The effects of alpha$_2$-adrenergic agonist, dexmedetomidine, in the spinal nerve ligation model of neuropathic pain in rats. *Anesth Analg.* 1998;86:355-360
108. Cunningham FE, Baughman VL, Tonkovich L, et al. Pharmacokinetics of dexmedetomidine in patients with hepatic failure (abstract). *Clin Pharmacol Ther.* 1999;65:128
109. De Wolf AM, Fragen RJ, Avram MJ, Fitzgerald PC, Rahimi-Danesh F. The pharmacokinetics of dexmedetomidine in volunteers with severe renal impairment. *Anesth Analg.* 2001;93:1205-1209.
110. Venn RM, Bradshaw CJ, Spencer R, et al. Preliminary UK experience of dexmedetomidine, a novel agent for postoperative sedation in the intensive care unit. *Anaesthesia.* 1999;54:1136-1142
111. Talke P, Chen R, Thomas B, et al. The hemodynamic and adrenergic effects of perioperative dexmedetomidine infusion after vascular surgery. *Anesth Analg.* 2000;90:834-839
112. Berkenbosch JW, Tobias JD. Development of bradycardia during sedation with dexmedetomidine in an infant concurrently receiving digoxin. *Pediatr Crit Care Med.* 2003;4:203-205

113. Hall JE, Uhrich TD, Barney JA, Arain SR, Ebert TJ. Sedative, amnestic, and analgesic properties of small-dose dexmedetomidine infusions. *Anesth Analg.* 2000;90:699-705
114. Belleville JP, Ward DS, Bloor BC, Maze M. Effects of intravenous dexmedetomidine in humans. I. Sedation, ventilation, and metabolic rate. *Anesthesiology.* 1992;77:1125-1133
115. Talke P, Tong C, Lee HW, Caldwell J, Eisenach JC, Richardson CA. Effect of dexmedetomidine on lumbar cerebrospinal fluid pressure in humans. *Anesth Analg.* 1997;85:358-364
116. Zornow MH, Scheller MS, Sheehan PB, Strnat MA, Matsumoto M. Intracranial pressure effects of dexmedetomidine in rabbits. *Anesth Analg.* 1992;75:232-237
117. Hoffman WE, Kochs E, Werner C, Thomas C, Albrecht RF. Dexmedetomidine improves neurologic outcome from incomplete ischemia in the rat. *Anesthesiology.* 1991;75:328-332
118. Kuhmonen J, Pokorny J, Miettinen R, et al. Neuroprotective effects of dexmedetomidine in the gerbil hippocampus after transient global ischemia. *Anesthesiology.* 1997;87:371-377
119. Freid EB, Bailey A, Valley R. Electrocardiographic and hemodynamic changes associated with unintentional intravascular injection of bupivacaine with epinephrine in infants. *Anesthesiology.* 1993;79:394-398
120. Wagner AM, Suresh S. Peripheral nerve blocks for warts: taking the cry out of cryotherapy and laser. *Pediatr Dermatol.* 1998;15:238-241
121. Wong K, Strichartz GR, Raymond SA. On the mechanisms of potentiation of local anesthetics by bicarbonate buffer: drug structure-activity studies on isolated peripheral nerve. *Anesth Analg.* 1993;76:131-143
122. Payne KA, Hendrix MR, Wade WJ. Caudal bupivacaine for postoperative analgesia in pediatric lower limb surgery. *J Pediatr Surg.* 1993;28:155-157
123. Berde CB. Convulsions associated with pediatric regional anesthesia. *Anesth Analg.* 1992;75:164-166
124. Berde CB. Toxicity of local anesthetics in infants and children. *J Pediatr.* 1993;122:S14-20
125. Groban L, Deal DD, Vernon JC, James RL, Butterworth J. Cardiac resuscitation after incremental overdosage with lidocaine, bupivacaine, levobupivacaine, and ropivacaine in anesthetized dogs. *Anesth Analg.* 2001;92:37-43
126. Chang DH, Ladd LA, Copeland S, Iglesias MA, Plummer JL, Mather LE. Direct cardiac effects of intracoronary bupivacaine, levobupivacaine and ropivacaine in the sheep. *Br J Pharmacol.* 2001;132:649-658

127. Badgwell JM, Heavner JE, Kytta J. Bupivacaine toxicity in young pigs is age-dependent and is affected by volatile anesthetics. *Anesthesiology.* 1990;73:297-303
128. Kohane DS, Sankar WN, Shubina M, Hu D, Rifai N, Berde CB. Sciatic nerve blockade in infant, adolescent, and adult rats: a comparison of ropivacaine with bupivacaine. *Anesthesiology.* 1998;89:1199-1208
129. Dony P, Dewinde V, Vanderick B, et al. The comparative toxicity of ropivacaine and bupivacaine at equipotent doses in rats. *Anesth Analg.* 2000;91:1489-1492
130. Da Conceicao MJ, Coelho L. Caudal anaesthesia with 0.375% ropivacaine or 0.375% bupivacaine in paediatric patients. *Br J Anaesth.* 1998; 80:507-508
131. Fernandez-Guisasola J, Andueza A, Burgos E, et al. A comparison of 0.5% ropivacaine and 1% mepivacaine for sciatic nerve block in the popliteal fossa. *Acta Anaesthesiol Scand.* 2001;45:967-970
132. Lonnqvist PA, Westrin P, Larsson BA, et al. Ropivacaine pharmacokinetics after caudal block in 1-8 year old children. *Br J Anaesth.* 2000;85: 506-511
133. Abouleish EI, Elias M, Nelson C. Ropivacaine-induced seizure after extradural anaesthesia. *Br J Anaesth.* 1998;80:843-844
134. Eledjam JJ, Gros T, Viel E, Mazoit JX, Bassoul B. Ropivacaine overdose and systemic toxicity. *Anaesth Intensive Care.* 2000;28:705-707
135. McLeod GA, Burke D. Levobupivacaine. *Anaesthesia.* 2001;56:331-341
136. Foster RH, Markham A. Levobupivacaine: a review of its pharmacology and use as a local anaesthetic. *Drugs.* 2000;59:551-579
137. Giaufre E, Dalens B, Gombert A. Epidemiology and morbidity of regional anesthesia in children: a one-year prospective survey of the French-Language Society of Pediatric Anesthesiologists. *Anesth Analg.* 1996;83:904-912
138. Ivani G, De Negri P, Lonnqvist PA, et al. A comparison of three different concentrations of levobupivacaine for caudal block in children. *Anesth Analg.* 2003;97:368-371
139. Huang YF, Pryor ME, Mather LE, Veering BT. Cardiovascular and central nervous system effects of intravenous levobupivacaine and bupivacaine in sheep. *Anesth Analg.* 1998;86:797-804
140. Raj PP, Ohlweiler D, Hitt BA, Denson DD. Kinetics of local anesthetic esters and the effects of adjuvant drugs on 2-chloroprocaine hydrolysis. *Anesthesiology.* 1980;53:307-314

141. Henderson K, Sethna NF, Berde CB. Continuous caudal anesthesia for inguinal hernia repair in former preterm infants. *J Clin Anesth.* 1993;5:129-133
142. Corbett JV. EMLA cream for local anesthesia. *Am J Matern Child Nurs.* 1995;20:178
143. Chang PC, Goresky GV, O'Connor G, et al. A multicentre randomized study of single-unit dose package of EMLA patch vs EMLA 5% cream for venipuncture in children. *Can J Anaesth.* 1994;41:59-63
144. Gourrier E, Karoubi P, el Hanache A, Merbouche S, Mouchnino G, Leraillez J. Use of EMLA cream in a department of neonatology. *Pain.* 1996;68:431-434
145. Stevens B, Johnston C, Taddio A, et al. Management of pain from heel lance with lidocaine-prilocaine (EMLA) cream: is it safe and efficacious in preterm infants? *J Dev Behav Pediatr.* 1999;20:216-221
146. Lander J, Brady-Fryer B, Metcalfe JB, Nazarali S, Muttitt S. Comparison of ring block, dorsal penile nerve block, and topical anesthesia for neonatal circumcision: a randomized controlled trial. *JAMA.* 1997;278:2157-2162
147. Eichenfield LF, Funk A, Fallon-Friedlander S, Cunningham BB. A clinical study to evaluate the efficacy of ELA-Max (4% liposomal lidocaine) as compared with eutectic mixture of local anesthetics cream for pain reduction of venipuncture in children. *Pediatrics.* 2002;109:1093-1099
148. Fisher R, Hung O, Mezei M, Stewart R. Topical anaesthesia of intact skin: liposome-encapsulated tetracaine vs EMLA. *Br J Anaesth.* 1998;81:972-973
149. Gesztes A, Mezei M. Topical anesthesia of the skin by liposome-encapsulated tetracaine. *Anesth Analg.* 1988;67:1079-1081

Chapter 3

Neuraxial Blockade: Epidural and Spinal Anesthesia/Analgesia

Stephen R. Hays, MD, FAAP
Joseph D. Tobias, MD, FAAP

Medications for Neuraxial Analgesia
- Local Anesthetic Agents
- Opioids and Adjuvant Agents

Epidural Analgesia Including Caudal Block
- Anatomy, General Considerations, and Dosing Regimens
- Special Considerations of Caudal Epidural Analgesia

Spinal Anesthesia and Analgesia
- Techniques of Spinal Anesthesia
- Combined Spinal and General Anesthesia

Adverse Effects of Neuraxial Anesthesia

Introduction

Use of neuraxial blockade in pediatric patients continues to increase in the operating room and beyond.[1-3] In infants and children, neuraxial anesthesia is most commonly administered with general anesthesia as a way to provide postoperative analgesia or as a combined general-regional anesthetic to limit the need for general anesthetic agents. However, neuraxial blockade also may be the sole surgical anesthetic in various clinical scenarios, such as in the former preterm infant at high risk for post-anesthetic apnea, in patients with concurrent medical conditions that increase the potential risks of general anesthesia, or in cooperative older pediatric patients who choose a regional anesthetic over general anesthesia. When performed preemptively before surgical incision, neuraxial blockade may ablate the surgical stress response, decrease postoperative analgesia requirements, and improve the postoperative course. Epidural and spinal techniques in children also have been used increasingly in the management of acute and chronic pain outside of the perioperative period. Additionally, the sympathetic blockade that may be induced by neuraxial techniques occasionally is used as a therapeutic tool to improve regional blood flow in cases of vascular insufficiency.[4] Epidural analgesia, including caudal block, involves the administration of medications (local anesthetic agents, opioids, and/or adjuvant agents such as clonidine) into the epidural space (the potential space between the ligamentum flavum and the dura mater). Spinal analgesia entails the administration of similar medications into the cerebrospinal fluid of the subarachnoid space. Either technique may be contraindicated in specific patient populations and clinical scenarios (Table 3-1). Only practitioners adept at neuraxial blockade in children should undertake these techniques. This chapter reviews local anesthetic agents, opioids, and adjuvant agents commonly used for pediatric epidural and spinal analgesia, and discusses the practical aspects of these techniques.

Table 3-1. Potential Contraindications to Neuraxial Blockage in Children

Localized infection at procedure site
Systemic infection (bacteremia or meningitis)
Coagulopathy, including thrombocytopenia or qualitative platelet disorder
Abnormal vascular fragility (Ehler-Danlos syndrome)
Hemodynamic instability
Increased intracranial pressure
Allergy to analgesic agent or local anesthetic
Anatomical deformity
Previous spinal instrumentation
Degenerative central nervous system disorder
Patient or guardian refusal

Medications for Neuraxial Analgesia

Local Anesthetic Agents

Local anesthetic agents bind to neuronal sodium channels, inducing conduction blockade and preventing neuronal depolarization. Based on their chemical structure, the local anesthetic agents are classified as either amides or esters (Table 3-2). A useful mnemonic for differentiating them is that the names of the amide local anesthetics all have at least one "i" in addition to the "i" in "caine" (eg, l*i*docaine, mep*i*vacaine) while the names of the ester local anesthetic agents do not (eg, tetracaine). Although the mechanism of action of the 2 classes of local anesthetics is identical in adults and children, the 2 classes have different metabolic fates. Amide local anesthetic agents undergo hepatic degradation, whereas ester local anesthetic agents undergo hydrolysis by plasma and tissue cholinesterases. The pharmacokinetics of amide anesthetic agents vary according to the age of the patient. In neonates and preterm infants, the immaturity of the hepatic enzyme system slows the metabolism of amide local anesthetic agents, leading to elevated plasma concentrations when compared with adults. The enzymes responsible for the metabolism of anesthetic agents of the ester class are present in the plasma body water and thereby increased in neonates and infants. Therefore, there is no clinically significant change in the pharmacokinetics of the esters among various age ranges. The pharmacodynamics of the amide local anesthetics also may vary across age ranges because a significant amount of the local anesthetic in the plasma is bound to plasma proteins (albumin, α_1 acid glycoprotein) with the remaining portion being unbound or free. It is the free fraction that is responsible for local anesthetic toxicity. In neonates and preterm infants, decreased serum protein levels can lead to an elevation in the percentage of the free fraction, thereby increasing the risk of toxicity.

Uptake of local anesthetic and, therefore, peak plasma concentration are dependent on several factors, most importantly the vascularity of the injection site. Different anatomical sites demonstrate markedly different absorption rates of local anesthetic (Table 3-3). Epidural blockade is associated with mid-range plasma concentrations. Addition of a vasoconstrictor such as epinephrine or phenylephrine to the local anesthetic may decrease absorption rate and lower the peak plasma concentration by 10% to 20%. Speed of injection and total dose administered

Table 3-2. Classification of Local Anesthetic Agents

Amides	Esters
Bupivacaine	Chloroprocaine
Etidocaine*	Cocaine†
Prilocaine	Procaine
Levobupivacaine	Tetracaine
Lidocaine	
Mepivacaine	
Ropivacaine	

*Causes preferential motor over sensory blockade: rarely used in clinical practice.
†Class II controlled substance used primarily in topical preparations.

Table 3-3. Rate of Absorption of Local Anesthetic From Various Administration Sites

Site of Administration by Rate of Absorption (Fastest to Slowest)	
Intrapleural	Fastest
Intercostal	↑
Caudal epidural	
Thoracic epidural	
Lumbar epidural	
Brachial plexus	
Spinal	
Sciatic, femoral	
Distal peripheral nerve	↓
Subcutaneous	Slowest

also influence uptake and peak serum concentration. To avoid toxicity from bolus administration of local anesthetic, the practitioner must be aware of the total dose administered in mg/kg and the maximum recommended dose (Table 3-4). This is especially important in younger patients, particularly neonates and preterm infants, in whom local anesthetic toxicity is more likely because of increased unbound agent and decreased metabolism. The recommendations in Table 3-4 are for single bolus dosing only. Other recommendations are necessary when continuous infusion techniques are used (Table 3-5).[5]

Bupivacaine is one of the most frequently used local anesthetic agents in neuraxial anesthesia because of its relatively long duration of action and its relative selectivity for sensory, rather than motor, blockade. However, bupivacaine is also one of the most cardiotoxic local anesthetics. Because the thresholds for cardiac and neurologic toxicity with bupivacaine are similar, cardiac toxicity may occur before neurologic toxicity is observed. Therefore, a warning sign (seizure) does not necessarily occur before the onset of cardiotoxicity. Bupivacaine binds avidly to myocardial sodium channels and, in toxic doses, can precipi-

Table 3-4. Maximum Recommended Bolus Doses of Local Anesthetic Agents

Local Anesthetic Agent	Dose Without Epinephrine	Dose With Epinephrine
Bupivacaine	3 mg/kg	3.5 mg/kg
Chloroprocaine	12 mg/kg	15 mg/kg
Levobupivacaine	3 mg/kg	3.5 mg/kg
Lidocaine	5 mg/kg	7 mg/kg
Mepivacaine	5 mg/kg	7 mg/kg
Prilocaine	7 mg/kg	9 mg/kg
Procaine	10 mg/kg	12 mg/kg
Ropivacaine	4 mg/kg	4 mg/kg
Tetracaine	1.5 mg/kg	2 mg/kg

Table 3-5. Maximum Recommended Continuous Infusion Doses of Local Anesthetics

Local Anesthetic Agent	Newborn to 6 Months	Older Than 6 Months
Bupivacaine	0.2 mg/kg/h	0.4 mg/kg/h
Levobupivacaine	0.2 mg/kg/h	0.4 mg/kg/h
Lidocaine	1.5 mg/kg/h	3 mg/kg/h
Ropivacaine	0.25 mg/kg/h	0.5 mg/kg/h

tate myocardial depression and ventricular dysrhythmias with resultant cardiovascular collapse.[6,7] Resuscitation following bupivacaine toxicity may be necessary for up to 60 minutes to allow sufficient time for the agent to be displaced from myocardial sodium channels (Table 3-6). Extracorporeal techniques such as dialysis are of no benefit in accelerating bupivacaine clearance, although extracorporeal support with cardiopulmonary bypass can be considered if available. Hypoxia, hypercarbia, and acidosis have been shown to potentiate local anesthetic toxicity. These derangements should be avoided whenever possible to decrease the likelihood of local anesthetic toxicity and should be corrected promptly if toxicity occurs (Table 3-6). Various pharmacologic approaches have been suggested in the treatment of bupivacaine-induced cardiotoxicity including bretylium, phenytoin, calcium channel blockers, lidocaine and, most recently, intralipid (Table 3-6).[8-10] The latter is thought to work through the binding of free local anesthetic in the plasma, thereby decreasing the free fraction. Given that none of these therapies is successful in a significant proportion of patients, the primary goal when using neuraxial techniques is to avoid toxicity by adhering to bolus and continuous infusion dosing guidelines, and to identify inadvertent intravascular injection by using appropriate test dosing (see following text).

Two newer local anesthetics, ropivacaine and levobupivacaine, have gained popularity as effective and potentially less toxic alternatives to bupivacaine. Ropivacaine has somewhat greater selectively for sensory over motor blockade than bupivacaine, with a somewhat higher threshold for cardiac toxicity. Levobupivacaine, the L-isomer of bupivacaine, causes conduction blockade similar to that of bupivacaine, but also has a lower potential for cardiotoxicity. Use of these newer, potentially less toxic, agents instead of bupivacaine has been limited somewhat by cost. Although the incidence of cardiotoxicity is exceedingly low, these agents may offer significant advantage over the older, potentially more toxic, agent bupivacaine.

Local anesthetic agents may be administered as a single bolus dose or as a bolus dose followed by continuous infusion for sustained neuraxial blockade. Although continuous spinal techniques occasionally are employed in adults, continuous neuraxial blockade with local anesthetic in children usually is undertaken as an epidural infusion. Preferential sensory over motor blockade is far easier to maintain with epidural than with spinal anesthesia. Moreover, the risk for inadvertent high block, with resultant respiratory and/or neurologic compromise, is lower with epidural techniques. Dosing of local anesthetic for continuous infusion requires more adjustment for age than does bolus injection (Table 3-5). Infants, neonates, and particularly premature infants,

Table 3-6. Management of Local Anesthetic Toxicity

Initial Therapy
Inciting Agent Discontinue local anesthetic administration *A, B, C* Assess adequacy of airway, breathing, and circulation *Supplemental O_2 and Assisted Ventilation* Supplemental oxygen, bag-mask ventilation, and/or endotracheal intubation as necessary *Intravascular Volume* Isotonic fluid to restore intravascular volume, vasoactive medications for hypotension and bradycardia, cardiopulmonary resuscitation may be necessary
Anticonvulsant Therapy
Diazepam 0.2 mg/kg IV/IO, maximum 10 mg (0.3 mg/kg PR, maximum 20 mg) *Midazolam* 0.1 mg/kg IV/IM/IO, maximum 10 mg *Lorazepam* 0.1 mg/kg IV/IO, maximum 4 mg *Thiopental* 4 mg/kg IV, maximum 500 mg *Propofol* 2 mg/kg IV, maximum 200 mg
Interventions for Ventricular Dysrhythmias: Avoid Lidocaine
Defibrillation 2 J/kg, may double to 4 J/kg, maximum 360 Joules, repeat prn *Epinephrine* 10-100 mcg/kg IV/ETT/IO, maximum 1 mg initial dose or 10 mg subsequent doses, repeat prn *Bretylium* 5 mg/kg IV, maximum 300 mg *Magnesium* 50 mg/kg IV, maximum 2 g *Phenytoin* 10-15 mg/kg IV, maximum 1 g (may use fosphenytoin at same dose) *Amiodarone* 2 mg/kg, maximum 150 mg

are at higher risk for local anesthetic toxicity when exposed to continuous infusions. They also will have higher concentrations of the free fraction of local anesthetic agents because of decreased plasma protein concentration and immature hepatic metabolism.

Lidocaine in a concentration of 0.1% to 0.5% has been used for continuous epidural infusion in children because of the theoretical advantage of being able to measure plasma lidocaine concentrations (methods to measure plasma concentrations of bupivacaine are not readily available in most institutions). In practice, this has proven to be of limited value because toxicity is uncommon if doses remain below recommended levels. Moreover, lidocaine is more likely to cause significant motor blockade. Therefore, bupivacaine, in concentrations ranging from 0.05% to 0.1%, remains the local anesthetic agent used most commonly for continuous epidural analgesia in children because of its longer duration of action and relative selectivity for sensory over motor blockade. Recommended doses for ropivacaine and levobupivacaine in children are largely extrapolated from adult data and from analogy to bupivacaine.

Even with appropriate caution and careful calculation, local anesthetic toxicity can occur, manifested by neurologic compromise including obtundation and seizures and/or as cardiovascular instability with dysrhythmias, hypotension, and potential circulatory collapse. Because neuraxial blockade in children is most commonly performed under general anesthesia, neurologic toxicity may not manifest itself, leaving cardiotoxicity as the first sign of systemic toxicity. Although local anesthetic toxicity may occur during continuous infusion techniques, particularly if the dose is not appropriately adjusted for patient age, most adverse reactions occur with bolus administration, during which there is a greater likelihood of rapidly reaching toxic serum levels. Local anesthetic toxicity may result from either accidental intravascular or intraosseous injection.

Before the administration of local anesthetic, aspiration to check for blood should be performed. Negative aspiration reduces, but does not eliminate, the risk of inadvertent systemic injection as inadvertent intraosseous injection may occur (generally during caudal epidural blockade) because of the cartilaginous nature of the lumbar and sacral vertebral bodies in neonates and infants. Following negative aspiration, a test dose of epinephrine-containing local anesthetic is injected (0.5-1 μg/kg of epinephrine, or 0.1-0.2 mL/kg of a solution containing epinephrine 1:200,000 or 5 μg/mL). After 30 to 60 seconds, during which time the patient is observed for hemodynamic changes suggestive of intravascular injection (eg, ST segment or T wave changes, increased heart rate, or hypertension), injection is continued. Even if no hemodynamic changes are noted, many practitioners administer the remainder of the dose slowly and in fractionated fashion, with repeated aspiration and observation after each subsequent dose.[11]

Should it occur, local anesthetic toxicity must be managed promptly (Table 3-6). Given the potential for toxicity, any administration of local anesthetic, including neuraxial blockade, must be performed with adequate age-appropriate resuscitation equipment immediately available. Adverse reactions from allergy to local anesthetics, although quite rare, also can occur. Allergy is more common with ester local anesthetics, the chemical structure of which is similar to that of para-amino benzoic acid (PABA), a known allergen. Allergy to amide local anesthetics is quite rare. Although it may be a true response to the preservative methylparaben (chemically similar to PABA), such "allergies" are usually a conscious patient's reaction to solutions containing epinephrine (eg, tachycardia and other systemic manifestations) and not a true allergy. Allergic reactions may range in severity from urticaria and pruritus, to bronchospasm and hypotension, to full-fledged anaphylaxis and cardiopulmonary arrest. Allergic reactions should be treated by discontinuing the inciting agent and appropriate supportive care.

Opioids and Adjuvant Agents

Opioids, either alone or in combination with other agents, are used frequently in pediatric neuraxial blockade. Neuraxial opioids bind to receptors in the dorsal horn of the spinal cord, inducing analgesia by modulating the synapses between first and second order sensory neurons. Unlike local anesthetics, opioids do not cause conduction blockade and, therefore, decrease pain sensation without affecting motor strength or sympathetic function. Because of the different mechanisms of action, opioids are synergistic with local anesthetics for neuraxial blockade, increasing the duration and improving the quality of analgesia. The addition of neuraxial opioids allows the use of lower doses and concentrations of local anesthetics, thereby lessening the potential for local anesthetic toxicity. This is particularly helpful with continuous techniques, for which the dose of local anesthetic must be adjusted for patient age. Neuraxial opioids also confer the advantage of causing fewer systemic side effects than would result from the higher doses of intravenous opioids required for comparable analgesia. This may be particularly beneficial in high-risk patients unlikely to tolerate systemic opioids, including preterm infants or children with other significant pulmonary disease.

Onset of action, duration of analgesia, and likelihood of adverse effects from cephalad spread are determined primarily by the relative hydrophilicity and lipophilicity of the neuraxial opioid administered. Fentanyl is a lipophilic agent that distributes rapidly into the lipid-rich neural elements of the central nervous system following neuraxial administration, resulting in a rapid onset of action (5-15 minutes) and comparatively brief period of analgesia (4-6 hours). Because very little fentanyl is absorbed into the cerebrospinal fluid, there is limited cephalad spread. This results in little or no analgesia beyond the dermatomes at which the agent is administered. There is also low risk of somnolence and respiratory depression from brainstem opioid effect and low risk of urinary retention from sacral spread. Given these properties, fentanyl is a popular choice for continuous neuraxial infusion. Morphine, by contrast, is a hydrophilic agent with significant solubility in cerebrospinal fluid, resulting in a delayed onset of action (20-60 minutes) and a prolonged period of analgesia (up to 24 hours) even after single-dose epidural or intrathecal administration. There is considerable cephalad spread and significant analgesia beyond the dermatomes at which the agent is administered. Caudal or lumbar epidural morphine can provide satisfactory analgesia for thoracic and even craniofacial procedures.[12,13] There is, however, risk of somnolence or respiratory depression from brainstem opioid effect and a higher incidence of urinary retention from sacral spread.

Hydromorphone is less lipophilic than fentanyl, but more so than morphine, with moderate solubility in cerebrospinal fluid. It has an intermediate onset of action (15-30 minutes) and duration of analgesia (6-12 hours) following neuraxial administration. There is some spread away from the dermatome at which it is administered, providing analgesia beyond that dermatome. There is an intermediate risk for somnolence, respiratory depression, and urinary retention. Lipophilic and hydrophilic opioids may be combined for bolus neuraxial administration to provide rapid onset of action and prolonged duration of analgesia. Fentanyl, hydromorphone, and morphine are the opioids most commonly used in the United States for pediatric epidural and spinal analgesia (Table 3-7). Numerous other opioids and adjuvant agents have been described for neuraxial administration in children (Table 3-8).

Other opioids are used less frequently for neuraxial anesthesia. Neuraxial diamorphine (heroin) has been shown to confer excellent analgesia in children with few side effects.[14] In the United Kingdom and other countries, caudal diamorphine is used almost as frequently as caudal fentanyl.[15] Medical use of diamorphine in the United States is limited because it is a Class I controlled substance. Historically, neuraxial meperidine has been used. Unlike the other opioids, when

Table 3-7. Recommended Dosing Ranges for Neuraxial Opioids

Dosing Range			
Agent	**Epidural, Bolus**	**Epidural, Infusion**	**Spinal, Bolus**
Fentanyl	0.5-1 μg/kg, maximum 50-100 μg	0.5-1 μg/kg/h, maximum 50-100 μg/h	0.25-0.5 μg/kg, maximum 25-50 μg
Hydromorphone	10-20 μg/kg, maximum 1 mg	2-5 μg/kg/h maximum 0.2-0.3 mg/h	1-2 μg/kg, maximum 0.1 mg
Morphine	30-60 μg/kg, maximum 4 mg	3-6 μg/kg/h, maximum 0.4 mg/h	3-6 μg/kg, maximum 0.4 mg

Table 3-8. Other Opioids and Adjuvant Agents for Neuraxial Analgesia

Dosing Range			
Agent	**Epidural, Bolus**	**Epidural, Infusion**	**Spinal, Bolus**
Diamorphine (Heroin)	30-60 μg/kg, maximum 4 mg	3-6 μg/kg/h, maximum 0.4 mg/h	15-30 μg/kg, maximum 2 mg
Meperidine	0.5-1 mg/kg, maximum 100 mg	0.125-0.25 mg/kg/h, maximum 25 mg/h	0.125-0.25 mg/kg, maximum 25 mg
Methadone	30-60 μg/kg, maximum 4 mg	*	*
Sufentanil	0.5-1 μg/kg, maximum 100 μg	0.1-0.2 μg/kg/h, maximum 10 μg/h	0.25-0.5 μg/kg, maximum 50 μg
Butorphanol	20-40 μg/kg, maximum 2 mg	*	*
Ketamine	0.5-1 mg/kg, maximum 100 mg	*	*
Clonidine	0.5-1 μg/kg, maximum 0.1 mg	0.25-0.5 μg/kg/h, maximum 50 μg/h	0.25-0.5 μg/kg, maximum 50 μg

*Agent not usually used.

administered as a neuraxial anesthetic, meperidine has significant local anesthetic effects in addition to its opioid effects. However, this agent is no longer favored as a first-line analgesic because of its adverse effect profile. The short-acting lipophilic opioid sufentanil is widely used in obstetric anesthesia because it is associated with a low risk of maternal and fetal respiratory depression, but offers few advantages over fentanyl in pediatric practice. Epidural butorphanol has been combined with epidural morphine to reduce side effects associated with neuraxial morphine including nausea, vomiting, and pruritus.[16] This combination offers the advantages of a single shot technique providing 18 to 24 hours of analgesia without the use of an indwelling catheter.

Nonopioid agents also are gaining popularity in caudal and epidural analgesia as a means of prolonging or intensifying the analgesia while limiting the dose and, therefore, the incidence of adverse effects with neuraxial opioids. The *N*-methyl-D-aspartate (NMDA) receptor antagonist, ketamine, has been used for bolus epidural analgesia in children.[17,18] Ketamine has been shown to prolong the duration of analgesia when added to the local anesthetic solution and to provide analgesia equivalent to that of a local anesthetic agent when used as the sole agent. However, ketamine for caudal administration is not currently available for routine clinical use in the United States. The α_2-adrenergic agonist, clonidine, has been used for epidural and spinal analgesia in children in conjunction with local anesthetic and more recently in combination with ketamine.[19-22] Preliminary studies in the pediatric population demonstrate superior and more prolonged analgesia with a combination of clonidine and a local anesthetic agent when compared with local anesthetic agents alone. Clonidine is available in the United States for epidural administration. Neuraxial clonidine can have systemic sedative effects, and anecdotal reports describe apnea in high-risk patients.[22] The risk of adverse effects (sedation, respiratory depression, bradycardia, hypotension) is greater with high dose (2 μg/kg) compared with low dose (0.5-1 μg/kg) regimens.

Although neuraxial opioids can provide effective analgesia, adverse effects may occur and often require specific therapy (Table 3-9). The risk of adverse effects due to cephalad spread of neuraxial opioids, including somnolence, respiratory depression, and urinary retention, is proportional to the hydrophilicity of the opioid. Fentanyl has the lowest, morphine the highest, and hydromorphone an intermediate risk. The duration of risk of such adverse effects also depends on opioid hydrophilicity and mirrors the duration of analgesia. Neuraxial fentanyl is unlikely to induce adverse effects after 4 to 6 hours, whereas respiratory depression may be seen up to 24 hours following neuraxial morphine. Because of the increased likelihood and prolonged period of risk for potentially serious adverse effects, patients should be monitored for respiratory depression for 24 hours after receiving neuraxial morphine. Although practices vary, many institutions do not use neuraxial opioids, including fentanyl, in outpatients.

Table 3-9. Management of Adverse Effects of Neuraxial Opioids

Adverse Effect	Treatment/Intervention
Somnolence (including respiratory depression)	*A, B, C* Assess adequacy of airway, breathing, and circulation *Supplemental O_2 and Assisted Ventilation* Bag-mask ventilation, endotracheal intubation as necessary *Naloxone* 0.5-1 µg/kg IV titrated prn *Naloxone* Infusion: 0.5-1 µg/kg/min IV to start and titrated prn *Dose Adjustment* Decrease or discontinue neuraxial opioid
Pruritus	*Diphenhydramine* 0.5-1 mg/kg PO/IV, maximum 25-50 mg, every 6 h prn *Hydroxyzine* 0.5-1 mg/kg PO/IV, maximum 25-50 mg, every 6 h prn *Nalbuphine* 50 µg/kg IV, maximum 5 mg, every 6 h prn *Naloxone* 0.5-1 µg/kg IV titrated every 2-3 minutes prn *Naloxone* Infusion: 0.5-1 µg/kg/h IV; higher doses may compromise analgesia *Dose Adjustment* Decrease or discontinue neuraxial opioid

Table 3-9. Management of Adverse Effects of Neuraxial Opioids, *cont.*

Adverse Effect	Treatment/Intervention
Nausea, emesis	*Ondansetron* 0.1 mg/kg IV, maximum 4 mg, every 6 h prn *Metoclopramide* 0.1 mg/kg IV, maximum 10 mg, every 6 h prn *Naloxone* 0.5-1 μg/kg IV every 2-3 minutes prn *Naloxone* Infusion 0.5-1 μg/kg/h IV; higher doses may compromise analgesia *Dose Adjustment* Decrease or discontinue neuraxial opioid
Urinary retention	*Naloxone* 0.5-1 μg/kg IV titrated prn *Naloxone* Infusion 0.5-1 μg/kg/h IV; higher doses may compromise analgesia *Urinary Catheter* Intermittent catheterization or indwelling catheter *Dose Adjustment* Decrease or discontinue neuraxial opioid

The adverse effects due to distal spread of neuraxial opioids may be treated with intravenous naloxone, either titrated by intermittent bolus dosing or by continuous infusion. The low dose of naloxone required (0.5-1 μg/kg/dose or 0.5-1 μg/kg/h by infusion) generally does not affect analgesia. Pruritus and nausea are fairly common with neuraxial opioids, especially hydrophilic agents such as morphine. Pruritus from a neuraxial opioid may respond to antihistamines, but is often more effectively treated with low-dose intravenous naloxone. Other options include the intravenous administration of mixed opioid agonist-antagonists such as nalbuphine or the combination of epidural butorphanol with morphine as previously mentioned.[16] Likewise, nausea and emesis from neuraxial opioid may be treated not only with conventional antiemetics, but also with low-dose naloxone infusions.

Epidural Analgesia Including Caudal Block

Anatomy, General Considerations, and Dosing Regimens

The spinal epidural space lies between the ligamentum flavum and the dura mater, extending from the base of the skull to the sacrococcygeal membrane at the base of the sacrum. To reach the epidural space, the needle must pass through the patient's skin, subcutaneous tissue, supraspinous ligament, interspinous ligament, and ligamentum flavum (Figure 3-1). The distance from the skin to the spinal epidural space varies depending on the age and body habitus of the patient. The spinal epidural space may be accessed at any vertebral level, although in pediatric practice, caudal block is most commonly performed, followed by lumbar, thoracic and, rarely, cervical epidural block. The vertebral level at which the epidural block is performed depends on the dermatomal distribution of the pain to be treated, and to some extent the size of the patient. The clinical experience of the practitioner may dictate the approach because significant experience is required to perform these techniques in children.

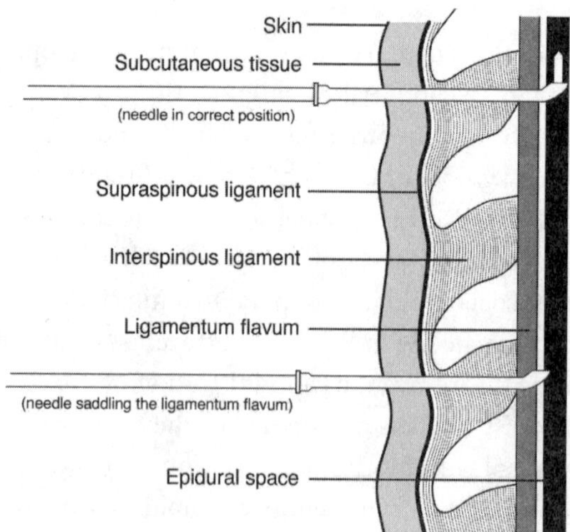

Figure 3-1
Anatomy of the epidural space.

Although hydrophilic neuraxial opioids such as morphine have considerable distal spread and may, therefore, provide analgesia at sites distant from the vertebral level at which the drug is administered, they also carry the highest risk of potentially serious side effects. The ability of hydrophilic opioids to travel in the cerebrospinal fluid after neuraxial administration is demonstrated by the efficacy of lumbar intrathecal morphine in providing analgesia following craniofacial procedures.[12,13] Lipophilic neuraxial opioids have limited spread from the site of administration and are, therefore, somewhat safer, but require delivery at or near the dermatomal level of the pain to be treated. Likewise, neuraxial local anesthetics induce conduction blockade only across the dermatomes at which they are administered and, therefore, provide analgesia only in this distribution. Although sometimes performed at sites distant from the surgical dermatomes for technical reasons, epidurals are optimally performed at the vertebral level corresponding to the dermatome at which maximal analgesia is desired.

Single bolus epidural techniques work well when pain is expected to last less than 24 hours. Even with neuraxial morphine, reliable analgesia will not persist beyond 24 hours. For pain expected to last longer than 24 hours, repeated bolus dosing or continuous infusion techniques with an indwelling epidural catheter are preferred. Although transient mid-thoracic analgesia can be achieved with bolus caudal administration of local anesthetic agents in young children and infants, the volume of local anesthetic required to maintain such a block is prohibitive, due to the certain risk of local anesthetic toxicity. For continuous techniques, it is necessary to approach the epidural space at the vertebral level corresponding to the dermatome at which maximal analgesia is desired. This allows the use of dilute neuraxial local anesthetic and/or low-dose neuraxial lipophilic opioid, or perhaps clonidine. These combinations provide optimal analgesia with the lowest risk of side effects and toxicities.

There remains controversy regarding the optimal technique for placing a catheter near the thoracic dermatomes for analgesia following thoracic and upper abdominal procedures. In infants and neonates, it may be possible to thread an epidural catheter from a caudal approach to the desired vertebral level. However, this technique is not uniformly successful, and even a styletted catheter may fail to advance, resulting in inadequate analgesia. Radiographic confirmation has been suggested by some authors to ensure cephalad advancement of the catheter from the caudal to the thoracic epidural space.[23-25] With the inherent problems of "blind" advancement from the caudal epidural space, Tsui et al[26,27] have suggested the use of either nerve stimulation or electrocardiographic guidance with specially adapted epidural catheters (Arrow International, Redding, PA). Alternatively, other authors have demonstrated the feasibility of direct placement of the catheter at the thoracic epidural level, thereby avoiding the need for advancement along multiple vertebral levels.[28]

Epidural anesthesia is performed under sterile conditions. Skin preparation with chlorhexidine rather than iodine-containing solutions may result in a lower risk of infectious complications.[29] Epidural anesthesia in children usually is performed under general anesthesia in the lateral decubitus position, although the sitting position may be used in cooperative older children and adolescents. Although the placement of epidural catheters in anesthetized adults is generally considered outside of the standard of care, given the difficulties that may be encountered with the performance of painful procedures in the awake infant, child, or adolescent, the consensus is that epidural catheters can be placed in the anesthetized pediatric patient.[30]

There are several commercially available kits for pediatric epidural anesthesia with 18- or 20-gauge Tuohy or Crawford needles with corresponding 19- or 20-gauge catheters. Three-inch or 3.5-inch needles, as in adult practice, are used for older children and adolescents, while 2-inch needles are available for use in younger children and infants. The authors prefer radiopaque catheters, given their ease in radiographic confirmation of catheter position without need for contrast injection (Figure 3-2). As expected, the distance from the skin to the epidural space is much shorter in children than in adults. Although formulas to predict this distance have been proposed, these formulas may be unreliable and, given interpatient variability, of limited practical use.[31] The needles for epidural analgesia are blunt to decrease the risk of inadvertent dural puncture. A skin nick before needle insertion allows easier passage of the epidural needle through the skin and subcutaneous tissue, avoids excessive forward pressure, and may decrease the risk of inadvertent excessive needle advancement. A loss-of-resistance technique with continuous or intermittent pressure on the plunger of a low-resistance syringe partially filled with normal saline is used to identify passage of the needle tip through the ligamentum flavum and into the epidural space. Although air has been used, saline is preferred, because using air for loss-of-resistance increases the risk of venous air embolism, intrathecal air injection if inadvertent dural puncture occurs, and patchy blockade if significant air is injected into the

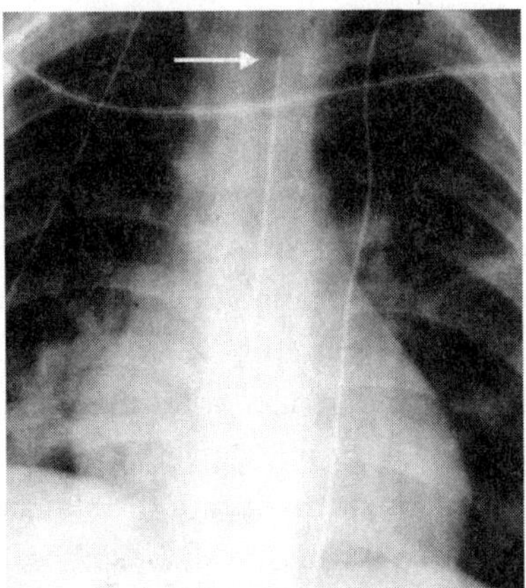

Figure 3-2
Radiographic confirmation of thoracic placement of a radiopaque epidural catheter.

epidural space. A patchy block resulting from use of air for loss-of-resistance is thought to be related to the presence of an air bubble over a nerve root that prevents contact with the local anesthetic/opioid solution. Alternatively, entry into the epidural space may be identified with a hanging-drop technique where a small amount of fluid is placed at the hub of the needle. Given the negative atmospheric pressure that is present within the epidural space, the drop of fluid will be drawn into the needle on entry into the epidural space. Entry into the epidural space is often subtle in children in whom ligaments are less calcified and more pliable. The characteristic "pop" usually noted in adults as the needle enters the epidural space may not be evident in children.

When needle entry into the epidural space is noted, a few milliliters of saline are injected to confirm loss of resistance and to open the space to facilitate catheter placement if a continuous technique is being used. After the injection of saline, fluid may drip back from the needle hub, because the epidural space is a potential space with a finite compliance. Brisk flow of clear fluid signals inadvertent dural puncture. Confirmation of the presence of cerebrospinal fluid (CSF) can be provided by detecting glucose using standard glucose test strips. After the epidural space is identified, careful aspiration for blood or CSF is then performed. After negative aspiration, a test dose of epinephrine-containing solution is injected. The test doses contains 0.5-1 μg/kg epinephrine (0.1-0.2 mL/kg of a local anesthetic solution containing epinephrine 1:200,000). After 30 to 60 seconds of observation for hemodynamic changes suggestive of intravascular injection (eg, ST or T wave changes, tachycardia, hypertension), the remainder of the dose is injected slowly in fractionated increments of 0.2 mL/kg, with repeated aspiration and observation after each subsequent dose of the local anesthetic solution. If a continuous technique is being used, an epidural catheter may be placed immediately after locating the epidural space or after the initial injection. Following placement, the catheter is aspirated for blood or

CSF. Temporarily holding the proximal catheter tip below the level of the insertion site may demonstrate flow of blood or CSF that was not observed with aspiration. If no blood or CSF is noted, a test dose of epinephrine-containing solution is given through the catheter, again with 30 to 60 seconds of observation for electrocardiogram and hemodynamic changes. Epidural catheters will not reliably thread to a vertebral level distant from the insertion site. Advancement of the catheters farther than 3 to 5 cm beyond the needle tip may cause the catheter to coil in the epidural space.[32] After the epidural space is accessed, administering an appropriate volume of medication ensures analgesic success (Table 3-10). The volume of medication depends on the size of the patient, the site of epidural access, and the dermatomal distribution over which analgesia is required.[33] Epidural medication is dosed on a mL/kg basis in children weighing less than 30 to 40 kg. Patients who weigh more than 30 to 40 kg may be dosed by adult parameters (Table 3-10). Caudal administration of 1 to 1.25 mL/kg of local anesthetic will result in adequate analgesia extending to mid-thoracic dermatomes in patients weighing less than 30 kg. Patients

Table 3-10. Suggested Volumes for Epidural Administration

Dose	Caudal	Lumbar	Thoracic	Cervical
Initial bolus	0.75-1.25 mL/kg, maximum 20-30 mL	0.5-0.75 mL/kg, maximum 15-20 mL	0.25-0.5 mL/kg, maximum 10-15 mL	0.1 mL/kg, maximum 5 mL
Additional bolus	0.4-0.5 mL/kg, maximum 15-20 mL	0.3-0.4 mL/kg, maximum 10-15 mL	0.2-0.3 mL/kg, maximum 5-10 mL	0.05 mL/kg, maximum 3 mL
Infusion	0.4-0.5 mL/kg/h, maximum 15-20 mL/h	0.3-0.4 mL/kg/h, maximum 10-15 mL/h	0.2-0.3 mL/kg/h, maximum 5-10 mL/h	0.05 mL/kg/h, maximum 3 mL/h

These dosing regimens are for volume only. Maximum bolus doses and continuous infusions must also consider the maximum dose in terms of mg/kg and mg/kg/h depending on the specific agent used.

weighing more than 30 kg are dosed with a finite volume (30 mL) and, therefore, will experience a progressively lower level of dermatomal coverage depending on their size. In adults, volumes of 30 mL will provide only sacral coverage. In younger patients, the caudal administration of 0.75 mL/kg of local anesthetic solution will provide analgesia extending to low thoracic or high lumbar dermatomes. These volumes are generally effective in providing analgesia following inguinal herniorrhaphy while 0.5 mL/kg provides only lumbosacral analgesia, effective for penoscrotal procedures such as circumcision.

Dermatomal coverage following the administration of lumbar or thoracic epidural medication is more difficult to predict. A widely used formula suggests that for bolus lumbar and thoracic epidural administration, the volume of medication required per dermatomal segment is approximately one tenth of the patient's age in years, up to 1 to 1.5 mL per dermatome.[33] The volume of the epidural space decreases, moving cephalad along the vertebral column. Lower volumes are required to provide the same dermatomal spread when comparing the thoracic to the lumbar to the caudal space. For continuous infusions, the volume of medication required per dermatomal segment is significantly less than that required for bolus administration (Table 3-5).

After the volume for epidural administration has been determined, an appropriate solution is prepared, and doses of local anesthetic (Tables 3-4 and 3-5), opioid (Table 3-7), and adjuvant agent are verified (Table 3-8). When considering the initial bolus injection, the total dose of local anesthetic (bupivacaine, levobupivacaine, or ropivacaine) should not exceed 3 to 4 mg/kg. Therefore, in smaller pediatric patients in whom the volume of epidural medication required may be as high as 1.3 mL/kg, the concentration of the local anesthetic may be as low as 0.1% to 0.2%. Although bupivacaine and levobupivacaine concentrations of 0.1% will provide effective analgesia, ropivacaine concentrations of 0.2% generally are necessary (Table 3-11).[34]

Despite the fact that optimal epidural analgesia ideally requires an individualized regimen, certain agents and combinations are commonly used for bolus and continuous epidural analgesia in children (Table 3-12). Continuous infusions may be delivered via patient-controlled analgesia (PCA) devices, in which case an intermittent bolus dose

Table 3-11. Bolus and Local Anesthetic Agents for Epidural Analgesia in Children*

Local Anesthetic	Dose	Approximate Maximum Dose
Bupivacaine 0.25%	2.5 mg/mL	1.3 mL/kg
Levobupivacaine 0.25%	2.5 mg/mL	1.3 mL/kg
Lidocaine 1%	10 mg/mL	0.7 mL/kg
Ropivacaine 0.2%	2 mg/mL	2 mL/kg

*Initial bolus; epinephrine usually added to detect intravascular administration.

Additional bolus generally 25%-50% of initial concentration, 50%-75% of initial volume; additional opioid and/or adjuvant agent added as desired. (See Tables 3-7 and 3-8.)

Table 3-12. Continuous Infusion: Local Anesthetic and/or Opioid and/or Adjuvant Agent

Local Anesthetic	Opioid/Adjuvant Agent	Approximate Maximum Dose
Bupivacaine 0.0625%-0.125%	Fentanyl 2-5 μg/mL (0.5-1 μg/kg/h)	For bupivacaine 0.0625%, 0.4 mg/kg/h = 0.6 mL/kg/h
-OR-	-OR-	
Levobupivacaine 0.0625%-0.125%	Hydromorphone 5-20 μg/mL (2-5 μg/kg/h)	For levobupivacaine 0.0625%, 0.4 mg/kg/h = 0.6 mL/kg/h
-OR-	-OR-	
Lidocaine 0.5%	Morphine 5-20 μg/mL (3-6 μg/kg/h)	For lidocaine 0.5%, 3 mg/kg/h = 0.6 mL/kg/h
-OR-	-AND/OR-	
Ropivacaine 0.1%-0.2%	Clonidine 0.5-1 μg/mL (0.25-0.5 μg/kg/h)	For ropivacaine 0.1%, 0.5 mg/kg/h = 0.5 mL/kg/h

Maximum dose for local anesthetic infusion is ~50% of the above in neonates and premature infants. The infusion rate and/or local anesthetic concentration must be adjusted accordingly.

(often 10%-20% of the basal infusion) may be provided every 30 to 60 minutes as needed. Bolus dosing is particularly useful before potentially painful activities, including ambulation and pulmonary toilet. Additional PCA-delivered doses must be considered in the total hourly dose to avoid potential systemic toxicity.

Special Considerations of Caudal Epidural Analgesia

The most commonly performed pediatric epidural technique is the caudal epidural block. First described for pediatric use in 1933,[35] caudal epidural analgesia involves accessing the epidural space through the sacrococcygeal ligament via the sacral hiatus at the base of the sacrum. The technique is relatively easy to perform and combines a high success rate with a low risk of complications. It is particularly popular in pediatric practice because of the ability to provide analgesia extending to the mid-thoracic dermatomes using doses of 1.3 to 1.5 mL/kg in infants and young children while approaching the epidural space below the level of the spinal cord. A caudal epidural block may be considered for any procedure or process below the umbilicus. Caudal block in children is most commonly performed in combination with a general anesthetic, but may be the sole technique in former preterm infants at high risk for post-anesthetic apnea. Caudal block is performed with the patient in the lateral or prone position.

The sacral hiatus is identified above the coccyx, at or near the superior aspect of the gluteal crease by palpation of the 2 sacral cornua (Figure 3-3). The sacral cornua represent the posterior bony elements of the S5 vertebral body. The sacrococcygeal membrane represents the most inferior aspect of the ligamentum flavum surrounding the spinal epidural space. Using appropriate sterile technique, a needle is inserted midway between and slightly inferior to the 2 sacral cornua at a 45° angle to the skin. The needle angle may be decreased immediately after passing through the skin or after encountering bone, representing the posterior wall of the ventral sacral elements. The needle is advanced, readjusting the angle as needed, until a characteristic "pop" indicating passage through the sacrococcygeal membrane, is appreciated (Figure 3-4). Potential sites of improper needle placement include intraosseous, subdural, in an epidural vein, and under the sacral ligament (Figure 3-5).

Recent controversy has developed regarding the type of needle to use—standard or styletted.[36] Advocates of a styletted needle voice concern with coring, or the removal of a tissue plug, which, theoretically, could be carried into the epidural space and develop into an epidermoid tumor. Goldschneider and Brandom[36] demonstrated residual material in 54% of cases when a non-styletted needle was used. In 33% of the cases, the core included epidermal tissue. This issue remains to be resolved because many institutions continue to use standard, short bevel, non-stylleted needles, while others use styletted needles such as a standard spinal needle.

After negative aspiration for blood or CSF, the same process as outlined previously for dosing an epidural block at the lumbar or thoracic level is followed, including the use of a test dose and fractionating the entire dose of local anesthetic solution. The volume administered depends on the desired area level of analgesia.

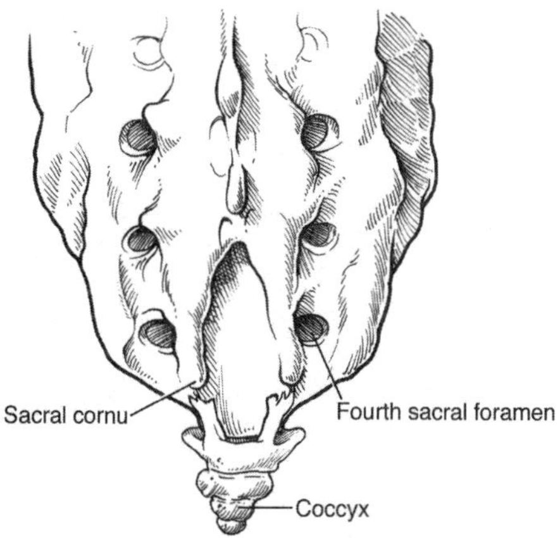

Figure 3-3
Anatomy of the sacrum and coccyx with identification of the sacral cornu.

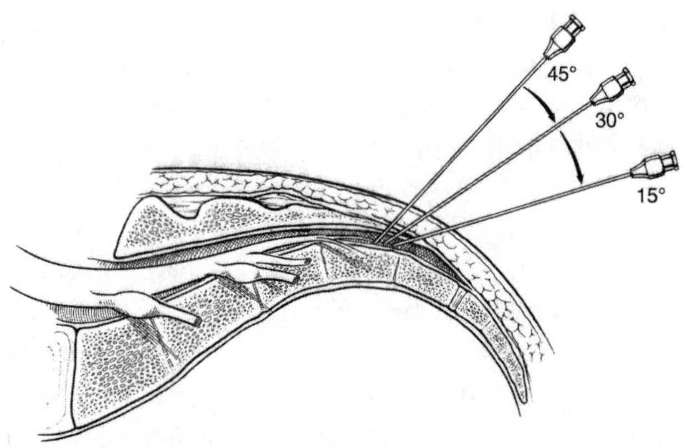

Figure 3-4
Coronal view of the sacrum with correct needle placement. The needle is inserted midway between and slightly inferior to the 2 sacral cornua at a 45° angle to the skin. The needle angle may be decreased immediately after passing through the skin or after encountering bone representing the posterior aspect of the anterior sacral elements. The needle is advanced, readjusting the angle as needed, until a characteristic "pop," indicating passage through the sacrococcygeal membrane, is appreciated.

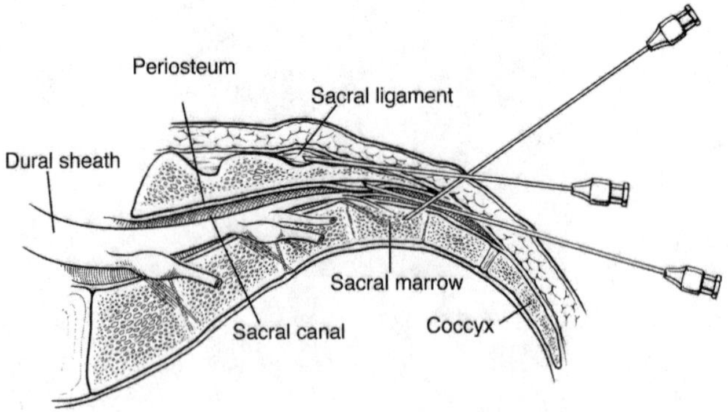

Figure 3-5
Diagram demonstrating the sites of potential misplacement of the needle during caudal epidural block, including subperiosteal, subdural (under the sacral ligament), and intraosseous.

Bupivacaine (0.125%-0.25%), levobupivacaine (0.125%-0.25%), and ropivacaine (0.2%) are the local anesthetics most commonly used for bolus caudal epidural administration (Table 3-11). Bupivacaine, levobupivacaine, and ropivacaine, when used in concentrations of 0.2% to 0.25%, will provide surgical anesthesia for 60 to 120 minutes with persistent analgesia for up to 6 to 12 hours thereafter. Analgesia at more distant sites or for longer periods may be achieved by adding opioid and/or adjuvant agents (Tables 3-7 and 3-8).

Although caudal block is most commonly performed as a "single shot" bolus technique, postoperative analgesia can be provided by a continuous caudal infusion following placement of a caudal epidural catheter as is performed for lumbar or thoracic epidural analgesia. Several commercially prepared kits are available for caudal anesthesia, or standard epidural kits may be used with a Crawford or other end-hole needle. Alternatively, a standard 20-gauge epidural catheter may be threaded through an 18-gauge intravenous catheter that has been placed into the caudal epidural space.

Regional anesthesia, either spinal or caudal block, with the patient awake occasionally is performed for surgical procedures below the umbilicus in children at high risk for post-anesthetic apnea, particularly former preterm infants. Avoiding general anesthesia may decrease the likelihood of postoperative respiratory complications, including apnea. Awake regional anesthesia generally uses only local anesthetic agents because adding a neuraxial opioid and/or adjuvant agent may confer the same risk for post-anesthetic apnea as does general anesthesia. Either caudal epidural or spinal anesthesia may be used (Table 3-13, see next section for a discussion of spinal anesthesia). Topical anesthesia is provided by skin infiltration or local anesthetic cream before block placement. Numerous regimens have been suggested for awake caudal anesthesia with volumes ranging from 1 to 1.5 mL/kg of bupivacaine in concentrations varying from 0.2% to 0.375%.[37] For these techniques, a higher volume is needed to provide high thoracic block

Table 3-13. Comparison of Caudal Epidural and Spinal Anesthesia in Children

Factor	Caudal Epidural	Spinal
Technique	Easier	More difficult
Success rate	Higher	Lower
Dose of local anesthetic	Higher (3 mg/kg*)	Lower (0.6-1 mg/kg*)
Speed of onset	Slower (15-20 minutes)	Faster (2-5 minutes)
Duration	Longer (90 minutes)	Shorter (<60 minutes)
Motor block	Partial	Complete
Influence of patient position	Minimal	Significant

*Dose of local anesthetic is listed in mg/kg when using bupivacaine.

while a higher concentration (0.2%-0.375% bupivacaine) of local anesthetic is needed to improve surgical anesthesia. Limitations of these techniques include incomplete motor block with resultant unfavorable surgical conditions and duration of anesthesia less than 90 minutes. Additionally, the combination of a high volume and a higher concentration of local anesthetic agent approaches or, in some suggested regimens, exceeds the recommended doses of bupivacaine. These concerns and the need to prolong anesthesia beyond 90 minutes in some cases have resulted in the use of 3% chloroprocaine by continuous infusion. Successful anesthesia can be provided for 2 to 3 hours in the awake neonate using a regimen of 1.5 to 2 mL/kg of 3% chloroprocaine as the initial bolus, followed by an infusion of 1.5 to 2.0 mL/kg/h.[38,39] Despite the high volume and high concentration of local anesthetic agent, serum concentrations have been shown to be insignificant even in the neonatal population.[40] This technique also has been shown to be effective as a combined technique with general anesthesia for abdominal surgical procedures in neonates, thereby allowing immediate tracheal extubation by avoiding high concentrations of an inhalational anesthetic agent and eliminating the need for parenteral opioids.[41]

Spinal Anesthesia and Analgesia

The use of spinal anesthesia in children dates back to 1909; however, the technique never gained popularity in pediatric anesthesia until the 1980s, when it was reintroduced as an alternative to general anesthesia in the high-risk, former preterm neonate. In this population, spinal anesthesia was suggested as a means of limiting the incidence of postoperative complications, including apnea and postoperative respiratory dysfunction.[42-47] In addition to inguinal herniorrhaphy, additional uses of spinal anesthesia have included general surgical, lower extremity orthopedic, and urological procedures (hydrocelectomy, orchidopexy, and circumcision).[48] See Reference 48 for a full review of the reports outlining the use of spinal anesthesia in infants and children for various types of surgical procedures.

While most reports regarding the use of spinal anesthesia include surgical procedures below the umbilicus, other investigators have reported the use of spinal anesthesia as the sole anesthetic for major procedures, including closure of meningomyelocele or repair of gastroschisis,[49,50] and combined with endotracheal intubation and general anesthesia for cardiothoracic surgical procedures.[51,52] Although these techniques should be undertaken only by those with significant experience in the use of regional anesthesia in neonates, such reports provide preliminary clinical evidence of the efficacy of such techniques.

Techniques of Spinal Anesthesia

The literature has described several variations in the technique of spinal anesthesia. These variations include positioning of the patient (both the sitting and lateral decubitus position), use of needles of various sizes and lengths, and variations in the agent and its dose. The authors' preference for the unsedated, awake neonate or infant is the sitting position. The lateral position may be easier for older patients who generally receive intravenous sedation. In neonates and infants, regardless of the position used, careful attention should be directed at maintaining patency of the airway, which can be compromised with overzealous positioning. Supplemental oxygen should be administered during the procedure and consideration given to the use of end-tidal carbon dioxide monitoring via nasal cannula to ensure ongoing airway patency.

Specific anatomical variations exist between neonates and infants compared with the adult population. In neonates, the spinal cord ends at L3, as opposed to L1 in adults. A line connecting the top of the iliac crests crosses the spinal axis at the L4-5 level in neonates and infants and the L3-4 level in older children and adolescents. The actual techniques used for spinal anesthesia in neonates, infants, and children are much the same as those used in adults. Superficial dermal analgesia may eliminate or decrease the need for intravenous sedation during performance of the lumbar puncture. Topical analgesia can be achieved using any of the available topical local anesthetic creams over the lumbar region 30 to 60 minutes before the procedure. When necessary in older patients, deeper analgesia may be obtained with the infiltration of local anesthetic. Various sizes of spinal needles are available. In older patients who may be at risk for a post-dural puncture headache, a 25- or 26-gauge needle can be used. The use of needles without stylets (ie, standard intravenous catheters or butterfly needles) is not recommended because epithelial tissue can be deposited in the intrathecal space and is a possible etiological factor in the subsequent development of epidermoid tumors of the neural axis. While some authors have advocated placing the intravenous cannula in an anesthetized lower extremity after placing the subarachnoid block, the authors' preference is to place it before placing the block. Although cardiorespiratory compromise is unlikely following spinal anesthesia in children (see following text), adverse cardiorespiratory complications may occur and the presence of a patent intravenous cannula may allow for more rapid intervention. Additionally, given the propensity of neonates and infants to develop bradycardia from any noxious stimulus, the administration of atropine before positioning and performing the spinal anesthetic is recommended.

Various dosing regimens have been suggested in the literature.[48] Higher doses than commonly used in adults are necessary given the larger volume of CSF per kilogram in neonates and infants compared with adults (4-6 mL/kg in a neonate vs 2 mL/kg in an adult). Most information on dosing refers to the neonatal and infant population, with more limited data on patients older than 6 to 12 months. In neonates and infants, dosing of tetracaine ranges from 0.2 to 0.6 mg/kg, whereas bupivacaine dosing ranges from 0.3 to 0.6 mg/kg. In patients older than 6 months, tetracaine dosing ranges from 0.2 to 0.4 mg/kg. Our unpublished experience suggests that isobaric levobupivacaine (0.5%) also can be used in patients ranging in age from 4 to 16 years in a dose of 1 mg/year up to a maximum dose of 15 mg. Despite the wide range of doses, the duration and level of anesthesia has been remarkably adequate and consistent for the desired procedures without a significant number of reports of excessively high levels resulting in cardiorespiratory compromise. The authors' preference is to use tetracaine crystals diluted in D10W to a final concentration of 1% or 10 mg/mL. A tuberculin syringe (1 mL) is used to draw up the desired amount of tetracaine. Prior to drawing up the tetracaine, an "epi wash" can be added to the solution. This is performed by drawing up epinephrine (1 mL of a 1 mg/mL solution) into the tuberculin syringe and then squirting out as much epinephrine as possible. This technique leaves a small amount in the hub and coating the sides of the syringe. The local anesthetic solution is then drawn up. Once the spinal needle is placed in the intrathecal space, the syringe is attached, gentle aspiration is performed to confirm intrathecal placement, and the local anesthetic solution is injected. A common mistake is failing to attach the syringe firmly to the hub of the needle so that some of the local anesthetic solution is lost during injection. Additionally, it is easy to displace the spinal needle while attaching the syringe, so careful aspiration must be performed after attaching the syringe to ensure that the needle is still within the intrathecal space. At the completion of the injection, cerebrospinal fluid is again aspirated (a volume of 0.2-0.3 mL) and reinjected to clear the dead space of the needle. Once the medication is injected, the sterile Betadine solution is wiped off the patient's back, the Bovie pad is placed, and the infant is positioned supine on the operating table. It is our preference to have the Bovie pad ready to be placed after completing the procedure to ensure that the infant's legs are not lifted to gain access to the back. After positioning on the table, a piece of tape is placed across the infant's legs, the blood pressure cuff is positioned on the lower extremity, and the procedure is started. Intermittent inflation of the blood pressure cuff can disturb a sleeping infant, so the cuff is placed on the lower extremity, which is anesthetized. The infant is then allowed to suck on a pacifier. In neonates and infants at risk for post-operative apnea, supplemental sedation is avoided because it entails the same risks for postoperative apnea as general anesthesia. Despite the decreased risk of apnea following a pure spinal anesthetic technique, apnea still may occur, so patients are monitored for 12 to 24 hours postoperatively to ensure adequate respiratory function.[53]

In addition to the reports outlining the technique and successes of spinal anesthesia, other investigators have attempted to answer specific clinical questions. Hirabayashi et al[54] compared the differential sensory spread of spinal anesthetic in adolescents versus adults. One hundred and thirty patients undergoing minor orthopedic and lower abdominal procedures comprised the cohort for the study. They were divided into 2 groups based on age, consisting of 21 patients ranging from 12 to 16 years and 111 patients ranging from 17 to 82 years. There was no difference in height and weight between the 2 groups. Spinal anesthesia was performed using 8 mg of hyperbaric amethocaine injected at the L3-4 interspace using a 25-gauge needle. The highest sensory level achieved in the younger population group was significantly greater ($P<.0001$) (range T4 to C5) compared with the older group (range T9 to C7). The authors speculated that the difference may have been related to the increased flexibility of the spine in younger patients, thereby limiting the normal thoracic kyphosis, which causes pooling of the solution below the level in older patients. This decreased kyphosis would, therefore, allow greater cephalad spread of the solution.

Clinically relevant information is also provided by Rice et al,[55] who evaluated the duration of anesthesia provided by various spinal regimens in 100 infants ranging in age from 1 month to 1 year. The duration was measured from the time of injection until the recovery of hip flexion and was 56 ± 2.3 minutes with lidocaine (3 mg/kg) plus epinephrine, 86 ± 4 minutes with tetracaine (0.4 mg/kg), and 128 ± 3 minutes with tetracaine plus epinephrine. Eighty-three infants required supplemental sedation during the procedures.

Three studies have formally evaluated the effect of the addition of epinephrine to the spinal solution.[55-57] Abajian et al[56] reported a prolongation of the duration of spinal anesthesia with the addition of epinephrine to tetracaine (0.22-0.32 mg/kg) from 84 ± 7.2 minutes (range 50-135 minutes) to 128 ± 3.3 minutes (range 80-145 minutes) in neonates and infants. Rice et al[55] noted similar findings with the addition of epinephrine prolonging tetracaine spinal anesthesia from 86 ± 4 minutes to 128 ± 3.3 minutes. Fosel et al[57] reported prolongation of the duration of anesthesia from a mean of 50 minutes (range 37-85 minutes) to 95 minutes (range 60-120 minutes) with the addition of epinephrine to bupivacaine. While these studies demonstrate a prolonged effect with the addition of epinephrine, any study dealing with the duration of spinal anesthesia must be examined closely because different criteria are used to define the "duration of spinal anesthesia." While it may be most helpful to examine the duration of surgical anesthesia (ie, the duration of sensory blockade of the dermatomes of the surgical procedure), most studies have examined other criteria, such as the time to return of motor function in lower extremities, assessed by return of hip flexion or movement of the toes or feet.

Combined Spinal and General Anesthesia

Although most reports outline the use of spinal anesthesia for surgical procedures below the umbilicus and the lower extremities, spinal anesthesia, either single shot or continuous, also has been combined with general anesthesia and tracheal intubation. In these cases, the technique is used as a means to avoid the use of systemic opioids, thereby limiting the postoperative respiratory depressant effects and allowing for earlier tracheal extubation. The spinal anesthetic also can combine a local anesthetic for surgical anesthesia with a small dose of intrathecal opioid to provide prolonged postoperative analgesia, provided that appropriate postoperative monitoring is available.

Payne and Moore[58] described the use of continuous spinal anesthesia combined with general anesthesia and tracheal intubation in 10 patients ranging in age from 2 to 59 months and weighing from 2 to 21 kg. The surgical procedures included ileostomy repair, pull-through procedure for Hirschsprung's disease, resection of an intra-abdominal mass, and an incisional hernia repair. General anesthesia included tracheal intubation with halothane followed by isoflurane (inspired concentration 1%-1.5%) in air and oxygen. An intrathecal catheter was then placed at either the L4-5 or L5 to S1 level using a 22-gauge spinal needle and a 28-gauge catheter. Spinal anesthesia was provided by intermittent doses of 0.5% bupivacaine (0.2 mL/kg to a maximum of 1 mL). Infants younger than 1 year required repeat dosing at 45- to 60-minute intervals, whereas patients older than 1 year required redosing at 60- to 80-minute intervals. Intrathecal catheters, left in for postoperative analgesia in the first 3 patients, were removed because there was significant leakage of CSF around the insertion site. The authors also noted that, following their report, there had been an association of arachnoiditis with the use of a microcatheter and they no longer recommended the technique. However, a single shot technique combined with a general anesthetic still can be used in neonates and infants undergoing major abdominal procedures. By doing this, surgical anesthesia is provided by the spinal anesthetic technique thereby eliminating the need for parenteral opioids, which may allow for earlier tracheal extubation in the neonatal population.

Finkel et al[52] reported their prospective experience with the combination of general and spinal anesthesia during cardiovascular surgery in infants and children. Following anesthetic induction and tracheal intubation, spinal anesthesia was administered in the lumbar intrathecal area in 30 children (aged 7 months-13 years). Surgical procedures included 18 atrial septal defect repairs, 8 ventricular septal defect repairs, 2 right ventricle-pulmonary artery conduits, 1 Fontan procedure, and 1 Glenn shunt. Spinal anesthesia included morphine (dose not specified) and tetracaine. The tetracaine dose was based on the patient's age (2 mg/kg in the 6-month to 1-year range, 1 mg/kg in the 1- to 3-year range, and 0.5 mg/kg in patients 4 years or older). Following placement of the spinal block, the patients were placed in the Trendelenburg position. No clinically significant hemodynamic changes were noted in any of the patients, although there was a statistically significant decrease in heart rate. The combination of the spinal with general anesthesia allowed for the use of low concentrations of inhalational anesthetic agents during the case. All patients were extubated in the operating room.

Table 3-14. Technical Complications of Neuraxial Blockade

Failure of technique—inadequate analgesia, need to convert to general anesthesia
Discomfort if procedure performed with patient awake, need to convert to general anesthesia
Infection including meningitis and epidural abscess
Bleeding including epidural hematoma
Inadvertent dural puncture with total spinal blockade or post-dural puncture headache
Traumatic nerve injury including intraneural injection

Adverse Effects of Neuraxial Anesthesia

Adverse effects related to medications administered for epidural analgesia and treatment algorithms have been reviewed previously (Table 3-9). Other potential adverse sequelae of neuraxial techniques include those related to needle insertion or catheter placement (Table 3-14). The technique may fail, necessitating conversion to general anesthesia or resulting in inadequate analgesia during the postoperative period. When analgesia seems to be inadequate, a prompt evaluation must be performed to avoid protracted periods of pain for the patient. Dosing the catheter with 3% chloroprocaine will result in a demonstrable level of anesthesia if the catheter is in the epidural space. If the patient's pain is resolved, the concentration of the local anesthetic agent can be increased (as dosing guidelines permit), the concentration of the opioid increased, or an adjuvant agent (clonidine) added. In some cases, the catheter may be in the epidural space, but at a level too far below the dermatomes involved to provide effective analgesia. In such cases, switching to a more hydrophilic opioid may be effective. Alternatively, if adequate analgesia is not achieved, the catheter should be removed and a different analgesic regimen instituted.

Infection is a risk of any interventional technique. However, even with caudal catheters, infectious complications are exceedingly rare with infusions up to 3 days.[59] If needed, epidural catheters may safely remain in place for up to 5 to 7 days, provided the patient is appropriately monitored and the epidural site inspected daily. Alternatively, subcutaneous tunneling of the catheter has been suggested for prolonged epidural analgesia in children.[60] Potential infectious complications include meningitis and epidural abscess. Fever, acute back pain, and new neurologic deficits should prompt an aggressive evaluation for potential abscess formation, which requires emergent neurosurgical consultation. Despite its widespread use, reports of infectious complications related to spinal anesthesia have been rare. Meningitis following spinal anesthesia may be related to hematogenous spread, contamination of the equipment and/or medications, or a break in sterile technique. A case of aseptic meningitis following spinal anesthesia in a high-risk former preterm neonate has been reported.[61] Despite the low incidence of infectious complications, prompt evaluation with possible repeat lumbar puncture is indicated in patients who develop fever following a neuraxial technique.

The epidural space is highly vascular with numerous epidural veins with the potential to bleed and result in epidural hematoma formation. Presentation of epidural hematoma is similar to that of epidural abscess, but without fever. Again, an aggressive evaluation is suggested with emergent surgical intervention as needed. The risk of hemorrhagic complications from epidural analgesia is higher in patients with abnormal coagulation function of any etiology. Given the risks of epidural hematoma formation, epidural anesthesia is contraindicated in patients with altered coagulation function, including qualitative platelet disorders, thrombocytopenia (platelet count less than 100,000/mm^3), or an international normalized ratio of 1.5 or greater. Inadvertent dural puncture may result in intrathecal medication administration and resultant spinal analgesia. Given the larger volumes and higher doses of local anesthetics used for epidural analgesia, total spinal blockade with apnea and hemodynamic instability may ensue, requiring aggressive supportive care until the block has resolved. Inadvertent dural puncture also carries a risk of subsequent post-dural puncture headache (PDPH).[62]

Post-dural puncture headache, although frequently thought of as an adult disease, has been documented in children, especially in patients older than 8 to 10 years. Kokki and Hendolin[63] reported an incidence of 5% in patients older than 11 years when a 22-gauge spinal needle was used. A subsequent study by the same group prospectively evaluated the incidence and influence of needle type on PDPH in 200 children, aged 2 to 128 months, undergoing spinal anesthesia.[64] In half of the cases, a cutting needle was used, while a pencil-point needle was used in the remaining patients. Seventeen (9%) of the children developed a headache; 10 (5%) were classified as PDPH. Eight patients described their headaches as mild, 2 described their headaches as moderate, while no patients described their headaches as severe. None required a blood patch. A cutting needle was used on 7 patients with headache, whereas a pencil-point needle was used on 3 patients with headache. Wee et al[65] investigated the occurrence of PDPH following lumbar puncture in 97 children with oncological diseases. Post-dural puncture headache occurred in none of 70 children younger than 10 years, 2 of 17 (11.8%) aged 10 to 12 years, and 5 of 10 aged 13 to 18 years.

Although the incidence of PDPH is assumed to be greater in older children, it is difficult to accurately assess such problems in preverbal infants and children. Preliminary information suggests that many of the same factors that govern the incidence of PDPH in adults, such as type and size of spinal needle, also apply to children. Therefore, whenever feasible, especially in the older pediatric patient, small gauge needles (25-26 gauge) with a non-cutting (pencil) point are suggested. A PDPH headache usually will resolve within 48 to 72 hours. Suggested supportive care, which has not necessarily been proven to be effective in prospective clinical trials, includes bed rest, hydration, and caffeine administration. Bed rest will decrease the pain of PDPH, but will not hasten its resolution. In cases where the pain is debilitating, placement of an epidural blood patch may be necessary.

Because neuraxial anesthetic techniques in children usually are performed under general anesthesia, it has long been held that unrecognized traumatic nerve injury, including intraneural injection, is a potential complication, particularly with lumbar and thoracic epidural techniques. Transient neurologic deficit possibly secondary to traumatic spinal cord injury during epidural analgesia in a child under general anesthesia has been reported recently.[66] Fortunately, serious complications of epidural analgesia in children remain rare when performed by experienced practitioners in appropriate settings, and the potential benefits from such techniques are considerable. As with any intervention, however, the risks and benefits of epidural analgesia must be considered in each patient.

Thoracic levels of epidural or spinal blockade may result in sympathetic blockade with vasodilatation, decreased preload, and decreased afterload, resulting in hypotension. Higher thoracic blockade (T1-4) also can result in blockade of the sympathetic cardioacceleratory fibers and bradycardia. This is rare in neonates and infants, given the relative immaturity of their sympathetic nervous system. In the absence of hypovolemia or underlying myocardial dysfunction, these complications are of limited clinical significance in most pediatric patients. Hypotension is generally easily treated with fluid administration or the use of a direct-acting α-adrenergic agonist such as phenylephrine.

Neuraxial anesthesia with a high sensory and motor level above the T1 dermatome can result in respiratory failure and/or apnea, requiring assisted ventilation until the block recedes. Often, this is not related to excessive dosing, but rather confounding factors, such as the legs being lifted after the spinal had been inserted for placement of the Bovie pad. To limit the risk, as mentioned previously, the Bovie pad should be placed after the spinal block is placed, then a piece of tape should be secured across the legs after the infant or child is positioned on the operating table.

Summary

Interest in pediatric neuraxial blockade continues to grow, with increasing applications of epidural and spinal analgesia in children. Neuraxial blockade in children entails placement of medications in the spinal epidural or intrathecal subarachnoid space. Medications used may include the combination of local anesthetic agent, opioid, and/or adjuvant agents such as ketamine or clonidine. Although the epidural space may be accessed at any vertebral level, caudal block is most common in pediatric practice. Unless a hydrophilic opioid such as morphine is used, epidural analgesia optimally requires an approach at the vertebral level corresponding to the dermatome at which maximal analgesia is desired. Epidural analgesia may entail a single bolus administration or a continuous infusion via an epidural catheter. Three options are available for prolonged analgesia (up to 24 hours): 1) caudal epidural injection of a hydrophilic opioid such as morphine, with butorphanol to limit the adverse effects of morphine; 2) lumbar intrathecal morphine, which has been shown to be effective for thoracic and craniofacial procedures; and 3) an indwelling epidural catheter with a continuous infusion of a combination of the agents outlined in this chapter.

Spinal anesthesia continues to gain acceptance as an alternative to general anesthesia in children. In most cases, spinal anesthesia has been used instead of general anesthesia when specific underlying patient factors are thought to increase the risks. However, accumulated experience suggests that it also may be viewed as an equal alternative to general anesthesia in healthy outpatients. To date, most experience has been during lower abdominal surgery in the former preterm neonate or infant. There also has been an increased use of spinal anesthesia for other surgical procedures, including lower extremity orthopedic procedures as well as specific surgical procedures above the umbilicus and in patients outside the neonatal age range. Some authorities have reported experience with spinal anesthesia for major surgical procedures, including repair of gastroschisis, meningomyelocele repair, and scoliosis surgery. Most of the reports describe a single shot technique, thereby limiting application to procedures lasting 90 minutes or less. Given the success of neuraxial analgesia, as well as the favorable adverse effect profile, its use is expected to continue to increase.

References

1. Dalens B. Regional anesthesia in children. *Anesth Analg.* 1989;68:654-672
2. McNeely JK, Farber NE, Rusy LM, Hoffman GM. Epidural analgesia improves outcome following pediatric fundoplication. *Reg Anesth.* 1997;22:16-23
3. Broadman LM. Pediatric regional anesthesia. *Clin Anesth Updates.* 1992;3:1-14
4. Tobias JD. Therapeutic applications of regional anesthesia. *Paediatr Anaesth.* 2002;12:272-277
5. Berde CB. Convulsions associated with pediatric regional anesthesia. *Anesth Analg.* 1992;75:164-166
6. McCloseky JJ, Haun SE, Deshpande JK. Bupivacaine toxicity secondary to continuous caudal epidural infusion in children. *Anesth Analg.* 1992;75:287-290
7. Agarwal R, Gutlove DP, Lockhart CH. Seizures occurring in pediatric patients receiving continuous infusion of bupivacaine. *Anesth Analg.* 1992;75:284-286
8. Kasten GW, Martin ST. Bupivacaine cardiovascular toxicity: comparison of treatment with bretylium and lidocaine. *Anesth Analg.* 1985;64:911-916
9. Haasio J, Pitkanen MT, Kytta J, Rosenberg PH. Treatment of bupivacaine-induced cardiac arrhythmias in hypoxic and hypercarbic pigs with amiodarone or bretylium. *Reg Anesth.* 1990;15:174-179
10. Weinberg G, Ripper R, Feinstein DL, Hoffman W. Lipid emulsion infusion rescues dogs from bupivacaine-induced cardiac toxicity. *Reg Anesth Pain Med.* 2002;28:198-202
11. Tobias JD. Caudal epidural block. A review of test dosing and recognition of systemic injection in children. *Anesth Analg.* 2001;93:1156-1161
12. Tobias JD, Deshpande JK, Wetzel R, et al. Postoperative analgesia: use of intrathecal morphine in children. *Clin Pediatr.* 1990;29:44-48
13. Tobias JD, Mateo C, Ferrer MJR, et al. Intrathecal morphine for post-operative analgesia following repair of frontal encephaloceles in children: comparison with intermittent, on-demand dosing of nalbuphine. *J Clin Anesth.* 1997;9:280-284
14. Moriarty A. Postoperative extradural infusions in children: preliminary data from a comparison of bupivacaine/diamorphine with plain ropivacaine. *Paediatr Anaesth.* 1999;9:423-427
15. Sanders JC. Paediatric regional anaesthesia: a survey of practice in the United Kingdom. *Br J Anaesth.* 2002;89:707-710
16. Lawhorn CD, Brown RE Jr. Epidural morphine with butorphanol in pediatric patients. *J Clin Anesth.* 1994;6:91-94

17. Weber F, Wulf H. Caudal bupivacaine and s(+)-ketamine for postoperative analgesia in children. *Paediatr Anaesth.* 2003;13:244-248
18. Marhofer P, Krenn CG, Plochl W, et al. S(+)-ketamine for caudal block in paediatric anaesthesia. *Br J Anaesth.* 2000;84:341-345
19. Sharpe P, Klein JR, Thompson JP, et al. Analgesia for circumcision in a paediatric population: comparison of caudal bupivacaine alone with bupivacaine plus two doses of clonidine. *Paediatr Anaesth.* 2001;11:695-701
20. Kaabachi O, Ben Rajeb A, Mebazaa M, et al. Spinal anesthesia in children: comparative study of hyperbaric bupivacaine with or without clonidine. *Ann Fr Anaesth Reanim.* 2002;21:617-621
21. Hager H, Marhofer P, Sitzwohl, et al. Caudal clonidine prolongs analgesia from caudal S(+)-ketamine in children. *Anesth Analg.* 2002;94:1169-1172
22. Bouchut JC, Dubois R, Godard J. Clonidine in preterm infant caudal anesthesia may be responsible for postoperative apnea. *Reg Anesth Pain Med.* 2001;26:83-85
23. Bosenberg AT, Bland BA, Schulte-Steinberg O, et al. Thoracic epidural anesthesia via the caudal route in infants. *Anesthesiology.* 1988;69:265-269
24. Valairucha S, Seefelder C, Houck CS. Thoracic epidural catheters placed by the caudal route in infants: the importance of radiographic confirmation. *Paediatr Anaesth.* 2002;12:424-428
25. Gunter JB, Eng C. Thoracic epidural anesthesia via the caudal approach in children. *Anesthesiology.* 1992;76:935-938
26. Tsui BC, Seal R, Koller J. Thoracic epidural catheter placement via the caudal approach in infants by using electrocardiographic guidance. *Anesth Analg.* 2002;95:326-330
27. Tsui BC, Gupta S, Finucane B. Confirmation of epidural catheter placement using nerve stimulation. *Can J Anaesth.* 1998;45:640-644
28. Tobias JD, Lowe S, O'Dell N, et al. Thoracic epidural anesthesia in infants and children. *Can J Anaesth.* 1993;40:879-882
29. Kinirons B, Mimoz O, Lafendi L, et al. Chlorhexidine versus povidone iodine in preventing colonization of continuous epidural catheters in children: a randomized, controlled trial. *Anesthesiology.* 2001;94:239-244
30. Krane EJ, Dalens BJ, Murat I, et al. The safety of epidurals placed during general anesthesia. *Reg Anesth Pain Med.* 1998;23:433-438
31. Uemura A, Yamashita M. A formula for determining the distance from the skin to the lumbar epidural space in infants and children. *Paediatr Anaesth.* 1992;2:305-307
32. Lim YJ, Bahk JH, Ahn WS, et al. Coiling of lumbar epidural catheters. *Acta Anaesthesiol Scand.* 2002;46:603-606

33. Schulte-Steinberg O, Rahlfs VW. Spread of extradural analgesia following caudal injection in children. A statistical study. *Br J Anaesth.* 1977;49:1027-1034
34. Luz G, Innerhofer P, Haussler B, Oswald E, Salner E, Sparr H. Comparison of ropivacaine 0.1% and 0.2% with bupivacaine 0.2% for single-shot caudal anaesthesia in children. *Paediatr Anaesth.* 2000;10:499-504
35. Campbell MF. Caudal anesthesia in children. *J Urol.* 1933;30:245-249
36. Goldschneider KR, Brandom BW. The incidence of tissue coring during the performance of caudal injection in children. *Reg Anesth Pain Med.* 1999;24:553-556
37. Gunter JB, Watcha MF, Forestner JE, et al. Caudal epidural anesthesia in conscious premature and high-risk infants. *J Feder Surg.* 1991;26:9-14
38. Tobias JD, Lowe S, O'Dell N, Pietsch JB, Neblett WW III. Continuous regional anesthesia in infants. *Can J Anaesth.* 1993;40:1065-1068
39. Tobias JD, Hersey S. Continuous caudal anaesthesia during inguinal herniorrhaphy in an awake, 1440 gram infant. *Paediatr Anaesth.* 1994;4:187-189
40. Henderson K, Sethna NF, Berde CB. Continuous caudal anesthesia for inguinal repair in former preterm infants. *J Clin Anesth.* 1993;5:129-133
41. Tobias JD, Rasmussen GE, Holcomb GW III, Brock JW III, Morgan WM III. Continuous caudal anaesthesia with chloroprocaine as an adjunct to general anaesthesia in neonates. *Can J Anaesth.* 1996;43:69-72
42. Harnik EV, Hoy GR, Potolicchio S, Stewart DR, Siegelman RE. Spinal anesthesia in premature infants recovering from respiratory distress syndrome. *Anesthesiology.* 1986;64:95-99
43. Mahe V, Ecoffey C. Spinal anesthesia with isobaric bupivacaine in infants. *Anesthesiology.* 1988;68:601-603
44. Welborn LG, Rice LJ, Hannallah RS, Broadman LM, Ruttiman VE, Fink R. Postoperative apnea in former preterm infants: prospective comparison of spinal and general anesthesia. *Anesthesiology.* 1990;72:838-842
45. Webster AC, McKishnie JD, Kenyon CF, Marshall DG. Spinal anaesthesia for inguinal hernia repair in high-risk neonates. *Can J Anaesth.* 1991;38:281-286
46. Sartorelli KH, Abajian JC, Mreutz JM, Vane DW. Improved outcome utilizing spinal anesthesia in high-risk infants. *J Pediatr Surg.* 1992;27:1022-1025
47. Krane EJ, Haberkern CM, Jacobson LE. Postoperative apnea, bradycardia, and oxygen desaturation in formerly premature infants: prospective comparison of spinal and general anesthesia. *Anesth Analg.* 1995;80:7-13

48. Tobias JD. Spinal anaesthesia in infants and children. *Paediatr Anaesth.* 2000;10:5-16
49. Vane DW, Abajian JC, Hong AR. Spinal anesthesia for primary repair of gastroschisis: a new and safe technique for selected patients. *J Pediatr Surg.* 1994;29:1234-1235
50. Viscomi CM, Abajian JC, Wald SL, et al. Spinal anesthesia for repair of myelomeningocele in infants. *Anesth Analg.* 1995;81:492-495
51. Williams RK, Abajian JC. High spinal anaesthesia for repair of patent ductus arteriosus in neonates. *Paediatr Anaesth.* 1997;7:205-209
52. Finkel JC, Boltz MG, Conran AM, et al. Hemodynamic changes during spinal anesthesia in children undergoing open heart surgery. *Paediatr Anaesth.* 2003;96:48-52
53. Tobias JD, Burd RS, Helikson MA. Apnea following spinal anaesthesia in two former preterm infants. *Can J Anaesth.* 1998;45:985-989
54. Hirabayashi Y, Shimizu R, Saitoh K, et al. Spread of subarachnoid hyperbaric amethocaine in adolescents. *Br J Anaesth.* 1995;74:41-45
55. Rice LJ, DeMars PD, Whalen TV, Crooms JC, Parkinson SK. Duration of spinal anesthesia in infants less than one year of age. *Reg Anesth.* 1994;19:325-329
56. Abajian JC, Mellish RWP, Browne AF, Perkins FM, Lambert DH, Mazuzan JE Jr. Spinal anesthesia for surgery in the high-risk infant. *Anesth Analg.* 1984;63:359-362
57. Fosel T, Wilhelm W, Gruness V, Molter G. Spinal anesthesia in infancy using 0.5% bupivacaine: the effect of an adrenaline addition on duration and hemodynamics. *Anesthetist.* 1994;43:26-29
58. Payne KA, Moore SW. Subarachnoid microcatheter anesthesia in small children. *Reg Anesth.* 1994;19:237-242
59. Kost-Byerly S, Tobin SR, Greenberg RS, Billett C, Zahurak M, Yaster M. Bacterial colonization and infection rate of continuous epidural catheters in children. *Anesth Analg.* 1998;86:712-716
60. Aram L, Krane EJ, Kozloski LJ, Yaster M. Tunneled epidural catheters for prolonged analgesia in pediatric patients. *Anesth Analg.* 2001;92:1432-1438
61. Easley RB, George R, Connors D, Tobias JD. Aseptic meningitis after spinal anesthesia in an infant. *Anesthesiology.* 1999;91:305-307
62. Tobias JD. Postdural puncture headache in children: etiology and treatment. *Clin Pediatr.* 1993;33:110-113
63. Kokki H, Hendolin H. Comparison of spinal anaesthesia with epidural anaesthesia in paediatric surgery. *Acta Anaesthesiol Scand.* 1995;39:896-900

64. Kokki H, Hendolin H, Turnen M. Postdural puncture headache and transient neurologic symptoms in children after spinal anaesthesia using cutting and pencil point paediatric needles. *Acta Anaesthesiol Scand.* 1998;42:1076-1082
65. Wee LH, Lam F, Cranston AJ. The incidence of post dural puncture headache in children. *Anaesthesia.* 1996;51:1164-1166
66. Kasai T, Yaegashi K, Hirose M, Tanaka Y. Spinal cord injury in a child caused by accidental dural puncture with a single shot thoracic epidural needle. *Anesth Analg.* 2002;96:65-67

Chapter 4

Peripheral Regional Blockade

Allison Kinder Ross, MD
Santhanam Suresh, MD, FAAP

General Techniques
Upper Extremity Blockade
- Anatomy of the Brachial Plexus
- Axillary Approach to the Brachial Plexus
- Parascalene Approach to the Brachial Plexus
- Nerve Block at the Wrist

Lower Extremity Blockade
- Femoral Nerve Block
- Fascia Iliaca Compartment Block
- Lumbar Plexus Block
- Sciatic Nerve Block
  - Posterior Approach to the Sciatic Nerve at the Hip
  - Raj Approach to the Sciatic Nerve
  - Popliteal Fossa Approach to the Sciatic Nerve
- Ankle Block

Digital Block
Continuous Peripheral Nerve Catheters
Blockade of the Thorax and Abdomen
- Interpleural Analgesia
- Intercostal Block
- Paravertebral Block
- Ilioinguinal/Iliohypogastric Nerve Block

Head and Neck Blockade

Introduction

Peripheral nerve blocks are used to provide analgesia specifically to the surgical site.[1] The practice of peripheral nerve blockade continues to improve and increase with the development of age-appropriate equipment and with the addition of safer, long-acting local anesthetic agents. The safety of peripheral nerve blockade in children has been established in large-scale studies and has been recommended in place of central blockade when appropriate.[2,3] Although most peripheral nerve blockade is performed in the perioperative arena by experienced anesthesia providers, there are several blocks, such as femoral nerve, digital, and intercostal that may be useful in emergency department or intensive care settings. This chapter outlines the more commonly used peripheral nerve blocks and describes blocks that are more unique to children.

General Techniques

The success of placing peripheral nerve blocks requires knowledge of the human anatomy, proper equipment, and an understanding of the risks involved with regional blockade in pediatric patients. Given the developmental status of infants and children, these blocks are performed with either sedation or general anesthesia. For most of the blocks presented in this chapter, an insulated needle and peripheral nerve stimulator are recommended. For a nerve stimulator to accurately locate a peripheral nerve or plexus, the child must not have received neuromuscular blocking agents that would inhibit the intensity of muscle contractions. The first step in placing a peripheral nerve block is to determine that the nerve stimulator is functioning properly. The device should be set initially at 1.0 to 1.2 mA and 2 Hz. The negative electrode is attached to the needle and the positive electrode is attached to the patient using a standard electrocardiogram pad. The needle should be placed on the skin to demonstrate that there is a complete circuit as indicated when the flashing light on the nerve stimulator box changes to a continuous light. The needle is then advanced until appropriate muscle contractions are elicited as a result of placing the needle near the appropriate nerve. The voltage is decreased and the location of the needle adjusted until there is persistent muscle stimulation at less than 0.5 mA. A local anesthetic solution is injected and the muscle stimulation will immediately cease. The local anesthetic should not be injected if there is intense muscle contraction near 0.2 mA, which may indicate that the tip of the needle is intraneural. Other signs of intraneural injection in an anesthetized child include immediate tachycardia or resistance to injection.

To determine the success of the block in an anesthetized child, the voltage of the nerve stimulator is increased while the needle is still in place. If the local anesthetic was injected in the correct location, there should be no stimulation. It also is possible to determine success of a peripheral block by checking limb flaccidity and comparing the muscle tone of the blocked limb to that of the opposite limb. Vasodilation and/or temperature changes may be subtle in children, but may be a reliable indicator if present. Response to surgical incision is typically the most reliable determinant of success of a peripheral block.

Dosing of peripheral nerve blocks requires the same considerations as dosing of central blocks due to the increased risks of toxicity from local anesthetic agents in children. Infants in particular are at risk from toxicity due to their lower levels of plasma proteins such as albumin and α_1-acid glycoprotein that are necessary for protein binding of the commonly used amide local anesthetics.[4]

To reduce the risks of toxicity, several recommendations should be followed. Of primary importance is following maximal allowable dosing guidelines for single injection and continuous blockade.[5] These guidelines are summarized in Table 4-1. For bolus dosing, lower concentrations of local anesthetics (0.2%-0.25%) should be used in neonates, infants, and preschool children. Once a child is 5 to 8 years old, higher concentrations (0.5%) may be used with caution. Regardless of the concentration used, it is imperative to use less than the maximum recommended dose as outlined in Table 4-1. The toxicities of 2 local anesthetics are additive and, when combinations of local anesthetics are used, reduced doses of each should be used to stay well below toxic levels.[2,5]

Adding epinephrine in a 1:200,000 concentration (5 µg/mL) to the local anesthetic mixture may increase its safety. First, the addition of epinephrine may alert the practitioner to inadvertent intravascular injection of the solution.[6,7] During sevoflurane anesthesia, following the injection of epinephrine (0.5 µg/kg or 0.1 mL/kg of the local anesthetic solution containing 1:200,000 epinephrine), a heart rate increase of 10 or more beats per minute or ST-T wave changes are indicative of intravascular injection and the need to stop the injection.[6-8] A T-wave amplitude change of 25% or greater from baseline is as reliable as heart rate changes in identifying a positive intravascular injection.[9] In addition, when epinephrine is added to the local anesthetic for peripheral nerve block, it may not only significantly decrease the peak plasma concentration of local anesthetic, but it also may delay the absorption time.[10]

Table 4-1. Suggested Dosing Guidelines for Local Anesthetic Agents

Local Anesthetic	Single Dose	Continuous Infusion Rate (Infants >6 mos)	Continuous Infusion Rate (Infants <6 mos)
Bupivacaine	3 mg/kg	0.3-0.4 mg/kg/h	0.2-0.25 mg/kg/h*
Levobupivacaine	3 mg/kg†	0.3-0.4 mg/kg/h	0.2-0.25 mg/kg/h*
Ropivacaine	3 mg/kg†	0.3-0.4 mg/kg/h	0.2-0.25 mg/kg/h*
Lidocaine	5 mg/kg	1.6 mg/kg/h	0.8 mg/kg/h
Lidocaine with epinephrine‡	7 mg/kg	N/A	N/A

*Rate should be reduced by additional 30% after 48 hours in infants.
†Maximal allowable dose may be up to 4 mg/kg (under investigation).
‡Epinephrine added to local anesthetic at 5 µg/cc or 1:200,000.
N/A = not applicable.

Upper Extremity Blockade

Anatomy of the Brachial Plexus

The brachial plexus is formed from the anterior branches of spinal roots C5 through T1 and provides motor and sensory innervation for most of the upper extremity. The shoulder also receives sensory innervation from the descending branches of the cervical plexus and the posterolateral aspect of the upper arm has input from the intercostobrachial nerve, a branch of the second intercostal nerve. In the neck, the brachial plexus is enclosed in a fascial sheath that runs between the anterior and middle scalene muscles. The branches of the spinal roots form 3 trunks (superior, middle, and inferior) that exit the interscalene groove and run posterior to the subclavian artery. As they exit the interscalene groove, these trunks split into anterior and posterior divisions, then unite to form 3 cords (lateral, posterior, and medial) named according to their position in relation to the axillary artery. These cords then give rise to the various nerves of the brachial plexus.

There are several approaches to placing a block along the brachial plexus from the neck to the axilla.[11] These include the interscalene and parascalene techniques in the neck, supraclavicular and infraclavicular approaches at the level of the clavicle, and the axillary approach. The choice is determined by the location of surgery as well as the experience and expertise of the health care provider performing the block. In adult practice, interscalene blockade is used frequently because it provides anesthesia of the shoulder and arm as well as blockade of the musculocutaneous nerve, which may be missed with the axillary approach (see following text). Disadvantages include the risk of pneumothorax (which may limit its use in pediatric practice); associated blockade of the phrenic nerve with ipsilateral paralysis of the hemidiaphragm, and limited anesthesia of the ulnar nerve (lateral aspect of the forearm). The ulnar nerve is a branch of the inferior trunk, which lies deepest from the skin in the interscalene groove and, hence, may be exposed to a lesser volume of local anesthetic agent. Therefore, in pediatric practice, parascalene and axillary approaches are most common.

Axillary Approach to the Brachial Plexus

The axillary block is the most commonly performed brachial plexus block. It is used for procedures on the arm and hand, such as open reduction with internal fixation of a forearm fracture, syndactyly repair, and finger reimplantation. The primary advantages of performing axillary blockade are its ease of placement and the low risk of complications. However, there is a 40% to 50% chance of missing the musculocutaneous nerve because of the proximal branching of the nerve, thereby placing it outside of the sheath at the axillary level. To ensure effective analgesia during procedures that involve the lateral forearm, the musculocutaneous nerve can be blocked separately.

Although there have been several techniques reported for performing an axillary block, a single injection technique seems to be as effective as a multiple injection technique, with a decreased risk of distortion of anatomy from the first injection or inadvertent arterial puncture.[12] To perform a single injection axillary block, the patient is positioned with the arm abducted to 90° with the elbow flexed and hand above the head (Figure 4-1). The needle is inserted immediately adjacent and superior to the axillary artery high in the axilla at a 30° to 45° angle to the skin, pointing toward the midpoint of the clavicle. A "pop" or loss of resistance may be felt as the needle pierces the brachial plexus sheath and enters the neurovascular bundle. Using a nerve stimulator as outlined previously, once there is evidence of muscle stimulation in the hand, the local anesthetic agent (0.2-0.5 mL/kg) is injected. A longitudinal swelling may be evident beneath the skin as the local anesthetic solution fills the sheath. This should disappear quickly as the solution spreads proximally and should not be confused with subcutaneous swelling. Distal pressure should be held during and immediately following injection and the arm should be adducted to release the pressure of the head of the humerus from the fossa to facilitate proximal spread of solution, thereby facilitating anesthesia of the musculocutaneous nerve.

To directly block the musculocutaneous nerve, the needle is redirected into the belly of the coracobrachialis muscle and a biceps contraction is elicited. Local anesthetic solution (0.1-0.2 mL/kg) is then injected. In addition, if a surgical tourniquet is to be used and the child will require analgesia of the upper arm to prevent tourniquet pain, the intercostobrachial nerve may be blocked by placing a subcutaneous ring of local anesthetic high around the medial aspect of the arm.

Disadvantages of the axillary approach include the potential for ineffective analgesia of the radial and musculocutaneous nerves and the need for arm abduction. Complications of axillary block are rare, but include hematoma from vascular puncture. If the artery is inadvertently punctured, pressure should be held for at least 5 minutes to avoid possible vascular insufficiency from hematoma formation.[13] Although not frequently chosen as an approach, a technique for axil-

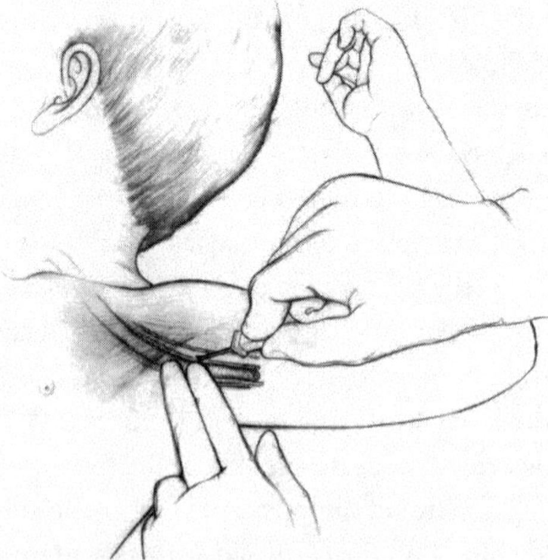

Figure 4-1
Technique for the axillary approach to the brachial plexus. The index finger is placed on the axillary artery and the needle inserted above the pulsation. Note that the musculocutaneous nerve is outside of the sheath at this level while the 3 cords of brachial plexus (lateral, medial, and posterior) surround the axillary artery. In this diagram, the needle is directed above the pulsation of the artery, directed toward the lateral cord.

lary blockade has been described whereby the axillary artery is intentionally punctured and half of the local anesthetic solution deposited posterior to the artery and half placed anterior to it. The advantage of this "transarterial" approach is more effective analgesia of the posterior cord (which gives rise to the radial nerve) because it lies directly behind the axillary artery.

Parascalene Approach to the Brachial Plexus

The parascalene approach to the brachial plexus is similar to the interscalene block without the risks of puncture of the vertebral artery or pneumothorax. This block will cover the arm and shoulder in its entirety with a reported success rate of 97% on the first or second attempt.[14] The child is positioned supine with a roll under the shoulders, head turned to the opposite side, and the arm adducted next to the trunk (Figure 4-2). A line is drawn between the transverse process of C6 and the midpoint of the clavicle. The stimulating needle is inserted perpendicular to the skin, at the junction of the upper two thirds and lower one third of this line. This point generally is near the external jugular vein. The needle is inserted somewhat posteriorly to avoid central structures. Once appropriate stimulation of the hand

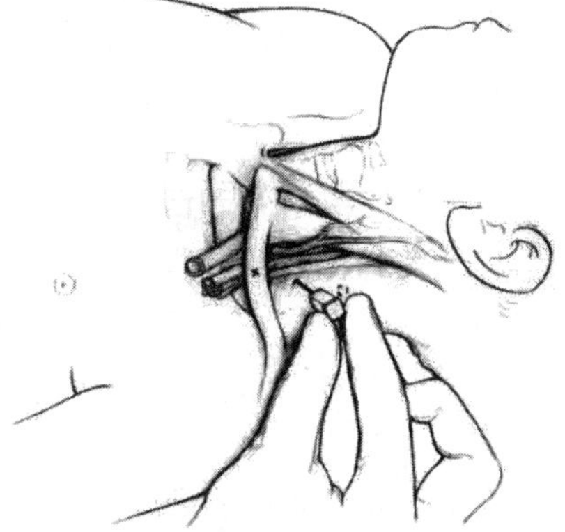

Figure 4-2

The parascalene approach to the brachial plexus. A line is drawn from the transverse process of C6 (small circle above the index finger) and the midpoint of the clavicle, which is marked with an "x." The needle is inserted at the junction of the upper two thirds and lower one third of this line.

or arm has been determined at low voltage, local anesthetic (0.2-0.4 mL/kg) may be injected. Complications of a parascalene block are rare, but may include venous puncture, Horner syndrome, or hemi-diaphragmatic paralysis from associated phrenic nerve blockade, as may occur with the interscalene approach. Advantages of this technique, compared with the axillary approach, include anesthesia of the shoulder, more effective anesthesia of the musculocutaneous nerve, and higher incidence of radial nerve (posterior cord) anesthesia. Additionally, it is not necessary to abduct the arm as with the axillary approach.

Nerve Block at the Wrist

Blocks of the median, ulnar, and radial nerves at the wrist may provide analgesia for distal extremity procedures. Similar to other distal blocks, no vasoconstrictors should be added to the local anesthetic solution. To block the median nerve, its course is identified on the volar aspect of the wrist between the palmaris longus and flexor carpi radialis tendons (Figure 4-3). A 25-gauge needle is inserted between the 2 tendons at a distance of 1 to 2 cm proximal to the first wrist crease. Local anes-

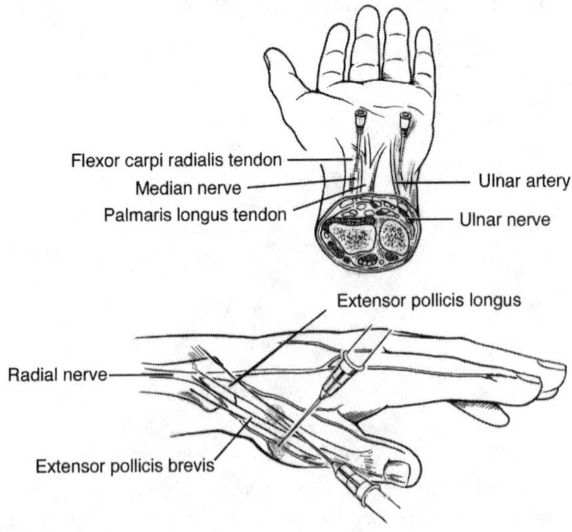

Figure 4-3
Anatomy for blockade of the ulnar, median, and radial nerves at the wrist.

thetic (0.5-3 mL or 0.5 mL/year of age) is injected after negative aspiration. The ulnar nerve is blocked on the volar aspect of the wrist by inserting a 25-gauge needle medial to the ulnar artery at the most proximal crease of the wrist (Figure 4-3). Local anesthetic solution (0.5-3 mL or 0.5 mL/year of age) is injected after negative aspiration. The radial nerve is blocked from the lateral aspect of the wrist with a subcutaneous injection near the base of the thumb extending along the extensor pollicis longus tendon and a second injection that runs perpendicular to the extensor pollicis brevis (Figure 4-3). Approximately 0.5 to 3 mL or 0.5 mL/year of age of local anesthetic solution should be delivered at each injection site.

Lower Extremity Blockade

The lumbar plexus and sacral plexus supply the lower extremity. Deciding which plexus to block depends on the location of desired analgesia.[15] The lumbar plexus is located in the psoas compartment and consists of lumbar nerves L1 to L4 and a small portion of T12. The femoral nerve, lateral femoral cutaneous nerve, and obturator nerve are branches of the lumbar plexus and supply most of the upper leg (Figure 4-4). The saphenous nerve, a small branch of the femoral

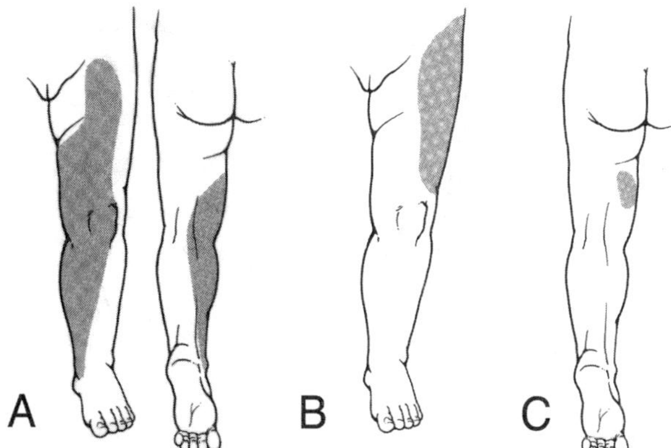

Figure 4-4
Cutaneous sensory distribution of the femoral nerve (A), lateral femoral cutaneous nerve (B), and obturator nerve (C).

nerve, provides some innervation below the knee to the medial aspect of the lower leg near the saphenous vein. The lower leg is otherwise supplied by the sacral plexus that is derived from the anterior rami of L4, L5, and S1 to S3. This plexus gives rise to the sciatic nerve, which innervates most of the lower leg via its 2 major branches: the common peroneal and posterior tibial nerves. The posterior cutaneous nerve of the thigh, as the name implies, supplies the posterior thigh and hamstring muscles.

Femoral Nerve Block

A femoral nerve block is appropriate for any procedure of the lower extremity above the knee, including the provision of analgesia following femur fracture.[15,16] A femoral nerve block may be performed with or without a nerve stimulator. A nerve stimulator should not be used, or should be set to very low amplitude, in a child with femur fracture so that pain does not occur from quadriceps muscle contraction.

The femoral nerve is blocked at its location immediately lateral to the femoral artery (Figure 4-5). With the child supine and the

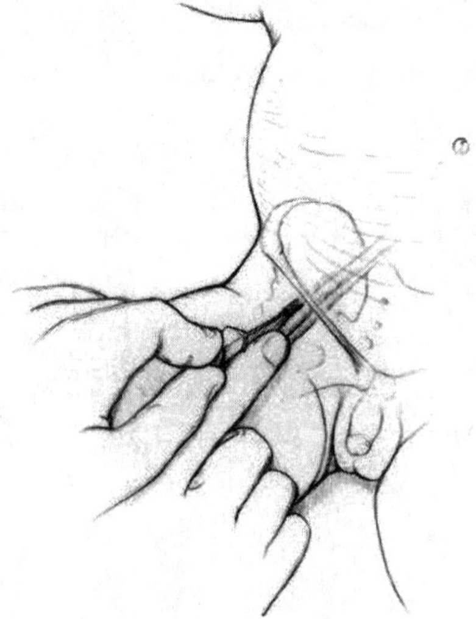

Figure 4-5
Technique for femoral nerve blockade. The tip of the index figure is placed on the femoral artery. The needle is inserted just lateral to the pulsation of the femoral artery.

foot rotated outward, the needle is inserted 0.5 to 1 cm below the inguinal ligament and 0.5 to 1 cm lateral to the femoral artery. The needle should be inserted in a slightly cephalad direction. As the needle pierces the fascia lata and fascia iliaca (the 2 fascial layers that cover the femoral nerve), a distinct "pop" should be felt and, if a nerve stimulator is used, the desired response is a "patellar kick" indicative of quadriceps contractions. Because of the close proximity of femoral vessels, continuous aspiration for blood should be performed during femoral blockade and prior to local anesthetic injection. In the event of femoral artery puncture, pressure should be held for at least 5 minutes to avoid hematoma formation.

A "3-in-1" block is essentially a femoral nerve block that attempts to anesthetize the femoral, lateral femoral cutaneous, and obturator nerves with a single injection by promoting proximal spread of the local anesthetic in the femoral sheath by holding pressure distal to the injection site and by increasing the volume of the local anesthetic solution. The 3-in-1 block has been shown to anesthetize the femoral nerve 100% of the time, but is only 20% effective in blocking all 3 nerves.[17] To block all 3 nerves more reliably, either a fascia iliaca or a lumbar plexus block should be used (see following text).

Fascia Iliaca Compartment Block

A fascia iliaca compartment block is 90% effective in blocking the femoral, lateral femoral cutaneous, and obturator nerves in children.[17] It is useful for any surgery that is performed on the lower extremity above the knee and may be successfully employed for postoperative analgesia or instead of general anesthesia in muscle biopsies of the thigh for malignant hyperthermia or other diagnostic testing. This block also may anesthetize the genitofemoral nerve that provides sensory innervation to Scarpa's triangle.

A fascia iliaca block delivers local anesthetic deep to the fascia iliaca and superficial to the iliacus muscle where the 3 distal nerves of the lumbar plexus emerge from the psoas muscle. With the child in the supine position, the inguinal ligament should be identified and a line drawn from the pubic tubercle to the anterior superior iliac spine. At the junction of the lateral one third and medial two thirds of this line, the needle is inserted 0.5 to 2 cm inferiorly at a perpendicular angle to the skin (Figure 4-6). A blunt needle should be used, but there is no need for a nerve stimulator because the needle is placed lateral to the femoral nerve. The goal is to bathe the nerves by injecting local anesthetic behind the fascia iliacus rather than to locate a specific nerve. Two pops will be felt as the needle pierces the fascia lata and then the fascia iliaca. A slight loss of resistance should be evident if light pressure is held on the plunger of the syringe. After negative aspiration, local anesthetic (0.5-1 mL/kg) may then be injected. Because the 3 nerves must be blocked with 1 injection, higher volumes of local anesthetic solution are required.

There are no known significant complications with performing a fascia iliaca compartment block if the needle remains inferior to the inguinal ligament and appropriately lateral to the femoral vessels. If the needle is too medial, isolated femoral nerve block or inadvertent femoral artery puncture may occur.

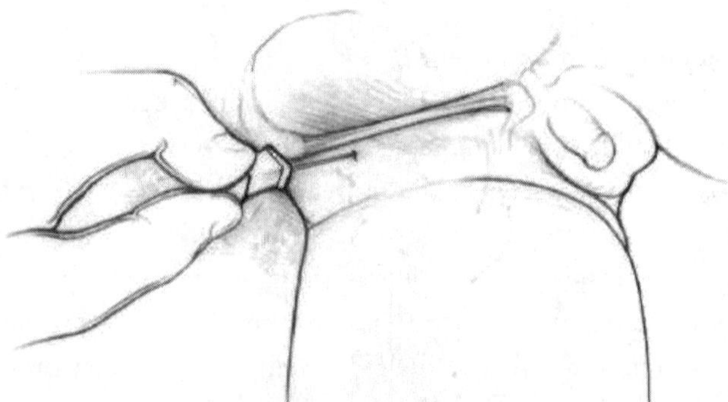

Figure 4-6
For a fascia iliaca block, the needle is inserted perpendicular to the skin, just below the inguinal ligament at a point of the junction of the middle two thirds and lateral one third of a line drawn from the anterior superior iliac spine and the pubic tubercle.

Lumbar Plexus Block

A lumbar plexus block will provide analgesia to the nerves of the lumbar plexus, including the femoral, lateral femoral cutaneous, and obturator nerves. This block also is effective for other procedures because it anesthetizes the distal branches of the lumbar plexus including the iliohypogastric, ilioinguinal, and genitofemoral nerves that innervate the groin area. The lumbar plexus lies in the psoas compartment between the 2 masses of the psoas muscle and is surrounded by fascia that is derived from the fascia iliaca. The approach that should be used in children is a modification of Winnie's approach and has been shown to be superior to other more medial approaches.[18] With the child in a lateral position, the 2 iliac crests are identified and a line drawn between them. Another line is drawn from the posterior superior iliac spine cephalad and parallel to the spinous processes on the side that is to be blocked (Figure 4-7). A nerve stimulator and an insulated needle are used for this block. The needle is inserted at the junction of these 2 lines, per-

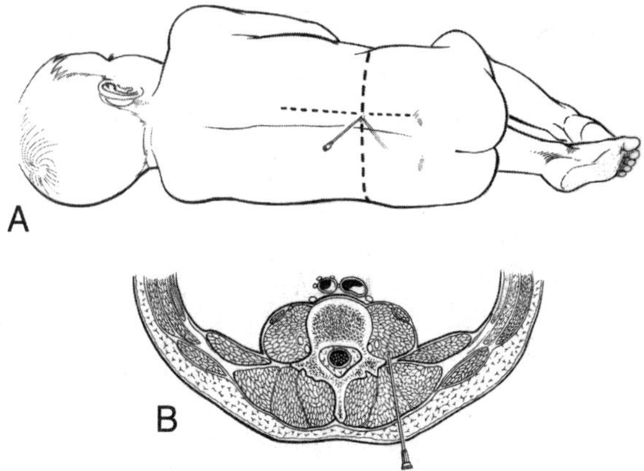

Figure 4-7
Technique of lumbar plexus blockade (A) and demonstration of internal needle location (B) for effective blockade. The lumbar plexus is deep to the quadratus lumborum muscle and within the body of the psoas muscle.

pendicular to the skin. Alternatively, the needle can be inserted at a point 1 to 2 cm more medial along the line connecting the 2 iliac crests. If this is done, the needle may contact the transverse process of the lamina of the vertebral column. When this occurs, the needle is walked off the lamina superiorly until a loss of resistance is felt and the patellar kick elicited. As it is inserted, the needle will traverse the quadratus lumborum muscle before reaching the lumbar plexus in the psoas muscle. When the lumbar plexus is identified, a strong "patellar kick" should be apparent. If hamstring contractions are observed, the needle should be directed more laterally and, if hamstring and quadriceps

Table 4-2. Suggested Dosing Guidelines for Peripheral Nerve Blocks

Regional Technique	Bolus Dose*†	Continuous Infusion
Axillary	0.2-0.5 mL/kg	0.1-0.2 mL/kg/h
Parascalene	0.2-0.4 mL/kg	0.1-0.2 mL/kg/h
Femoral or LFC	0.3-1mL/kg	0.15-0.3 mL/kg/h
Fascia iliaca	0.5-1 mL/kg	0.15-0.3 mL/kg/h
Lumbar plexus	0.5-1 mL/kg	0.15-0.3 mL/kg/h
Sciatic	0.3-1 mL/kg	0.15-0.3 mL/kg/h
ILIH	0.25-0.5 mL/kg	N/A
Penile block	0.1 mL/kg	N/A
Intercostal	0.1-0.15 mL/kg/level	N/A
Paravertebral	0.5 mL/kg	0.2-0.25 mL/kg/h

*Bupivacaine, levobupivacaine, or ropivacaine may be used. For bolus dosing, lower concentrations (0.2%-0.25%) are recommended in infants and young children, whereas concentrations of 0.375% to 0.5% can be used in children older than 5 to 8 years. For continuous infusions, lower concentrations such as 0.1% to 0.2% of all agents are acceptable with care taken to avoid exceeding 0.3 to 0.4 mg/kg/h in older children and 0.2 mg/kg/h in infants younger than 6 months.

†Epinephrine 1:200,000 should be added to single-shot peripheral nerve blocks except for penile block.

N/A=not applicable.

contractions are observed simultaneously, the needle should be directed more cephalad to isolate the lumbar plexus rather than sacral plexus. Volumes of up to 1 mL/kg may be required to adequately block the plexus in this approach (Table 4-2).

Complications with the lumbar plexus block are rare, but may be serious if the needle is advanced too deeply into the retroperitoneum. Retroperitoneal hematoma is a significant risk, and there should be constant aspiration for blood during performance of this block. A review of the depth to the lumbar plexus is essential because it can vary depending on the patient's age.[18,19]

Sciatic Nerve Block

Blockade of the sciatic nerve provides anesthesia of the posterior aspect of the thigh and the entire leg below the knee, except for a small portion along the medial aspect of the lower half of the leg over the medial malleolus and onto the medial aspect of the foot. This area is innervated by the saphenous nerve, a branch of the femoral nerve. The sciatic block can be combined with a femoral nerve block using one of the techniques outlined previously or more distal along the course of the femoral nerve (at the knee or ankle), depending on which area needs to be anesthetized. Such blockade is effective for procedures that involve the posterior thigh or the lower extremity below the knee. Several approaches to the sciatic nerve have been described and compared in children.[20]

Posterior Approach to the Sciatic Nerve at the Hip

A modified posterior approach to the sciatic nerve provides a good combination of ease of use and low risk of complications. With the child in the lateral position, the side to be blocked should be uppermost with the leg flexed at the hip and knee. A line is drawn from the tip of the coccyx to the greater trochanter of the femur. The needle is inserted at the midpoint of this line and directed toward the lateral ischial tuberosity (Figure 4-8). When using a nerve stimulator, the desired motor response should be seen in the foot with evidence of either plantar flexion (tibial nerve) or dorsiflexion (peroneal nerve). Once a response is elicited, local anesthetic in a dose of 0.3 to 0.7 mL/kg is injected after negative aspiration. Complications of the posterior approach are rare, but may include vascular puncture of the gluteal vessels. Continuous aspiration for blood should occur during performance of the block and local anesthetic injection.

Raj Approach to the Sciatic Nerve

The Raj approach blocks the sciatic nerve as it travels between the greater trochanter of the femur and the ischial tuberosity.[21] The advantage of this block is the simplicity of the landmarks and the ability to bring the sciatic nerve close to the skin with exaggerated hip flexion in obese children and adolescents. With the child in the supine position, the leg to be blocked should be flexed at the hip and knee. The

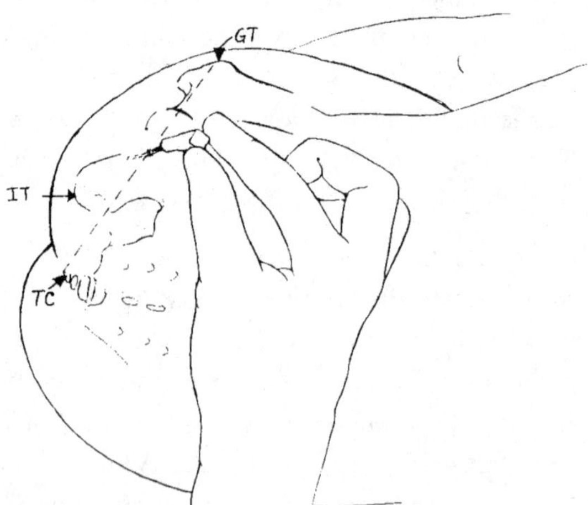

Figure 4-8
Technique for posterior approach to the sciatic nerve. The needle is inserted at the midpoint of the line connecting the greater trochanter of the femur and the tip of the coccyx. TC = tip of the coccyx, GT = greater trochanter, IT = ischial tuberosity.

needle is inserted at the midpoint between the ischial tuberosity and greater trochanter of the femur in the sciatic groove (Figure 4-9). Using a nerve stimulator, once appropriate muscle stimulation is seen in the foot, local anesthetic (0.3-0.7 mL/kg) is injected.

Popliteal Fossa Approach to the Sciatic Nerve

The sciatic nerve may be blocked as it courses through the popliteal fossa behind the knee for procedures of the distal lower extremity.[22,23] In the popliteal fossa, the sciatic nerve divides into the common peroneal nerve that runs anteriorly and wraps around the head of the fibula and the posterior tibial nerve that travels down the posterior aspect of the lower leg. Although in most patients the sciatic nerve branches near the popliteal fossa, 10% of patients will have branching of the sciatic nerve proximally. Despite this, even with a single injection, the success rate of popliteal fossa block in anesthetizing both branches is high, presumably because of a common epineural sheath that envelops the common peroneal and tibial nerves.[24] The landmarks of the superior triangle of the popliteal fossa are the semimembranosus and semitendinosus tendons medially, the biceps femoris tendon laterally, and the popliteal crease inferiorly. The distance above the popliteal crease

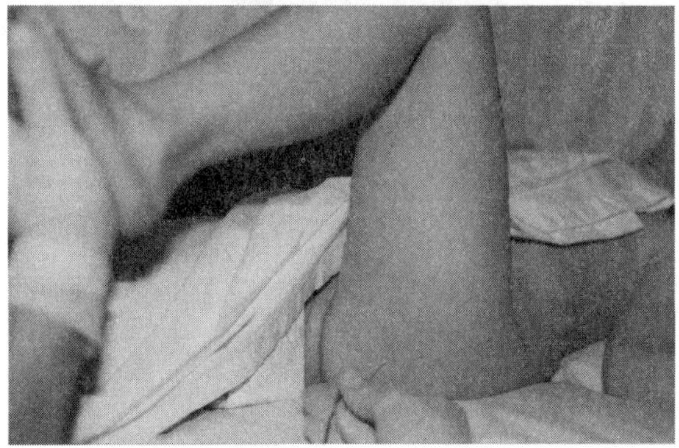

Figure 4-9
Raj approach to the sciatic nerve. The point of needle insertion is midway between the greater trochanter and ischial tuberosity.

to the point of needle insertion for popliteal fossa block may be estimated based on weight. The needle is moved cephalad in the midline of the triangle above the popliteal crease by 1 cm for each 10 kg of body weight.[25] Alternatively, this distance can be approximated by assuming it to be equal to the length of the popliteal crease between semimembranosus/semitendinosus and biceps femoris tendons. The needle is inserted at a 45° angle to the skin in a cephalad direction just lateral to the midline of the popliteal triangle (Figure 4-10). Once appropriate muscle contraction is seen in the foot at 0.5 mA, the local anesthetic solution is injected. Volumes of 0.75 to 1 mL/kg may be required to promote cephalad spread of the local anesthetic (Table 4-2). Complications during popliteal fossa block are rare, but may include vascular puncture due to the close proximity of the popliteal vessels to the site of injection.

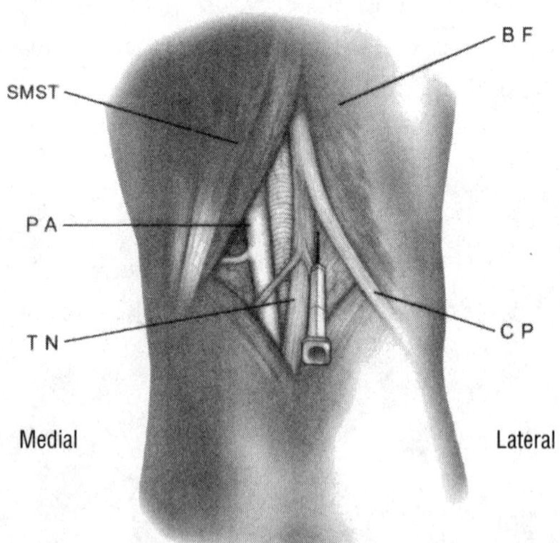

Figure 4-10
Popliteal fossa approach to the sciatic nerve at the knee. The suggested site of injection is illustrated by the needle and syringe. SMST = semimembranosus/semitendinosus, PA = popliteal artery, TN = tibial nerve, BF = biceps femoris, CP = common peroneal nerve.

Ankle Block

An ankle block may be used for procedures that are confined to the foot, such as toe amputation, foreign body removal, or simple distal reconstructive surgery. To successfully anesthetize the foot using an ankle block, 5 nerves must be anesthetized (Figure 4-11). Approximately 0.1 to 0.2 mL/kg up to a maximum of 5 mL of local anesthetic solution should be injected at each nerve. Because of the potential of local anesthetic solution to travel distally and cause vasoconstriction, epinephrine should **not** be added to the solution. The saphenous nerve, a branch of the femoral nerve, innervates the medial aspect of the ankle and foot. It is located on the medial side of the dorsum of the foot anterior to the medial malleolus. It may be blocked by injecting local anesthetic solution subcutaneously near the saphenous vein and over the medial malleolus. The 4 other nerves that must be blocked for total analgesia of the foot are branches of the sciatic nerve. The deep peroneal nerve innervates the first web space of the foot and is blocked by

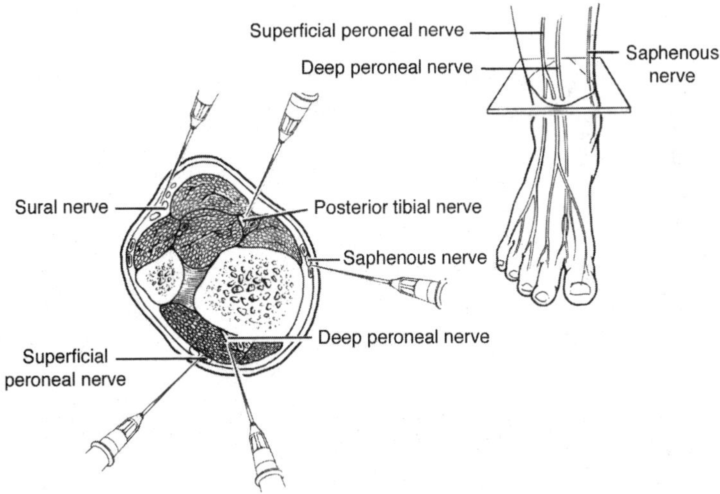

Figure 4-11
Technique for ankle blockade includes separately anesthetizing the 5 individual nerves that provide sensory innervation to the foot, including the saphenous, deep peroneal (anterior tibial), posterior tibial, superficial peroneal, and the sural nerves.

inserting the needle lateral to the extensor hallucis longus tendon near the tibial artery and advancing the needle until it contacts the tibia. The needle is then withdrawn slightly, and the local anesthetic solution is injected. The superficial peroneal nerve that supplies the dorsum of the foot is blocked by subcutaneous infiltration across the dorsum of the foot between the lateral malleolus and extensor hallucis longus tendon. The 2 remaining nerves to be blocked require that the patient's foot be positioned so that the posterior aspect of the ankle may be easily accessed. The tibial nerve innervates the plantar surface of the foot and is blocked midway between the medial malleolus and the calcaneus, with an injection posterior to the tibial artery. On the opposite side of the Achilles tendon (lateral aspect of the foot/ankle), the sural nerve may be blocked between the lateral malleolus and the calcaneus. The sural nerve supplies sensory innervation to the lateral aspect of the foot. Complications secondary to ankle block are rare; however, because of the proximity of the vessels to the nerves, frequent aspiration for blood should be performed during the blocks. As previously mentioned, the use of epinephrine is contraindicated in ankle blocks, particularly in infants and young children, because of the risk of decreased perfusion to the distal extremity and possible ischemia.

Digital Block

Digital blocks are simple to perform and provide effective analgesia for minor procedures of the digits (fingers or toes), such as ingrown toenail or foreign body removal. Because of the ability of a local anesthetic solution to improve circulation, digital blocks also have been used clinically to improve pulse oximetry readings in patients with poor perfusion. To perform a digital block, each of the 4 nerves of the digit must be anesthetized (Figure 4-12). After sterile preparation, a 25-gauge needle is inserted first on the lateral surface at the base of the finger or toe. Local anesthetic is injected anterior to the bone and posterior to the bone in a fan-like manner to reach the 2 nerves on the lateral side of the digit. This procedure is repeated on the medial side of the digit. Because a finger or toe has end-arterial vascular supply, vasoconstrictors such as epinephrine should not be added to the local anesthetic solution. Bupivacaine 0.25%, levobupivacaine 0.25%, ropivacaine 0.2%, or lidocaine 1% may be used for digital block. No significant complications occur from digital block when vasoconstrictors have not been added to the local anesthetic solution.

Continuous Peripheral Nerve Catheters

Continuous peripheral nerve catheters may be placed in children who undergo procedures or have associated conditions that will result in significant and prolonged postoperative pain or poor peripheral perfusion. A modification of the Seldinger technique can be used with placement of a wire through a needle followed by needle removal and placement of a catheter over the wire such as a 3F or 4F central line

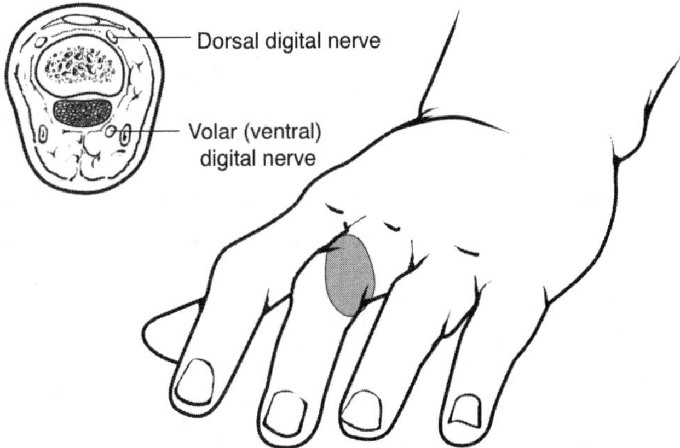

Figure 4-12
Technique for digital nerve block of either finger or toe. Each finger or toe has 4 nerves (2 along the ventral and 2 along the dorsal aspect of the digit).

catheter. For this purpose, a standard insulated needle with a nerve stimulator can be used, provided the wire will fit through the needle. Epidural catheters may also be used. Ideally, a commercially available kit should be used because it allows the use of a nerve stimulator to identify the nerve sheath prior to placement of the catheter. For pediatric patients, several manufacturers now provide insulated Tuohy needles with an appropriate-sized catheter.

Although continuous peripheral nerve catheters are not commonly used in children, there have been some reports of their use for postoperative pain management or therapeutic care. Continuous brachial plexus anesthesia has been effective in managing a child with epidermolysis bullosa simplex who required placement of an external fixator with adjustments.[26] The catheter was managed for 2 days with bolus injections of 0.125% bupivacaine (0.5 mL/kg) every 8 hours with success. Continuous catheters are used more often for lower extremity indications, particularly in the care of femur fracture.[27,28] Catheters also may be placed in the lumbar plexus or fascia iliaca compartments for total analgesia of the thigh.[29,30] Dosing recommendations include 0.1 to 0.2 mL/kg/h of either bupivacaine or levobupivacaine (0.125%-0.25%) or ropivacaine (0.15-0.2%) following the initial bolus dose (Table 4-1). The lower rates generally are used for upper extremity catheters and the higher rates for lower extremity plexus analgesia. Increases of the infusion rate may be made, as needed, with maximum infusion rates of 0.2 mg/kg/h in infants younger than 6 months and 0.4 mg/kg/h in children older than 6 months (Table 4-2). Disposable infusion pumps, which may be programmed to deliver local anesthetic based on a child's weight, currently are available and may offer a future option for outpatient pediatric pain control.[31]

Blockade of the Thorax and Abdomen

Interpleural Analgesia

Interpleural analgesia provides analgesia for patients after thoracotomy via a catheter in the paravertebral space between the visceral and parietal pleurae (Figures 4-13 and 4-14).[32,33] The technique involves the administration of local anesthetic through the catheter into the paravertebral space between the visceral and parietal pleura. The mechanism of action involves diffusion of the local anesthetic solution through the parietal pleura to provide blockade of multiple intercostal nerves, spinal roots, and the sympathetic chain. Although interpleural analgesia is superior to intravenous opioids after thoracotomy, it is less effective than thoracic epidural analgesia.[33] To place an intrapleural catheter, a standard epidural catheter may be used, preferably one that is radio-opaque so that the position may be verified by x-ray. The most common mode of insertion is under direct vision by a surgeon in the operative field. The catheter is inserted 1 to 2

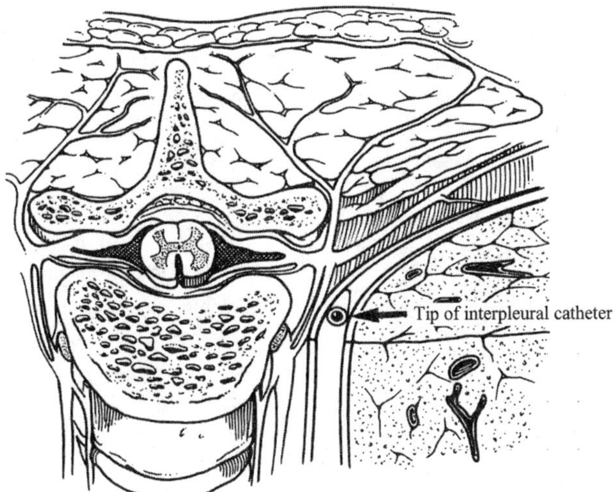

Figure 4-13
Transverse section through the intervertebral body with arrow showing location of an interpleural catheter in the paravertebral space between the visceral and parietal pleurae.

interspaces below the surgical incision and 4 to 8 cm from the posterior midline. The tip should be posterior and approximately 2 to 4 cm above the incision.

Dosing of an intrapleural catheter must take into account that there may be an increased risk of local anesthetic toxicity because of increased uptake when compared with other blocks.[32] An initial bolus dose of 0.2% ropivacaine or 0.25% bupivacaine with epinephrine (5 µg/mL) at a dose of 1 mL/kg to a maximum of 30 mL is recommended. Continuous infusion should be kept well below the maximum allowable dosing guidelines by starting at 0.1 mL/kg/h of either the 0.2% ropivacaine or 0.25% bupivacaine or levobupivacaine. To improve the analgesic efficacy of an interpleural catheter, the chest tube should be inserted anteriorly and clamped for approximately 1 hour after the initial bolus to avoid drainage of the local anesthetic solution from the thoracic cavity. Alterations of patient positioning, which cause the local anesthetic solution to move from the paravertebral space, can significantly affect the efficacy of the block.

Complications from inserting an interpleural catheter are rare when placing a catheter under direct vision. The primary risk of interpleural analgesia is the risk of local anesthetic toxicity from systemic absorption

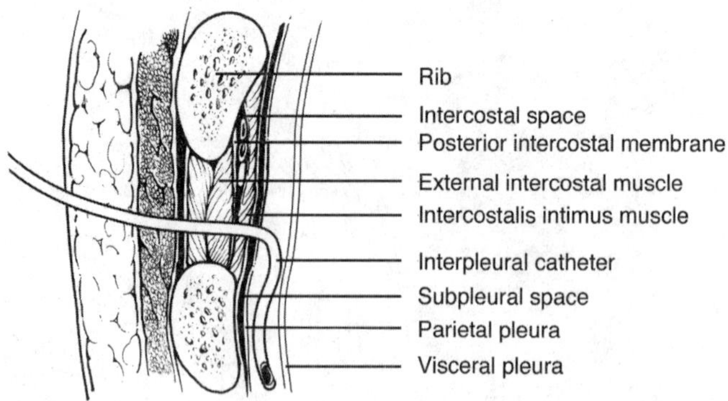

Figure 4-14
Cross section of an intercostal space showing percutaneous placement of an interpleural catheter over the top border of a rib and into the interpleural space with the tip of the catheter lying between the visceral and parietal pleurae.

by the rich pleural vasculature. In one study, 11 of 14 children who received between 1.25 and 2.5 mg/kg/h of bupivacaine via interpleural catheter had plasma bupivacaine levels greater than 2 μg/mL.[32] Because of the higher risk of systemic toxicity, infusion rates of local anesthetic should be well below maximum allowable dosing recommendations (Table 4-1).[5] Given the superiority of thoracic epidural analgesia and the potential risks related to local anesthetic toxicity, interpleural analgesia is used infrequently in current anesthetic practice.

Intercostal Block

Intercostal nerve block may be useful for providing analgesia after thoracotomy and upper abdominal procedures, and to alleviate pain from rib fractures and chest tubes. For these indications, intercostal block may be used perioperatively or in an emergency department or intensive care unit setting. Intercostal blocks are not effective for intraperitoneal procedures because they do not block the celiac plexus. The intercostal nerves arise paravertebrally from the thoracic spinal nerves and may be blocked in their position between the intercostal muscles in a groove that is found underneath the corresponding rib and shared with the intercostal vessels (Figure 4-15). Gray and white rami communicantes branch from the spinal nerves before entering

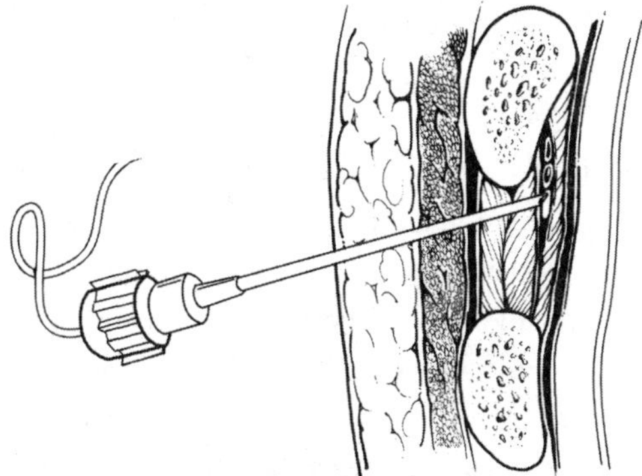

Figure 4-15
Cross section of an intercostal space showing correct needle placement for intercostal blockade. The needle is walked off the inferior border of the rib. Note the proximity of the neurovascular bundle to the needle tip.

the intercostal space and join the sympathetic ganglia to form the thoracic sympathetic chain. A second branch, the posterior cutaneous nerve, travels posteriorly innervating the paraspinous musculature. It may not be anesthetized by intercostal block.

Although an intercostal block may be performed at any location along the lower border of the rib, the most common approach is at the posterior axillary line. This approach will provide adequate analgesia for thoracotomy and is relatively simple to perform. The child should be in the lateral decubitus position with the arm elevated so that the posterior axillary line is easily accessed (Figure 4-16). Alternatively, the patient can be sitting upright (Figure 4-17); however, the lateral decubitus position is generally easier in the anesthetized or sedated patient. Blockade should be performed at the interspace of the surgical incision or injury and 2 interspaces above and below. After sterile preparation, a 22- or 25-gauge needle (length dependent on the age of child) is inserted through the skin, less than 1 cm below the lower border of the rib. The needle is directed cephalad until it contacts the rib. The needle is then withdrawn and advanced to "walk under" the inferior border of the rib until there is a slight loss of resistance as the external and internal oblique muscles are penetrated. After negative aspiration for blood, 0.1-0.15 mL/kg/interspace (maximum of 3 mL) of local anesthetic agent is injected. Bupivacaine 0.25%, levobupivacaine 0.25%, or ropivacaine 0.2% may be used and each can be expected to provide 8 to 12 hours of analgesia.

Complications of intercostal block include pneumothorax, vascular puncture, and epidural or spinal local anesthetic spread. A chest x-ray should be performed to rule out pneumothorax if a chest tube is not placed for surgery. Spread of local anesthetic to the epidural or spinal spaces may occur if the injection travels through a dural sleeve covering the spinal root. This is rare, but may be more common with the posterior approach compared to more anterior approaches. Another complication that must be considered during intercostal nerve blockade is the

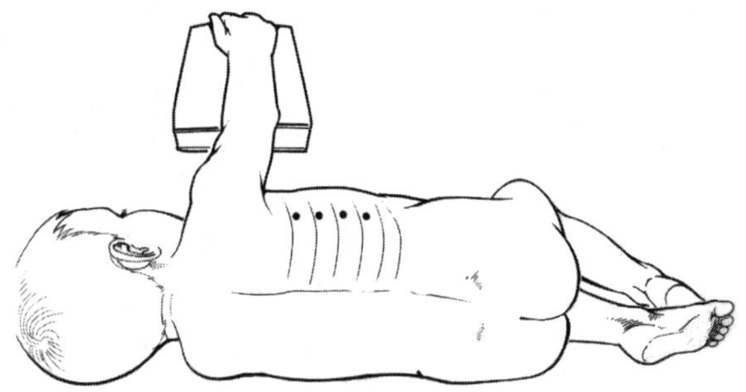

Figure 4-16
Lateral patient positioning for placement of intercostal blocks with needle entry at the posterior axillary line.

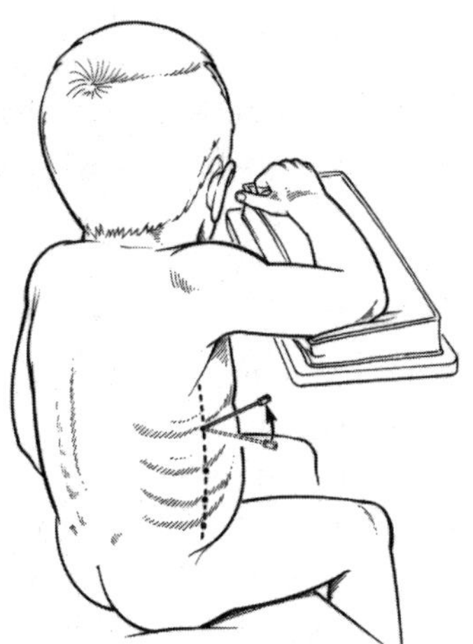

Figure 4-17
Alternatively, the patient may be placed in the sitting position; however, this positioning may be difficult in the heavily sedated or anesthetized patient.

risk of local anesthetic toxicity. Because of the proximity of vessels to the intercostal nerves, there may be increased risk of local anesthetic toxicity from systemic uptake or inadvertent vascular puncture compared with other peripheral nerve blocks. In fact, the peak blood concentration of the local anesthetic agent is second only to interpleural analgesia.

Paravertebral Block

Paravertebral nerve block can provide perioperative analgesia for unilateral procedures, including thoracotomy and upper abdominal surgery. The advantages of paravertebral block include the ability to provide unilateral analgesia without adverse effects that may be associated with central neuraxial techniques and a lower risk of systemic local anesthetic toxicity than interpleural analgesia.[34-36] Continuous paravertebral block has been shown to be superior to epidural anesthesia for unilateral renal surgery and also may be used for analgesia during inguinal surgery in children.[37-39] Although paravertebral blockade has a definite place in pediatric anesthesia, there are limited reports on its use. As with all regional anesthetic techniques, paravertebral blockade should be performed only by those who have experience in pediatric regional anesthesia, possess a thorough knowledge of the anatomy of the paravertebral space, and have used the technique in adults.

The paravertebral space is a wedge-shaped space along the vertebral column that is bound by the parietal pleura, the superior costotransverse ligament, and the intercostal membrane. It contains the intercostal nerve and dorsal ramus, rami communicantes, and sympathetic chain. There is free communication between adjacent levels of the paravertebral space, making it possible to achieve multiple levels of analgesia with the use of a continuous catheter technique or a single injection. The exception to the free communication is at the level of T12, where the insertion of the psoas muscle may inhibit flow to the lumbar areas of the paravertebral space.[40] This anatomical variant mandates a 2-injection technique for inguinal procedures, one above T12 and one below.[38]

To perform a paravertebral block, the patient is placed in the lateral position with the surgical side up. The spinous process of the desired primary dermatome to be blocked is identified. The point of needle insertion is lateral to midline across from this spinous process, at a distance that is equal to the distance from spinous process to spinous process. Alternatively, the approximate lateral distance in millimeters from the spinous process to the point of needle insertion equals (0.12 x body weight in kg) + 10.2.[41] After sterile preparation and draping, a short beveled needle (or Tuohy needle if a catheter is to be threaded) is inserted and advanced using a loss of resistance technique to saline. With the needle perpendicular to the skin, the transverse process of the lamina is contacted and the needle then walked over the cephalad margin of this process (Figure 4-18). The approximate depth from the skin to the paravertebral space in millimeters can be determined using the formula: (0.48 x body weight in kg) + 18.7. As the transverse process is passed, there should be a slight loss of resistance as entry is gained into the paravertebral space. Local anesthetic may be injected after negative aspiration for blood or cerebrospinal fluid, and a catheter threaded if desired. In infants and children, only 2 to 4 cm of the catheter should be threaded into the paravertebral space to avoid placing the tip laterally into an intercostal space, which would

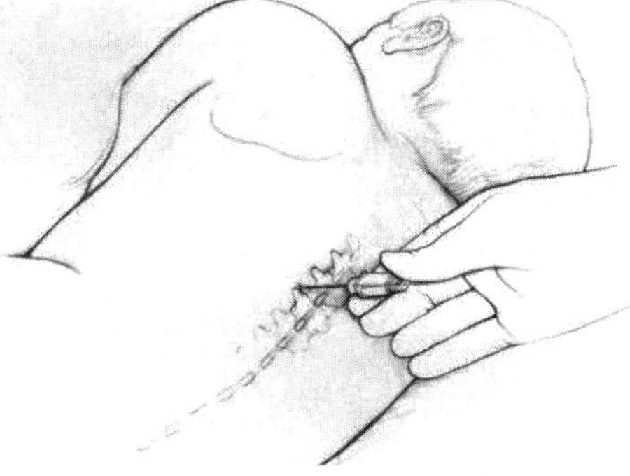

Figure 4-18
Technique of paravertebral block. The needle is inserted perpendicular to the skin until the lamina is contacted. The needle is walked off over the lamina until loss of resistance is noted.

result in analgesia of a single dermatome. An initial bolus dose of 0.5 mL/kg of local anesthetic will provide analgesia of approximately 4 to 5 dermatomes in a child.[42] Epinephrine 5 µg/mL should be added to the local anesthetic solution. Dosing of a continuous catheter for paravertebral analgesia should start at 0.25 mL/kg/h of a 0.1% solution for most children, but reduced to 0.2 mL/kg/h for infants.[43,44] Complications from paravertebral block in children are rare, but may include vascular puncture, pleural puncture, and pneumothorax. In older children or adults, hypotension also may occur from sympathectomy.

Ilioinguinal/Iliohypogastric Nerve Block

Ilioinguinal/iliohypogastric (ILIH) nerve block provides analgesia to the inguinal area for inguinal hernia repair, orchidopexy, and hydrocelectomy. This block may be as effective as a caudal block for these procedures.[45-48] An ILIH block cannot be used as the sole anesthetic for groin surgery because it does not block the stress response and visceral pain from peritoneal traction and manipulation of the spermatic cord.[49] The ilioinguinal (L1) and iliohypogastric (T12 and L1) nerves originate from the lumbar plexus and provide innervation to the scrotum and inner thigh. These nerves pierce the transversus abdominus muscle near the anterior superior iliac spine. If an ILIH block is performed before incision, a blunt (short beveled) 22- or 25-gauge needle is inserted 1 cm inferior and 1 cm medial to the anterior superior iliac spine after sterile preparation (Figure 4-19). The needle is directed toward the inner superficial lip of the ileum and local anesthetic injected while the needle is withdrawn. The needle is then redirected toward the inguinal ligament (but not into the inguinal ligament), and local anesthetic is injected after a pop is felt as the needle penetrates the external oblique muscle. A third injection is made in a longitudinal and medial direction from the needle insertion site (Figure 4-18).

Alternatively, an ILIH block may be performed under direct vision by the surgeons before wound closure. Bupivacaine, levobupivacaine, or ropivacaine, in a dose of 0.25-0.5 mL/kg, may be used. Lower concentrations should be used in infants and higher concentrations in older children, not to exceed maximal allowable dosing. (See Tables 4-1 and 4-2.)

Complications from ILIH block are rare; however, there have been reports of colon and small-bowel puncture.[50,51] An ILIH block also may result in motor block of the quadriceps muscle if the local anesthetic solution spreads below the inguinal ligament.[52]

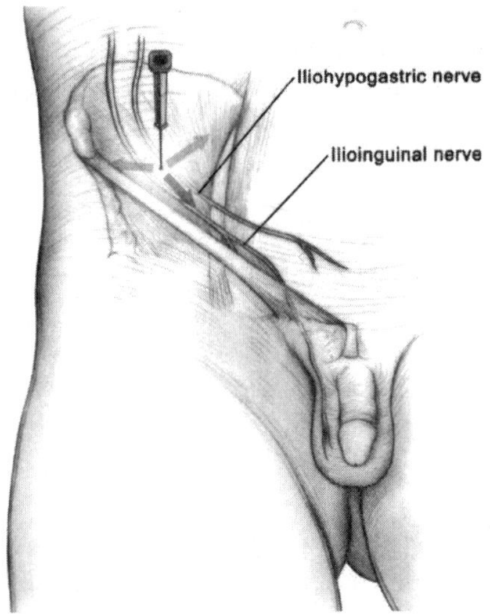

Figure 4-19
Technique for ilioinguinal/iliohypogastric nerve block. The needle is inserted 1 cm inferior to and 1 cm medial to the anterior superior iliac spine. The needle is directed toward the inner superficial lip of the ileum and local anesthetic injected while the needle is withdrawn. The needle is then redirected toward the inguinal ligament (but not into the inguinal ligament), and local anesthetic is injected after penetration of the external oblique muscle. A third injection is made medial to the needle insertion site.

Head and Neck Blockade

The scalp is innervated by 2 groups of nerves (Figure 4-20). The first group innervates the anterior part of the scalp, or forehead, and includes the first division of the trigeminal nerve, which divides into the supraorbital and supratrochlear nerves. The second group supplies the posterior part of the scalp and is derived from the cervical root of C2. Blocking those nerves provides pain relief for procedures performed on the head and neck.

Supraorbital and supratrochlear blocks may be used to provide pain relief for scalp excisions, frontal craniotomies, and frontal ventriculoperitoneal shunts.[53] To block the supraorbital nerve, the supraorbital notch is palpated, and a 27-gauge needle is inserted perpendicular to the skin into this notch. After negative aspiration, 1 to 2 mL of local anesthetic solution is injected. The supratrochlear nerve is blocked by withdrawing the needle to the skin level and directing it medially toward the tip of the nose. One milliliter of local anesthetic solution is injected after negative aspiration. Bupivacaine, levobupivacaine, or ropivacaine (0.2% to 0.25% with 1:200,000 epinephrine) may be used for all head and neck blocks discussed here.

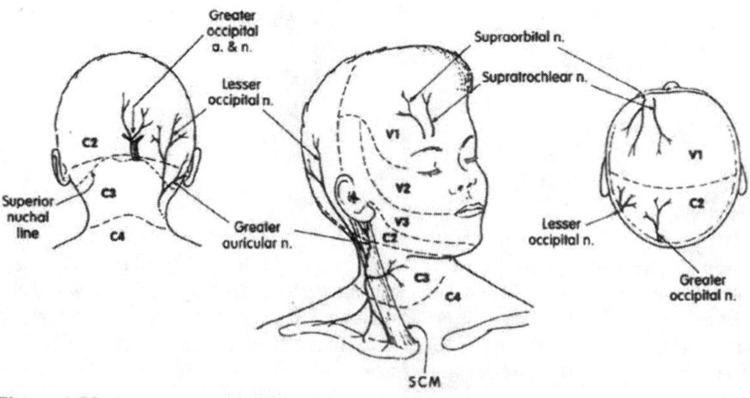

Figure 4-20
Innervation of the scalp by the greater auricular, lesser occipital, greater occipital, supratrochlear, and supraorbital nerves. SCM = sternocleidomastoid muscle.

Complications of these blocks include ecchymosis from the bleeding and dissection of the loose areolar tissue of the eyelid during injection of local anesthetic. Gentle pressure should be applied to the supraorbital area after block placement.

A greater occipital nerve block may be used to treat occipital pain after posterior fossa surgery or posterior shunt revisions. It also is useful for treating chronic pain secondary to occipital neuralgia. The cutaneous innervation to the major portion of the posterior scalp is provided by the dorsal rami of cervical spinal nerve C2, which ends in the greater occipital nerve (Figure 4-21). The child's head is turned to the side and the occipital artery palpated at the level of the superior nuchal line. One to 2 mL of local anesthetic solution should be placed medial to the occipital artery. Because of the proximity of the artery to the nerve, complications may include intravascular injection.

An infraorbital block can be used to provide analgesia for cleft lip repair, nasal reconstructive procedures including rhinoplasty, and endoscopic sinus surgery.[54-56] The infraorbital nerve is entirely sensory and is the termination of the second division of the trigeminal nerve.

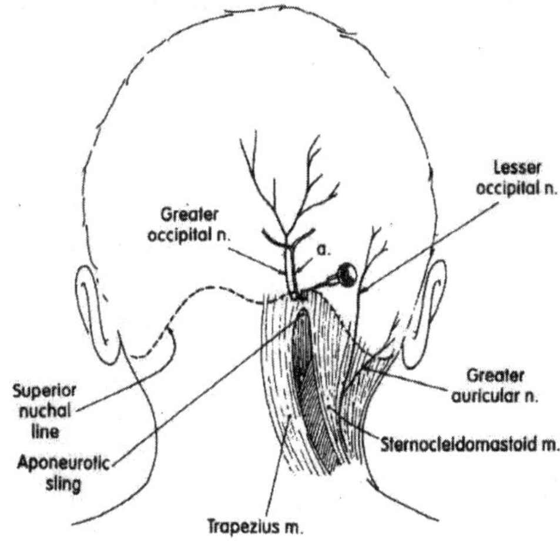

Figure 4-21
Innervation of the posterior aspect of the scalp by the greater and lesser occipital nerves.

It emerges in front of the maxilla through the infraorbital foramen and divides into the inferior palpebral, external nasal, internal nasal, and superior labial branches. This nerve may be blocked by using an intraoral approach (Figure 4-22). The infraorbital foramen is palpated and the upper lip folded back. A 27-gauge needle is inserted through the buccal mucosa parallel to the second maxillary molar. Once the tip of the needle is at the level of the infraorbital foramen, and after negative aspiration, 0.5 to 1 mL of local anesthetic solution is injected. Complications of an infraorbital block include ecchymosis and swelling due to the loose adventitious tissue. Care must be taken to prevent direct local anesthetic injection into the eye or orbit.

A greater auricular nerve block can be used to provide postoperative pain relief following mastoidectomy and otoplasty, and may reduce postoperative nausea and vomiting when compared with intravenous opioids for these procedures.[57,58] The greater auricular nerve is a branch of the superficial cervical plexus that wraps around the posterior belly

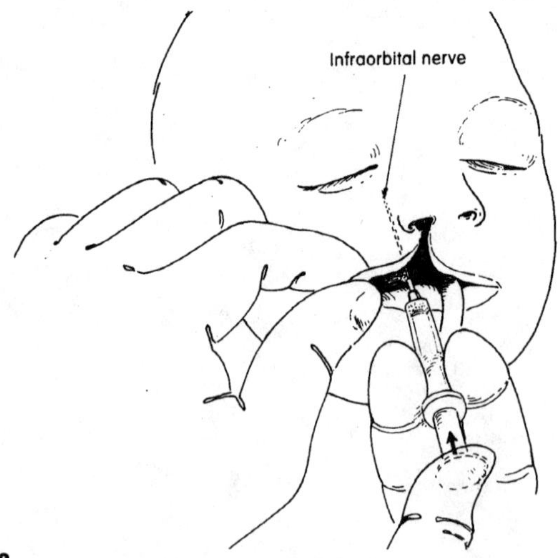

Figure 4-22
The technique for infraorbital nerve block. The infraorbital foramen is palpated and a needle is directed toward it through the mucosa parallel to the second molar.

of the sternocleidomastoid muscle (SCM) at the level of the cricoid cartilage and supplies sensory innervation to the mastoid and external ear. To block this nerve, a line is drawn from the superior margin of the cricoid cartilage to the posterior border of the SCM. Local anesthetic solution is injected superficially along this line over the belly of the SCM and also along the mid-portion of the posterior border of the SCM (Figure 4-23). Complications include Horner syndrome, phrenic nerve block, or subarachnoid block. Care should be taken to keep the needle superficial to avoid these complications.

Summary

Peripheral nerve blocks may be used in infants and children to provide postoperative analgesia and pain relief from acute and chronic pain conditions, and can be used as an alternative to general anesthesia for specific surgical procedures. Although most complications are rare and of little permanent clinical consequence, given the dose of local anesthetic used, the greatest life-threatening risk remains local anesthetic

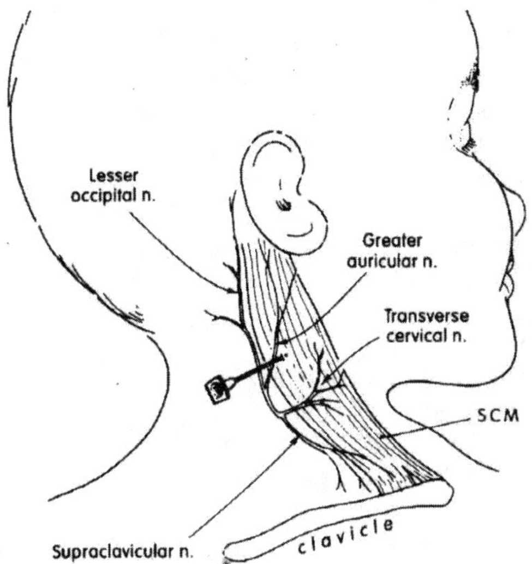

Figure 4-23
Technique of greater auricular nerve block. SCM = sternocleidomastoid muscle.

toxicity. As such, strict adherence to dosing guidelines for both single injection and continuous infusion techniques is recommended. When used appropriately, these techniques are safe and effective in many situations.

References

1. Ross AK, Eck JB, Tobias JD. Pediatric regional anesthesia: beyond the caudal. *Anesth Analg.* 2000;91:16-26
2. Giaufre E, Dalens B, Gombert A. Epidemiology and morbidity of regional anesthesia in children: a one-year prospective survey of the French-language society of pediatric anesthesiologists. *Anesth Analg.* 1996;83:904-912
3. Dalens BJ, Mazoit JX. Adverse effects of regional anaesthesia in children. *Drug Safety.* 1998;19:251-268
4. Lerman J, Strong HA, LeDez KM, Swartz J, Rieder MJ, Burrows FA. Effects of age on serum concentration of alpha-1 acid glycoprotein and the binding of lidocaine in pediatric patients. *Clin Pharm Ther.* 1989;46:219-225
5. Berde CB. Convulsions associated with pediatric regional anesthesia. *Anesth Analg.* 1992;75:164-166
6. Tanaka M, Nishikawa T. Simulation of an epidural test dose with intravenous epinephrine in sevoflurane-anesthetized children. *Anesth Analg.* 1998;86:952-957
7. Tobias JD. Caudal epidural block: a review of test dosing and recognition of systemic injection in children. *Anesth Analg.* 2001;93:1156-1161
8. Freid EB, Bailey AG, Valley RD. Electrocardiographic and hemodynamic changes associated with unintentional intravascular injection of bupivacaine with epinephrine in infants. *Anesthesiology.* 1993;79:394-398
9. Tanaka M, Nishikawa T. Evaluating t-wave amplitude as a guide for detecting intravascular injection of a test dose in anesthetized children. *Anesth Analg.* 1999;88:754-758
10. Doyle E, Morton NS, McNicol LR. Plasma bupivacaine levels after fascia iliaca compartment block with and without adrenaline. *Paediatr Anaesth.* 1997;7:121-124
11. Tobias JD. Brachial plexus anaesthesia in children. *Paediatr Anaesth.* 2001;11:265-275
12. Carre P, Joly A, Field BC, Wodey E, Lucas MM, Ecoffey C. Axillary block in children: single or multiple injection? *Paediatr Anaesth.* 2000;10:35-39

13. Merril DG, Brodsky JB, Hentz RV. Vascular insufficiency following axillary block of the brachial plexus. *Anesth Analg.* 1981;60:162-164
14. Dalens B, Vanneuville G, Tanguy A. A new parascalene approach to the brachial plexus in children: comparison with the supraclavicular approach. *Anesth Analg.* 1987;66:1264-1271
15. Tobias JD. Regional anaesthesia of the lower extremity in infants and children. *Paediatr Anaesth.* 2003;13:152-163
16. Ronchi L, Rosenbaum D, Athouel A, et al. Femoral nerve blockade in children using bupivacaine. *Anesthesiology.* 1989;70:622-624
17. Dalens B, Vanneuville G, Tanguy A. Comparison of the fascia iliaca com partment block with the 3-in-1 block in children. *Anesth Analg.* 1989;69:705-713
18. Dalens B, Tanguy A, Vanneuville G. Lumbar plexus block in children: a comparison of two procedures in 50 patients. *Anesth Analg.* 1988;67:750-758
19. Horlocker TT, Wedel DJ, Benzon H, et al. Regional anesthesia in the anticoagulated patient: defining the risks (The second ASRA consensus conference on neuraxial anesthesia and anticoagulation). *Reg Anesth Pain Med.* 2003;28:172-197
20. Dalens B, Tanguy A, Vanneuville G. Sciatic nerve blocks in children: comparison of the posterior, anterior, and lateral approaches in 180 pediatric patients. *Anesth Analg.* 1990;70:131-137
21. Raj PP, Parks RI, Watson TD, Jenkins MT. A new single-position supine approach to sciatic-femoral nerve block. *Anesth Analg.* 1975;54:489-493
22. Kempthorne PM, Brown TCK. Nerve blocks around the knee in children. *Anaesth Intensive Care.* 1984;12:14-17
23. Tobias JD, Mencio GA. Popliteal fossa block for postoperative analgesia after foot surgery in infants and children. *J Pediatr Ortho.* 1999;19:511-514
24. Vloka JD, Hadzik A, Lesser JB, et al. A common epineural sheath for the nerves in the popliteal fossa and its possible implications for sciatic nerve block. *Anesth Analg.* 1997;84:387-390
25. Konrad C, Johr M. Blockade of the sciatic nerve in the popliteal fossa: a system for standardization in children. *Anesth Analg.* 1998;87:1256-1258
26. Diwan R, Vas L, Shah T, Raghavendran S, Ponde V. Continuous axillary block for upper limb surgery in a patient with epidermolysis bullosa simplex. *Paediatr Anaesth.* 2001;11:603-606
27. Johnson CM. Continuous femoral nerve blockade for analgesia in children with femoral fractures. *Anaesth Intensive Care.* 1994;22:281-283

28. Tobias JD. Continuous femoral nerve block to provide analgesia following femur fracture in a paediatric ICU population. *Anaesth Intensive Care.* 1994;22:616-618
29. Sciard D, Matuszczak M, Gebhard R, Greger J, Al-Samsam T, Chelly JE. Continuous posterior lumbar plexus block for acute postoperative pain control in young children. *Anesthesiology.* 2001;95:1521-1523
30. Paut O, Sallabery M, Schreiber-Deturmeny E, Remond C, Bruguerolle B, Camboulives J. Continuous fascia iliaca compartment block in children: a prospective evaluation of plasma bupivacaine concentrations, pain scores, and side effects. *Anesth Analg.* 2001;92:1159-1163
31. Dadure C, Pirat P, Raux O, et al. Perioperative continuous peripheral nerve blocks with disposable infusion pumps in children: a prospective descriptive study. *Anesth Analg.* 2003;97:687-690
32. McIlvaine WB, Knox RF, Fennessey PV, Goldstein M. Continuous infusion of bupivacaine via intrapleural catheter for analgesia after thoracotomy in children. *Anesthesiology.* 1988;69:261-264
33. Tobias JD. Analgesia after thoracotomy in children: a comparison of interpleural, epidural, and intravenous analgesia. *Southern Med J.* 1991;84:1458-1461
34. Lonnqvist PA. Continuous paravertebral block in children: initial experience. *Anaesthesia.* 1992;47:607-609
35. Lonnqvist PA, MacKenzie J, Soni AK, Conacher ID. Paravertebral blockade. Failure rate and complications. *Anaesthesia.* 1995;50:813-815
36. Richardson J, Lonnqvist PA. Thoracic paravertebral block. *Br J Anaesth.* 1998;81:230-238
37. Lonnqvist PA, Olsson GL. Paravertebral vs epidural block in children: effects on postoperative morphine requirements after renal surgery. *Acta Anesthesiol Scand.* 1994;38:346-349
38. Eck JB, Cantos-Gustafsson A, Ross AK, et al. What's new in pediatric paravertebral analgesia. *Tech Reg Anesth Pain Management.* 2002;6:131
39. Eng J, Sabanathan S. Continuous paravertebral block for postthoracoto my analgesia in children. *J Pediatr Surg.* 1992;27:556-557
40. Lonnqvist PA, Hildingsson U. The caudal boundary of the thoracic paravertebral space. A study of human cadavers. *Anaesthesia.* 1992;47:1051-1052
41. Lonnqvist PA, Hesser U. Location of the paravertebral space in children and adolescents in relation to surface anatomy assessed by computed tomography. *Paediatr Anaesth.* 1992;2:285

42. Lonnqvist PA, Hesser U. Radiological and clinical distribution of thoracic paravertebral blockade in infants and children. *Paediatr Anaesth.* 1993;3:83
43. Cheung SL, Booker PD, Franks R, et al. Serum concentrations of bupivacaine during prolonged paravertebral infusion in young infants. *Br J Anaesth.* 1997;79:9-13
44. Karmaker MK, Booker PD, Franks R, Pozzi M. Continuous extrapleural paravertebral infusion of bupivacaine for post-thoracotomy analgesia in young infants. *Br J Anaesth.* 1996;76:811-815
45. Hannallah RS, Broadman LM, Belman AB, Ambramowitz MD, Epstein BS. Comparison of caudal and ilioinguinal/iliohypogastric nerve blocks for control of post-orchiopexy pain in pediatric ambulatory surgery. *Anesthesiology.* 1987;66:832-834
46. Casey WF, Rice LJ, Hannallah RS, Broadman L, Norden JM, Guzzetta P. A comparison between bupivacaine installation versus ilioinguinal/iliohypogastric nerve block for postoperative analgesia following inguinal herniorrhaphy in children. *Anesthesiology.* 1990;72:637-639
47. Fisher QA, McComiskey CM, Hill JL, et al. Postoperative voiding interval and duration of analgesia following peripheral or caudal nerve blocks in children. *Anesth Analg.* 1993;76:173-177
48. Splinter WM, Bass J, Komocar L. Regional anaesthesia for hernia repair in children: local vs caudal anaesthesia. *Can J Anaesth.* 1995;42:197-200
49. Somri M, Gaitini LA, Vaida SJ, et al. Effect of ilioinguinal nerve block on the catecholamine plasma levels in orchidopexy: comparison with caudal epidural block. *Paediatr Anaesth.* 2002;12:791-797
50. Amory C, Mariscal A, Guyot E, Chauvet P, Leon A, Poli-Merol ML. Is ilioinguinal/iliohypogastric nerve block always totally safe in children? *Paediatr Anaesth.* 2003;13:164
51. Johr M, Sossai R. Colonic puncture during ilioinguinal nerve block in a child. *Anesth Analg.* 1999;88:1051
52. Roy-Shapira A, Amoury RA, Ashcraft KW, Holder TM, Sharp RJ. Transient quadriceps paresis following local inguinal block for post-operative pain control. *J Pediatr Surg.* 1985;20:554-555
53. Suresh S, Wagner AM. Scalp excisions: getting "ahead" of pain. *Pediatr Dermatol.* 2001;18:74-76
54. Prabhu KP, Wig J, Gewal S. Bilateral infraorbital nerve block is superior to peri-incisional infiltration for analgesia after repair of cleft lip. *Scand J Plastic Reconst Surg Hand Surg.* 1999;33:83-87

55. Bosenberg AT, Kimble FW. Infraorbital nerve block in neonates for cleft lip repair: anatomical study and clinical application. *Br J Anaesth.* 1995;74:506-508
56. Molliex S, Navez M, Baylot D, Prades JM, Elkhoury Z, Auboyer C. Regional anesthesia for outpatient nasal surgery. *Br J Anaesth.* 1996;76:151-153
57. Suresh S, Barcelona SL, Young NM, Seligman I, Heffner CL, Cote CJ. Postoperative pain relief in children undergoing tympanomastoid surgery: is a regional block better than opioids? *Anesth Analg.* 2002;94:859-862
58. Cregg N, Conway F, Casey W. Analgesia after otoplasty: regional nerve blockade vs local anaesthetic infiltration of the ear. *Can J Anaesth.* 1996;432:141-147

Chapter 5

Managing Procedure-Related Pain and Anxiety

John W. Berkenbosch, MD, FAAP

Definitions
Pre-sedation Assessment
Preparation for Sedation
    Personnel
    Equipment
Monitoring During Sedation
    Comfort and Consciousness Monitoring
    Post-procedure Monitoring and Discharge Criteria
    Record Keeping
Choice of Agent
    Sedatives
        Chloral Hydrate
        Benzodiazepines
        α-adrenergic Agonists
    Analgesic Agents
        Opioids
        Ketamine
    Anesthetic Agents
        Barbiturates
        Propofol
        Nitrous Oxide
    Combination of Agents
        Lytic Cocktail
Opioid and Benzodiazepine Reversal Agents
    Opioid Antagonists
    Benzodiazepine Antagonists
Topical and Local Anesthetics
Non-pharmacologic Methods

Introduction

Invasive and noninvasive procedures remain a common and necessary component in managing acute and chronic diseases in children (Table 5-1). While adults may be able to tolerate such procedures without sedation, developmental issues such as stranger anxiety, fear during illness, previous experiences with painful procedures, fear of pain, and the inability to cooperate and/or remain motionless for prolonged periods often mandate the use of sedation in children.

Current opinion about pediatric procedural sedation has shifted and health care professionals are increasingly recognizing the negative consequences of inadequate sedation. Surveys of parents and patients with pediatric malignancies have shown that invasive procedures often are perceived as worse than the disease itself. Therefore, more children are being sedated for procedures, the depth of sedation achieved is increasing in certain environments, and the scope of practitioners performing sedations is widening, with an increasing number of sedations being

Table 5-1. Procedures Commonly Requiring Sedation in Children

Noninvasive	Invasive/Painful
Radiologic	Lumbar puncture
MRI (magnetic resonance imaging)	Bone marrow aspirate/biopsy
CT (computed tomography) scan	Flexible fiberoptic bronchoscopy
Nuclear medicine	Gastrointestinal endoscopy
Brainstem auditory evoked response	Gastroduodenoscopy
Electroencephalogram	Colonoscopy
	Botulinum toxin injections
	Electromyelogram/nerve conduction studies
	Vascular access
	Central venous catheter insertion
	Arterial line insertion
	Thoracentesis
	Thoracostomy tube insertion

performed by non-anesthesiologists. This chapter discusses procedural sedation in pediatric patients, including factors involved in making a decision to sedate, current guidelines for patient assessment before and monitoring during sedation, factors that determine the choice of sedative and/or analgesia, and some of the more commonly used sedative and analgesic agents in the pediatric population. While the principles discussed apply to both anesthesiologists and non-anesthesiologists, the focus of this chapter will be the non-anesthesiologist practitioner.

Definitions

In response to the expanding use of procedural sedation outside the traditional operating room setting, the American Academy of Pediatrics (AAP) published guidelines for preoperative evaluation/preparation, monitoring during the procedure, and observation following its completion.[1-3] The guidelines include pertinent information for providing procedural sedation and analgesia. The guidelines also stress important features of procedural sedation and the principle that depths of sedation occur along a continuum. The transition from one level to the next, including the changes in risks associated with each level, can occur very easily and often without the practitioner's awareness. The guidelines define 3 depths, or levels, of sedation.

Moderate sedation is defined as a "medically controlled state of depressed consciousness" that 1) allows protective reflexes to be maintained, 2) retains the patient's ability to maintain a patent airway independently and continuously, and 3) permits appropriate response of the patient to physical stimulation or verbal command (eg, "open your eyes").[3]

Deep sedation is defined as a "medically controlled state of depressed consciousness or unconsciousness from which a patient is not easily aroused. It may be accompanied by a partial or complete loss of protective reflexes, and includes the inability to maintain a patent airway independently and respond purposefully to physical stimulation or verbal command."[3]

General anesthesia is defined as a "medically controlled state of unconsciousness accompanied by a loss of protective reflexes, including the inability to maintain a patent airway independently and respond purposefully to physical or verbal stimulation." The Joint Commission on Accreditation of Healthcare Organizations (JCAHO) has dictated that its standards for sedation monitoring be based on the depth of sedation, with deeper levels of sedation mandating increased monitoring measures.[4]

These definitions raise several important points. First, there is significant overlap between each level of sedation, and knowing when a patient has passed from one level to the next may be difficult to ascertain, especially if ongoing medications are being administered. However, knowledge of the depth of sedation achieved is important because the risks of adverse events increase with increasing depth of sedation. The use of a specific medication does not ensure one particular level of sedation. Any of the medications used for sedation can result in any of the 3 levels described because of significant interpatient variability, thereby suggesting that the type and level of monitoring should be uniform any time "procedural sedation" is performed. Although we traditionally refer to the use of "moderate sedation" for pediatric procedures, this is somewhat of a misnomer; in many situations, what is really achieved is deep sedation, leading many institutions to abandon the use of the term "conscious sedation" and adopt the broader term "procedural sedation."

Pre-sedation Assessment

Ideally, the pre-sedation assessment should be performed by the practitioner who will be providing the sedation to ensure first-hand knowledge of the patient and his or her medical needs. This also allows the practitioner to address specific patient concerns before and during the procedure. The pre-sedation assessment is outlined in Table 5-2. A focused history and physical examination help determine the patient's fitness for sedation. The history should focus on the patient's current state of health as it relates to the reason for the procedure, as well as medical history to identify significant comorbidities. Because the primary risks associated with sedation include adverse respiratory (eg, apnea, hypoxemia, and upper airway obstruction) or cardiovascular (eg, hypotension, dysrhythmias) events, emphasis is placed on these systems. A complete upper airway assessment should be performed, which includes obtaining a history of sleep obstruction and an examination of the head and neck designed to identify the patient in whom endotracheal intubation may be difficult. This examination focuses on

Table 5-2. Components of the Pre-sedation Assessment

Table 5-2. Components of the Pre-sedation Assessment
Patient's name, age, weight, and gender
Medical history
Underlying medical conditions
Previous sedation/anesthetic history or problems
Allergies
Current medications
Family history of anesthetic complications
Dietary history (NPO status)
Pregnancy history
Physical examination
Baseline vital signs, including room air saturation
Airway examination
Cardiorespiratory examination
Laboratory (if appropriate)
Summary
American Society of Anesthesiologists status
Plan
Risks discussed
NPO history reviewed

neck mobility (flexion and extension), mouth opening, the size of the oral cavity, presence of macroglossia, and the thyromental distance (distance from the thyroid cartilage to the tip of the mandible). Limitations of any of these features may suggest difficulty in performing endotracheal intubation or bag-mask ventilation. An objective measure of the potential for difficult intubation is the Mallampati Classification. Specifically, if the patient is Mallampati Grade III or IV (tonsillar pillars and base of the uvula cannot be visualized with mouth opening and tongue protrusion), the trachea may be difficult to intubate. While the possibility of a difficult airway does not preclude the use of procedural sedation, pediatric anesthesiology consultation may be considered prior to the sedation and it may be prudent to ensure that anesthesiology backup is available when the procedure is performed. On completion of the history and physical examination, an American Society of Anesthesiologists (ASA) classification may be assigned (Table 5-3). Patients with ASA Classification III or IV are at higher risk of adverse events when sedated, and pediatric anesthesiology consultation also may be considered in these patients.

It also is important during the pre-sedation assessment to discuss the patient's previous experiences with procedural sedation, including effectiveness and the patient's and parent's perceptions of the experiences.

Table 5-3. American Society of Anesthesiologists (ASA) Classification System

ASA Class	Description
I	No underlying medical problems
II	Mild systemic illness Well-controlled asthma, corrected CHD
III	Severe systemic illness Sickle cell disease, severe asthma, uncorrected CHD
IV	Severe systemic illness that is a constant threat to life Uncorrected cyanotic CHD
V	Patient is unlikely to survive 24 hours with or without the procedure

CHD = congenital heart disease.

The practitioner should engage the patient and family in pre-sedation counseling during which the risks, benefits, and limitations of sedation and/or analgesia are discussed. This discussion should include a description of the agents chosen and specific effects and/or behaviors that the patient and/or parents can expect.

A final and important component of the pre-sedation assessment is establishing when the child last had any oral intake to decrease the possibility of aspiration if airway protective reflexes are lost. The ASA recommends that children be *nil per os* (NPO) for clear liquids, including human milk, for 2 to 3 hours and, for solids or infant formula, for 4 to 8 hours before undergoing sedation for elective procedures (Table 5-4).[5] These guidelines should be reviewed with the parents at the time the procedure is scheduled and should be repeated if a reminder phone call is made in the 24 to 48 hours before the scheduled procedure date.

The NPO guidelines have been increasingly challenged, particularly by those working in acute care environments where procedures may need to be performed more urgently. While clinical experience has failed to definitively show an effect of pre-procedure fasting on the incidence of adverse outcomes, this question has not been investigated systematically in an appropriate prospective trial. Until studies have adequately addressed this issue, adhering to the ASA guidelines as much as possible is prudent. At times, however, sedation will need to proceed without strict adherence to the NPO guidelines due to the

Table 5-4. Guidelines for NPO Status Prior to Elective Procedural Sedations

Age	Solids/Non-clear Liquids	Clear Liquids*
<6 mo	4-6 h	2 h
6-36 mo	6 h	2-3 h
>36 mo	6-8 h	2-3 h
Adults	6-8 h	2-3 h

*Human milk is considered a clear liquid; formula is a non-clear liquid.

emergent or urgent nature of the procedure. In some instances, such as a patient with altered mental status or impaired airway protective reflexes who has recently eaten, the safest way to proceed may be with a rapid sequence induction and endotracheal intubation to provide airway protection.

Preparation for Sedation

Personnel

The JCAHO has mandated that the use of deep sedation requires the same monitoring standards as are used during general anesthesia. Because deep sedation typically is used for pediatric procedures, special preparation of the sedation environment is required involving the personnel and equipment that must be available during the sedation. Because most of the adverse events that occur during procedural sedation involve respiratory depression with the potential loss of a patent airway, one of the most important requirements is that at least one person in attendance must be skilled in emergent airway management, including performing bag-valve-mask ventilation and endotracheal intubation. This person is solely responsible for observing the patient throughout the procedure, for performing sedation-related assessments and documentation, and should not be involved in the procedure itself. Finally, while it may not be specifically required, it is strongly encouraged that the person monitoring the patient retain current certification in pediatric advanced life support.[1-3]

In response to the JCAHO's standards, many institutions have implemented sedation credentialing procedures for non-anesthesiologists. While this process may satisfy regulatory bodies and may raise the level of awareness of those who go through the process, it may not ensure that the practitioner who earns the credential can safely attend to all aspects of sedation, including resuscitation. Therefore, individual practitioners must use good judgment and restrict their use of sedatives to agents with which they are both familiar and comfortable. They also should aim only to achieve depths of sedation from which they are proficient at rescuing a patient and should consider either seeking additional airway experience with their anesthesiology colleagues or abstain from providing sedation if they are not proficient.

Equipment

Necessary equipment and medications to perform resuscitation should be readily available in the procedure area. If patients are sedated in one area and moved to a second area for their procedure, a stocked equipment cart should either be available in both areas or a portable cart should be available to transport with the patient. Table 5-5 lists suggested emergency equipment and medications for procedural sedation.

Before administering any sedative agent, specific equipment should be within reach, including an appropriately sized bag-valve-mask device, Yankauer suction system, and monitoring devices. When moderate sedation is desired and oral medications are used, placing an intravenous catheter is optional. However, when deep sedation is planned, even if administered via the inhalation or oral route, a functioning intravenous catheter is suggested.

Monitoring During Sedation

The JCAHO mandates the use of general anesthesia standards for monitoring patients undergoing sedation with or without analgesia that may reasonably be expected to result in the potential for loss of airway protective reflexes. Sedation presents a risk of adverse events, most commonly cardiorespiratory, and appropriate monitoring may prevent a significant number of negative outcomes.[6] Malviya et al[7] evaluated the incidence of complications in 1,140 sedations performed by non-anesthesiologists. Complications other than inadequate sedation occurred in 98 patients (8.6%). Of those complications, 55 were primarily respiratory (4.8%) and 6 were primarily cardiac (0.5%). Fifteen patients (1.3%) were reported to have become oversedated. Risk factors for adverse events included age younger than 1 year and ASA classification III or IV. Similarly, in an analysis of 95 severe sedation-related adverse events, Cote et al[8] found that respiratory events accounted for more than 80% of complications.

Table 5-5. Suggested Emergency Equipment and Medications for Procedural Sedation

Airway
Portable or permanent suction apparatus
Oral and nasal airways—infant, child, small adult, medium adult, and large adult
Nasal cannula—infant, child, and adult sized
Face masks—infant, child, small adult, medium adult, large adult
Self-inflating bag-valve set—250 mL, 500 mL, 1000 mL
Laryngoscope handles (tested)
Laryngoscope blades (bulbs tested)
- Miller (straight)—sizes 0,1,2,3
- Macintosh (curved)—sizes 2,3,4

Endotracheal tubes
- Uncuffed (2.5, 3.0, 3.5, 4.0, 4.5, 5.0 mm ID)
- Cuffed (5.0, 5.5, 6.0, 6.5, 7.0, 8.0 mm ID)

Stylets—appropriately sized for endotracheal tubes
Suction catheters—appropriately sized for endotracheal tubes
Yankauer suction system and nasogastric tubes
Surgical lubricant
McGill forceps (optional)

Intravenous Equipment
Surgical gloves
Tourniquets
Alcohol swabs
Adhesive tape, steri-strips
Arm boards—small and medium sized
Sterile gauze (2x2 or 4x4)
Syringes: 60 mL, 10 mL, 5 mL, 3 mL, 1 mL
Needles: 18, 20, 22, 25 gauge
Intravenous catheters 18, 20, 22, 24 gauge
Intraosseous/bone marrow needle
Tubing/connectors including T-connectors, 3-way stopcocks, extension tubing (standard, microbore, and burette-type)
Isotonic intravenous fluids—lactated Ringer's or normal saline

Table 5-5. Suggested Emergency Equipment and Medications for Procedural Sedation, *continued*

Medications
Oxygen
Albuterol
Atropine
Calcium (chloride or gluconate)—10% solution
Dextrose—50%
Diphenhydramine HCl
Diazepam or lorazepam
Dopamine
Epinephrine—1:1,000 and 1:10,000
Flumazenil
Glycopyrrolate
Hydrocortisone or methylprednisolone or dexamethasone
Labetalol
Lidocaine (1% or 2%)
Naloxone
Phenylephrine
Racemic or L-epinephrine for nebulization
Rocuronium or vecuronium
Sodium bicarbonate (0.5 and 1 mEq/mL)
Succinylcholine
Note: Choice of specific emergency drugs in various classes may vary according to individual preference, need, and/or availability.
Monitoring Equipment
Precordial stethoscopes
Electrocardiogram pads
Blood pressure cuffs
Pulse oximetry probes
End-tidal CO_2 device with sampling tubing

Formal monitoring should include, at a minimum, continuous pulse oximetry and heart rate (via the pulse oximeter or electrocardiogram [ECG]) as well as documentation of respiratory rate and blood pressure at least every 5 minutes in a time-based record.[1-3] The frequency may be decreased as the patient regains consciousness during the recovery phase. To ensure patient safety, those monitoring vital signs should keep a vigilant watch over the patient and be able to anticipate the potential for respiratory compromise. The monitoring personnel should have an unobstructed view of the patient's face, mouth, and chest wall throughout the procedure. Drapes and barriers should not obstruct this view unless completely necessary (eg, upper central venous catheter insertion, magnetic resonance imaging [MRI] scanning). Because most respiratory events occur in the period immediately following the administration of medications, it is particularly important that the monitoring health care provider watch the patient for signs of hypoventilation, decreased chest wall movement, and airway obstruction because devices such as pulse oximeters may not detect problems until the patient has begun to have oxygen desaturation.

Pulse oximetry is the most widely used adjunct measure and has improved the ability to continuously evaluate a patient's oxygenation status. However, currently available oximeters are calibrated for SaO_2 values greater than 80% and lose their accuracy at values less than 75%.[9] While this is clinically unimportant for most patients, in whom SaO_2 values would normally be in the upper 90% range, this may become significant when sedating patients with residual cyanotic congenital heart disease where SaO_2 values of 70% to 80% are common. Also, patient movement may be interpreted as pulsatile flow, resulting in inaccurate readings, and has been documented in up to 25% of patients monitored with older oximeters,[10] so care should be used when relying on the oximeter to monitor heart rate. Ideally, pulse oximeters that display the plethysmography tracing should be used. If this is not possible or there are concerns about the accuracy of the oximeter, heart rate should be monitored directly with ECG recording. Placing the oximeter probe on cool extremities also has been associated with decreased accuracy, a factor that should be considered during invasive procedures in which the patient is partially disrobed. Newer pulse oximetry technologies such as Signal Extraction Technology[11] (Masimo, Irvine, CA) and forehead reflectance sensors[12] (Nellcor, Pleasantville, CA), seem to be more rapidly responsive and less sensitive to motion artifact and extremity temperature.

Intermittent recording of respiratory rate is best done manually to allow the monitoring health care provider to determine the effectiveness of the respiratory effort. When the chest must be obscured by drapes during the procedure (eg, central venous line insertion), or there is a reasonable risk of respiratory compromise (eg, flexible fiberoptic bronchoscopy), continuous respiratory monitoring using plethysmography may be implemented. While not required, monitoring ventilation via end-tidal carbon dioxide ($ETCO_2$) also should be considered, particularly under conditions where access to the patient is limited, such as during MRI scanning. With $ETCO_2$ devices, reports from the emergency department[13] and procedure suite[14] have documented the development of hypercarbia in the absence of clinically apparent respiratory depression or desaturation by pulse oximetry. These data suggest that $ETCO_2$ monitoring may facilitate the earlier detection of respiratory compromise and should, perhaps, be utilized more frequently than current practices suggest. With $ETCO_2$ monitoring, there is an immediate cessation of the waveform the instant air flow stops related either to apnea or upper airway obstruction, thereby providing a much earlier warning of respiratory compromise.

Comfort and Consciousness Monitoring

Ensuring patient comfort during procedures has become increasingly important, and the concept of pain as the fifth vital sign has gained popularity. Assessing pain during procedures may be difficult, especially in the preverbal or nonverbal patient in whom determining the cause of distress (pain vs irritation vs fear) may be difficult. Whereas scoring systems to assess post-procedure, particularly postoperative pain, have been well established, they remain limited for assessing pain during a procedure. While the lack of movement or struggling during a painful manipulation likely indicates the absence of significant pain, it would be inappropriate to expect that every patient undergoing painful procedures be sufficiently sedated as to lose all responsiveness.

Because a patient may slip from moderate to deep sedation to general anesthesia easily, accurately assessing and documenting the depth of sedation achieved throughout the procedure is critical. A variety of scales have been developed to measure sedation level. The Observers Assessment of Alertness and Sedation Scale has been validated in children, but is limited in its ability to differentiate among deeper levels of sedation.[15] Conversely, other scales, such as the Vancouver Sedative Recovery Scale, are better at differentiating deeper levels of sedation, but are too cumbersome to be used during short procedures.[16] More recently, Malviya et al[17] developed and validated the University of Michigan Sedation Scale (UMSS), which was designed to be used by a variety of health care providers as a simple and efficient tool to assess depth of sedation over the entire sedation continuum. It uses a simple scale of 0 to 4 (Table 5-6), with 0 being an awake, alert patient, and 4 indicating unresponsiveness.

A major drawback of all these tools is that they require patient stimulation. In patients who have been difficult to sedate or in whom movement during the assessment may interfere with the procedure, this may lead the assessor to inadequately stimulate the patient during the assessment and, therefore, overestimate the true depth of sedation. In such cases, the Bispectral Index (BIS) monitor (Aspect Medical, Newton, MA) may be more useful. The BIS monitor processes a modified electroencephalogram (EEG) to assess the sedative effects of anesthetic

Table 5-6. University of Michigan Sedation Scale

Score	Sedation Level
0	Fully awake and alert
1	Lightly sedated—appropriate response to verbal conversation and/or sound
2	Sedated—easily aroused with light tactile stimulus or simple verbal command
3	Deeply sedated—aroused only with significant physical stimulation
4	Unarousable

agents via a sensor placed on the patient's forehead, replacing the reliance on physiological parameters for determining the depth of anesthesia. The validity of the BIS for determining depth of anesthesia has been well documented in adults[18] and children.[19] More recently, the BIS also has been shown to accurately assess depth of sedation during mechanical ventilation in critically ill children.[20,21] To date, there are few published studies evaluating the BIS during procedural sedation. Gill et al[22] compared BIS values with Ramsay sedation scores in 37 adult patients receiving procedural sedation and/or analgesia in the emergency department. The authors reported a significant correlation between the BIS reading and the depth of sedation. However, there was variability of BIS values at similar sedation scores. They noted that the BIS was most effective at differentiating moderate-to-deep sedation from general anesthesia. McDermott et al[23] compared BIS values with UMSS scores in 86 children 12 years or younger. The authors reported a strong correlation between the BIS value and the sedation score, even in patients younger than 6 months. However, they reported that the correlation was agent dependent; they noted a poor correlation in patients receiving either ketamine or a combination of oral chloral hydrate, hydroxyzine, and meperidine. While further study is required, these studies suggest that the BIS monitor provides useful information, especially during lengthy procedures (nuclear medicine) or when drug infusions (vs intermittent dosing) are employed.

Post-procedure Monitoring and Discharge Criteria

While the greatest risk of adverse events occurs at the time sedation is administered, continued monitoring of cardiorespiratory and neurologic function in the post-procedure period remains important. Sedation-related nausea may occur during this period and, if it is sufficient to cause vomiting prior to the patient regaining consciousness, the risks of pulmonary aspiration may be increased. In addition, it is possible that sedative-induced respiratory depression lessens during painful procedures only to manifest after the stimulus of the procedure is removed.

Monitoring in the initial post-procedure period should include continuous pulse oximetry, heart rate monitoring, and intermittent recording of blood pressure and respiratory rate. Depth of sedation also should be assessed. As the patient regains consciousness, the frequency with which these assessments are done may be decreased, although it is recommended that pulse oximetry continue until the patient is at or near baseline. Discharge criteria established by the AAP and the ASA require that the patient return to his or her baseline from a neurologic standpoint and that his or her vital signs are normal (Table 5-7).[1-3,5] It also is prudent to ensure that the patient has been able to tolerate oral intake to limit the likelihood of dehydration from protracted vomiting. The phone number of a professional familiar with sedation practices and the management of post-sedation complications also should be provided to the family in the event that questions arise following discharge.

Record Keeping

All documentation from a procedure should be incorporated into the medical record. Many centers use a single-page sedation sheet with the preoperative assessment on one side and a time-based record for vital signs and medication administration on the other. This sheet also can include a space for documenting informed consent as well as a section to document post-procedure monitoring. Space for documenting that parents or caregivers have been given discharge instructions also should be included.

Table 5-7. Recommended Discharge Criteria

1 – Satisfactory and stable cardiovascular function and airway patency
2 – Patient is easily arousable and protective reflexes are intact
3 – Patient can talk (if age appropriate)
4 – Patient can sit up unaided (if age appropriate)
5 – Patient's level of responsiveness is near normal or as close to normal as possible in the preverbal or nonverbal patient
6 – Patient's state of hydration is adequate

Choice of Agent

The number of sedative agents available to the anesthesiologist and the non-anesthesiologist has significantly increased, and newer agents continue to be developed (Table 5-8). These agents generally can be grouped into 3 categories: sedatives, analgesics, and general anesthetic agents. Pure sedatives have no analgesic properties and should not be used alone for painful procedures. They often are combined with an analgesic agent.

Deciding which sedative agent(s) to use is based on several factors, including 1) the procedure being performed (type and duration), 2) the depth of sedation required, 3) the need for intravenous access, 4) the patient's previous experiences with sedation or anesthesia, 5) risk factors identified in the pre-sedation assessment, and 6) the health care professional's experience and comfort with specific medications.

Health care professionals must realize that there is no magic medication that works in all patients. For example, the medication choice for an MRI evaluation or lumbar puncture may be very different in an otherwise healthy 10-year-old compared with a 4-year-old with developmental delays. In addition, there may be considerable variation among patients in the dose of a particular drug required to achieve a specific depth of sedation. Therefore, dosage ranges should be considered guidelines and the drug should be titrated to the desired effect based on the guidelines. (See Table 5-8.)

The route of delivery of the sedative drug is also extremely important, particularly in children who do not require intravenous access for the procedure itself. In those situations, nonparenteral administration may be appropriate because many children view having an intravenous administration started or an intramuscular injection as invasive as the procedure itself. For example, chloral hydrate is a popular choice for radiologic procedures. Many physicians are familiar and comfortable with it, it has a good safety profile, and doses of 75 to 80 mg/kg (orally

Table 5-8. Procedural Sedation Agents, Doses, and Indications

Agent	Route	Dose	Indications/Applications
Chloral hydrate	PO/PR	50-100 mg/kg	Noninvasive radiologic procedures BAER, EEG
Midazolam	IV PO IN/SL	0.05-0.1 mg/kg 0.5-0.7 mg/kg 0.2-0.4 mg/kg	Noninvasive radiologic procedures Need analgesia for painful procedures
Dexmedetomidine	IV	Induction: 0.5-1.0 μg/kg over 5-10 min; maintenance: 0.5-0.7 μg/kg/h	Noninvasive radiologic procedures BAER, EEG
Morphine*	IV	0.05-0.15 mg/kg	Short, painful procedures (eg, LP, EMG, thoracentesis)
Fentanyl*	IV	1-2 μg /kg	Short, painful procedures (eg, LP, EMG, thoracentesis)
Remifentanil*	IV	Infusion: 0.05-0.1 μg/kg/min	Short painful procedures Flexible bronchoscopy
Ketamine*	IV IM PO	0.5-1.0 mg/kg 4-6 mg/kg 10 mg/kg	Short radiologic procedures Painful procedures (eg, central venous catheter, bronchoscopy GI endoscopy)
Methohexital	PR IV	20-30 mg/kg 0.75-1.0 mg/kg	Noninvasive radiologic procedures
Thiopental	PR	25-50 mg/kg	Noninvasive radiologic procedures
Propofol	IV	Bolus: 1-2 mg/kg q 2-3 min: Infusion: 50-100 μg/kg/min	Noninvasive radiologic procedures, bronchoscopy, GI endoscopy Need analgesia adjunct for painful procedures (eg, LP, BMA)
Nitrous oxide	Inhalation	30%-70% with oxygen	Dental procedures Short painful procedures (eg, burn debridement, laceration repair)

*Often combined with a sedative (midazolam, propofol).
PO = oral, PR = rectal, BAER = brainstem auditory evoked response, EEG = electroencephalogram, IV = intravenous, IN = intranasal, SL = sublingual, LP = lumbar puncture, EMG = electromyelogram, IM = intramuscular, GI = gastrointestinal, BMA = bone marrow aspirate.

or per rectum) are effective in up to 90% of patients. Onset of sedation varies from 15 to 60 minutes and, although most children are awake and responsive within 60 to 90 minutes, sedation may be prolonged and last more than 6 hours. Such variability in sedation duration must be taken into consideration especially for short procedures (computed tomography [CT] imaging). It may be reasonable for the patient and family to conclude that the inconvenience of intravenous administration is an acceptable compromise for the ability to use a short-acting intravenous medication. Topical anesthetic agents to facilitate intravenous placement (see following text) are available, making this option even more attractive.

Sedation During Cardiac Catheterization

Many sedative and analgesic agents may alter cardiovascular parameters such as heart rate, blood pressure, or vascular resistance of either the systemic or pulmonary beds. It is imperative to consider the underlying cardiac lesion and determine how such changes might affect both the child's hemodynamic status as well as the data obtained during the procedure. Most diagnostic, noninterventional catheterizations are performed with procedural sedation. In infants and young children, this may include an initial dose of chloral hydrate (75-100 mg/kg) supplemented with intermittent doses of a benzodiazepine (midazolam 0.05 mg/kg) or an opioid (morphine 0.05 mg/kg). Sedation may be combined with a topical anesthetic cream to the groin to minimize discomfort during vessel cannulation. Alternative agents for patients who cannot be adequately sedated with the previously discussed agents include ketamine, propofol, or the intramuscular mixture of chlorpromazine, meperidine, and promethazine. Because of its negative inotropic properties, propofol should be used only in patients with stable cardiovascular function. Due to limited patient accessibility during cardiac catheterization, it also may be wise to secure the airway if this agent is used, making general anesthesia a more appropriate choice.

Sedatives

Chloral Hydrate

Chloral hydrate is an alcohol-based sedative-hypnotic agent with no analgesic properties. Because of its ease of administration and safety profile, it remains one of most popular sedative agents used in the pediatric population. Recommended doses range from 30 to 100 mg/kg (maximum dose of 2 g), although the likelihood of sedation failure increases with doses less than 60 mg/kg.[24] Chloral hydrate may be administered either orally or rectally. While efficacy and onset of action seem to be more predictable with oral administration, rectal administration may be required in some children due to the unpalatable taste of the drug and the potential to cause gastrointestinal (GI) upset. It is used most commonly for sedation during radiologic or echocardiographic evaluations.

Chloral hydrate is rapidly absorbed from the GI tract and metabolized to the active compound trichloroethanol, which is further metabolized by the liver to the inactive trichloroacetic acid. The mean time to onset of sleep is 25 minutes, although a wide range (5-120+ minutes) has been reported.[24,25] Similarly, the mean duration of sleep is 60 to 90 minutes, but may last more than 6 hours. While it has been generally felt that chloral hydrate produces a relatively lighter depth of sedation compared with other agents, Malviya et al[17] reported, during a more formal evaluation of depth of sleep, that a significant number of patients sedated with chloral hydrate (50-75 mg/kg) became deeply sedated.

One of the most often discussed advantages of chloral hydrate is its favorable cardiorespiratory profile, with most reports confirming few adverse respiratory or hemodynamic events. However, significant hypoxemia from obstruction during sleep and death from respiratory depression have been reported.[26] Due to its long half-life, children should be monitored following their procedure until fully awake because mortality has been reported in patients discharged home before being fully awake after receiving chloral hydrate.[27] Ventricular dysrhythmias also have been reported, particularly when administered with other pro-dysrhythmic drugs (eg, phenothiazines or tricyclic antidepressants), and are believed to be related to trichloroethanol, which is a halogenated hydrocarbon and sensitizes the myocardium to the arrhythmogenic effects of endogenous catecholamines. More common adverse events include GI upset/vomiting (6%-7%), ataxia (17%), and paradoxical agitation (2%-18%).[24,25] The latter reaction can be particularly upsetting for parents and health care providers. Paradoxical agitation has been associated with increasing age (older than 5-6 years), and underlying neurologic disorders. As such, it may be advisable to use alternative agents in these patient populations.

Benzodiazepines

Benzodiazepines are anxiolytic, sedative-hypnotic agents. They produce antegrade and retrograde amnesia, muscle relaxation, and sedation, but have no analgesic properties. They induce sedation via potentiation of chloride currents via neuroinhibitory γ-aminobutyric acid (GABA) receptors. They are used commonly as sole agents for both anxiolysis and/or sedation during non-painful procedures or in combination with other agents (eg, opioids, ketamine) for painful procedures.

There are 3 commonly used benzodiazepines: lorazepam, diazepam, and midazolam. While all 3 are effective, lorazepam and diazepam have a relatively longer duration of action, and diazepam causes pain on injection due to the propylene glycol in which it is dissolved. Conversely, midazolam is water-soluble, so there is no pain with intravenous administration. Midazolam has multiple effective delivery routes, and a shorter elimination half-life than diazepam and lorazepam. Therefore, it has become the benzodiazepine of choice for procedure-related applications. Due to its rapid onset of action and short duration, midazolam should be administered intravenously if intravenous access is already present. Sedation and anxiolysis are produced within minutes of administration and the duration of action is 30 to 60 minutes. Starting doses of 0.05 mg/kg (maximum dose 2 mg) can be administered intravenously every 2 to 3 minutes and titrated to achieve the desired effect.

For minor procedures for which intravenous access is not required (or desired) non-parenteral routes may be used. Oral administration of 0.5 to 0.7 mg/kg produces anxiolysis in 15 to 20 minutes and is currently the preferred agent for premedication in the operating room. The mean duration of action is 60 minutes (range 45-120 minutes).[28] The primary disadvantage of oral administration is that the commonly used intravenous preparation (5 mg/mL) contains the preservative benzyl alcohol, which gives the drug a very bitter taste. Mixing the drug in a strong fruit-flavored drink, acetaminophen elixir, or other syrupy sweet solutions may mask the taste. Concern has been raised regarding the potential for altering the absorption characteristics of midazolam based on the solution in which it is mixed. Alternatively, a commercially available preparation of midazolam in a cherry-flavored solution for oral administration is available (Versed syrup, Roche Laboratories Inc, Nutley, NJ). Because of the control of pH by the manufacturers, preliminary data suggest that effective sedation can be achieved with doses as low as 0.25 mg/kg compared with the 0.5 to 1.0 mg/kg doses reported when using the intravenous preparation diluted in other solutions.[29]

Alternative non-parenteral administration routes include intranasal and sublingual administration. The dose (0.2-0.4 mg/kg) is lower compared with the oral route. Midazolam is absorbed rapidly across mucosal surfaces and sedation occurs within 5 to 10 minutes. Patients may object to intranasal administration because the benzyl alcohol may burn the nasal mucosa. This is avoided in sublingual administration, but issues of taste and patient cooperation may limit the usefulness of this route.

When midazolam is used as a sole sedative agent, cardiorespiratory suppression is rare and sedation tends to be lighter, with many patients remaining awake, calm, and cooperative. While this may limit the use of midazolam in younger children for procedures in which movement cannot be tolerated, it is an ideal agent for older children who simply require anxiolysis. When administered with other agents, particularly opioids, respiratory depression can occur.[30,31] Similarly, hypotension is uncommon with midazolam alone, but can occur when combined with opioids. Paradoxical excitement or delirium can occur with lower doses, particularly if pain is present.

α-adrenergic Agonists

While α_2-adrenergic agonists have been in clinical use for some time, they have not played a major role in procedural sedation. However, a recently developed specific α_2-adrenergic agonist, dexmedetomidine, has been shown to provide effective sedation during mechanical ventilation in adults[32] and children.[33] Dexmedetomidine is primarily a sedative/anxiolytic agent, although it has been shown to decrease opioid requirements during the perioperative period, thereby demonstrating analgesic or opioid-sparing properties as well.[32]

Because it is a specific α_2-adrenergic agonist, dexmedetomidine provides sedation with fewer cardiovascular effects compared with other α_2-adrenergic agonists, such as clonidine. It also causes less respiratory depression compared with other sedative/analgesic agents[34] and has a relatively short elimination half-life (2 hours). Given these advantages, dexmedetomidine is being used for sedation during MRI and other non-painful radiologic examinations. Sedation is effectively induced with a loading dose of 0.5 to 1.0 μg/kg and then maintained with an infusion of 0.5 to 0.75 μg/kg/h. The loading dose is administered over 5 to 10 minutes because more rapid infusions may cause significant bradycardia, hypotension, or even hypertension (from peripheral α_1-adrenergic agonism).[35] The development of bradycardia may be exaggerated when taken concurrently with other negative chronotropic agents, such as digoxin.[36] Sedation develops without the agitation that often accompanies sedation with chloral hydrate or sodium pentobarbital and recovery is generally smooth and rapid. While further data are needed, dexmedetomidine seems to offer a safe, effective, and appealing option during noninvasive procedures.

Analgesic Agents

Opioids

Opioids provide analgesia and varying degrees of sedation without amnesia. Therefore, they frequently are combined with a benzodiazepine for procedural sedation. As has been discussed previously, this combination may cause significant respiratory depression, so appropriate monitoring must be used and resuscitative equipment be readily available during these sedations. The risks of respiratory depression are similar with equipotent doses of any of the opioid drugs.

The most commonly used opioids for procedural sedation are morphine, meperidine, and fentanyl. The effects of morphine and meperidine last relatively long (2-4 hours), which increases the risk for adverse respiratory events for a significant period after the procedure when there is little patient stimulus and when vigilance and monitoring may be more relaxed.[37] However, a longer duration of action also provides prolonged analgesia, which is beneficial in some circumstances (eg, fracture reduction).

Fentanyl is a synthetic opioid with a potency 100 times greater than morphine. It is a pure analgesic with no sedative properties. It is highly lipid-soluble, which allows rapid penetration across the blood/brain barrier and a rapid onset of action. It is rapidly metabolized with a duration of action of 20 to 30 minutes, making it an attractive option for short procedures such as lumbar puncture or fracture reduction. Fentanyl is administered in increments of 0.5 to 1.0 μg/kg every 2 to 3 minutes and titrated to effect. Rapid administration, especially of higher doses, may cause chest wall rigidity and impair respiratory function. This can be treated with naloxone or neuromuscular blocking agents and controlled ventilation. An additional concern with fentanyl is the risk of inadvertent overdose because it is available only as a 50 μg/mL preparation.

Fentanyl was available previously in a transmucosal preparation with the drug incorporated into a raspberry flavored lozenge called the fentanyl Oralet. Sedation resulted from direct transmucosal absorption because gastric bioavailability was limited (5%-10%). Onset of analgesia and sedation generally occurred in 10 to 15 minutes. It was most frequently used as a preoperative medication in doses of 10 to 20 μg/kg, although later applications included oncologic procedures[38] and laceration repair.[39] Effective sedation was reported, although at the higher doses, adverse effects, including pruritus (65%), nausea and vomiting (31%), and desaturation (7%) were common.[38] While the fentanyl Oralet is no longer commercially available, a newer preparation, Actiq (Cephalon, West Chester, PA), is now available, which also provides fentanyl in a similar formulation. It is available in dosages of 200, 400, 600, 800, 1,200, and 1,600 μg. Currently, it is approved only for use in treating cancer-related pain and it is not recommended for procedure-related use.

Remifentanil is an ultra–short-acting synthetic opioid, metabolized by plasma esterases with a half-life of 8 to 10 minutes. Although popular for intraoperative use when rapid awakening is desired, interest has developed in using this agent for procedural sedation. Dosing regimens include an infusion of 0.05 to 0.2 μg/kg/min, with or without an induction bolus of 0.2 to 1 μg/kg over 2 to 5 minutes. Because remifentanil has no amnestic properties, it is combined with midazolam[31] or propofol[40,41] to provide sedation for lumbar punctures, fracture reductions, and flexible fiberoptic bronchoscopy. These regimens provide effective sedation with rapid recovery (5-20 minutes). However, the reported incidence of respiratory depression or desaturation is relatively high (20%-25%), which may limit widespread use of this drug. Other reported adverse effects include nausea, vomiting, and pruritus.

Ketamine

Ketamine is a dissociative anesthetic chemically related to phencyclidine.[42] Unlike the previously mentioned agents, it provides sedation, analgesia, and amnesia. It is metabolized in the liver and has an active metabolite (norketamine), which has one third of the analgesic potency of the parent drug. Interestingly, analgesia with orally administered ketamine occurs at a lower plasma level than with intramuscular administration, likely as a result of higher concentrations of norketamine being produced from first-pass hepatic metabolism with oral administration.

The advantages of ketamine include a relatively short duration of action (15 to 30 minutes), multiple routes of administration, and the provision of both amnesia and analgesia, as well as a favorable cardiorespiratory profile. Ketamine produces minimal respiratory depression and has bronchodilating properties, making it an attractive agent for patients with reactive airway disease. Because it stimulates the release of endogenous catecholamines, ketamine causes an early and transient elevation of heart rate and blood pressure. Cardiovascular depression is uncommon and should occur only in patients with catecholamine-depleted states. Due to the excellent analgesia produced, ketamine has become a popular agent for painful or invasive procedures, including fracture reductions, invasive line insertions, oncologic procedures, and endoscopies.[43-45] Experience with ketamine administration via the nasal, oral, or intramuscular routes has been positive also.[46,47] As with midazolam, when the intravenous solution is used, burning may occur with contact to mucous membranes, whereas oral administration requires diluting the solution in a liquid to mask its unpleasant taste and the use of larger doses (5-10 mg/kg) due to decreased oral bioavailability.

Despite providing excellent sedation and analgesia, ketamine may, in rare cases, cause specific adverse effects such as apnea, laryngospasm, and loss of protective airway reflexes. Therefore, it should be used with the same NPO guidelines as the other sedative/analgesic agents. Apnea seems to be more common in younger children, which has prompted some to exclude children younger than 3 months from ketamine protocols. However, a recent report describes the safe and effective use of ketamine during flexible bronchoscopy in infants.[48] Ketamine increases the production of upper airway secretions and should, therefore, be administered with an antisialagogue (glycopyrrolate). Nausea and vomiting are not infrequent and premedication with an antiemetic should be considered, particularly in patients with a history of vomiting.

The most frequently discussed adverse effects of ketamine are emergence delirium and/or hallucinations. These occur more commonly if ketamine is used alone and in older patients. While many patients will still experience dysphoria during recovery, the concurrent administration of a benzodiazepine (eg, midazolam) with ketamine is very effective in eliminating the occurrence of true delirium or hallucinations. While early reports suggested that ketamine increases intracranial pressure (ICP), more recent reports have demonstrated that the ICP response can be blunted or obliterated when a benzodiazepine is added,[49] allowing ketamine to remain an option for sedation during lumbar puncture when an opening pressure is desired. The effect of ketamine on patients with seizures remains unclear and controversial. Although seizures have been reported following its administration in at-risk patients, ketamine also has been used to treat refractory status epilepticus.

Intravenous use is preferred if intravenous access is available because the onset of action is rapid (1-2 minutes) and the recovery time is short (30-60 minutes). Midazolam (0.05-0.1 mg/kg), and glycopyrrolate (5 to 10 μg/kg) are administered 3 to 5 minutes before ketamine. The initial dose of ketamine is 0.5 to 1 mg/kg. Additional doses of 0.5 mg/kg may be administered every 2 to 3 minutes to achieve and maintain the desired levels of sedation and analgesia. The initial dose for intramuscular administration is 4 to 6 mg/kg. The 100 mg/mL preparation of ketamine should be used to limit the injected volume, and glycopyrrolate, 5 to 10 µg/kg, may be mixed with the ketamine prior to injection. Additional injections of 2 to 4 mg/kg of ketamine may be administered after 5 to 10 minutes if adequate sedation is not achieved. For oral administration, 10 mg/kg is used. The drug may be mixed in a small amount of a clear fluid to make it more palatable. Moderate to deep sedation occurs in 30 to 45 minutes. Emergence reactions have not been a significant problem with either intramuscular or oral ketamine, even without concomitant administration of midazolam.

Anesthetic Agents

Barbiturates

Barbiturates remain commonly used agents for intravenous induction of anesthesia. They are potent respiratory depressants, so appropriate airway management skills and monitoring for deep sedation are required. The 3 most commonly used agents are methohexital, thiopental, and pentobarbital. Like the benzodiazepines, barbiturates provide sedation and amnesia without analgesia. Consequently, they are useful for non-painful procedures, especially radiologic procedures such as CT scanning or MRIs.

Methohexital is a short-acting oxybarbiturate with a long history of use as a *per rectum* induction agent in children. It also has been used extensively as a sedative for CT scans and MRIs with reported success rates of 80% to 85%.[50] The standard rectal dose is 20 to 30 mg/kg. Onset of sleep is rapid (6-10 minutes) with recovery to baseline occurring by 1.5 to 2 hours after administration. Adverse effects are uncommon; mild respiratory depression responsive to repositioning and/or supplemental oxygen occurs in up to 4% of patients. The duration of action with intravenous use (0.75-1.0 mg/kg) is approximately 10 minutes, making the drug attractive for short procedures such as CT scans. However, the incidence of respiratory depression is greater with this route of administration, which may limit its usefulness. Methohexital has been reported to precipitate seizures in patients with underlying seizure disorders.

Thiopental is another short-acting barbiturate and is the most commonly used barbiturate for intravenous induction of anesthesia. Like all barbiturates, thiopental has negative inotropic and vasodilatory properties that can result in hypotension, especially in patients with hypovolemia or underlying cardiovascular dysfunction. Rapid redistribution accounts for its short duration of action (5-10 minutes) after intravenous administration. It is a potent anticonvulsant and may be safely administered to patients with seizure disorders. It also has been used as a rectal agent for sedation for radiologic procedures in doses of 25 to 50 mg/kg.[51,52] The depth of sedation achieved is somewhat deeper than with methohexital and reported success rates for procedures are somewhat higher (>90%). The onset of action is slightly longer (15-30 minutes) with a similar duration of action (60-90 minutes) compared with methohexital.

Sodium pentobarbital is a longer-acting barbiturate than either methohexital or thiopental and remains a popular choice for intravenous sedation during radiologic procedures, especially MRIs. Multiple delivery options are available including intravenous, intramuscular, and enteral; although intravenous delivery is used most commonly. For intravenous administration, pentobarbital should be given in increments of 1 to 2 mg/kg every 3 to 5 minutes until sleep is induced (average total dose 4-5 mg/kg).[53] The average duration of sleep after induction is 60 to 90 minutes, which is adequate to perform most routine MRI evaluations. Respiratory depression and hypotension may occur, especially with rapid intravenous administration. A drawback to pentobarbital sedation is that recovery time may be long (2-4 hours) and emergence problems, including agitation, may occur.

Propofol

Propofol is an anesthetic agent with sedative and hypnotic properties. It is available only for intravenous administration. It has a rapid onset and a short duration of action (5-10 minutes) allowing for early discharge. Given its short duration of action, an infusion or repeated bolus doses generally are needed for all but the briefest procedures. Propofol also provides a beneficial antiemetic effect. It decreases the cerebral metabolic rate for oxygen and ICP, making it an attractive agent in patients with intracranial hypertension, provided that airway control and mechanical ventilation are in place.

Adverse effects associated with propofol are similar to those of other sedatives. Propofol can cause cardiovascular depression and hypotension, related to both negative inotropic and vasodilatory properties.[54] Respiratory depression is dose-dependent and apnea easily can be induced with excessive or rapid bolus dosing. Other reported central nervous system (CNS) effects include opisthotonus, myoclonus, and other movement disorders. To date, there is no EEG documented seizure activity during propofol administration and given its anticonvulsant properties, propofol remains in many of the treatment algorithms for refractory status epilepticus.[55] Administration of propofol is associated with a high incidence of pain, particularly when injected into the small veins on the dorsum of the hand.[56] Administering a small dose of fentanyl (0.5-1 μg/kg), lidocaine (0.2-0.5 mg/kg), or ketamine (0.5 mg/kg) before injection, or cooling the solution, may decrease the likelihood of pain. Propofol remains restricted to use by anesthesia personnel in some institutions, primarily due to its cardiorespiratory effects.

For all but the shortest procedures, propofol generally is administered as a bolus induction dose followed by an infusion. For radiologic or non-painful procedures, propofol may be used as a single agent. For short, painful procedures, such as lumbar punctures, the addition of an analgesic agent such as fentanyl (1 μg/kg), remifentanil, or ketamine should be considered. Because individual responses vary from patient to patient, sedation should be induced using intermittent boluses of 0.5 to 1 mg/kg every 1 to 2 minutes until adequate sedation is achieved (usually 1-3 mg/kg total). For brief procedures, continued use of intermittent bolus doses (0.5 - 1 mg/kg) may be used; whereas, for longer procedures, sedation may be maintained with an infusion of 60 to 300 µg/kg/min.[57] Alternatively, there is recent clinical experience with mixing ketamine (1-3 mg/mL) or remifentanil (15-20 µg/mL) in a single syringe with propofol. For such purposes, ketamine can be added to propofol in a concentration of 1 to 3 mg/mL.

Nitrous Oxide

Nitrous oxide has a rapid onset of action, is relatively easy and inexpensive to use, and its effects dissipate rapidly once discontinued. Its solubility characteristics allow rapid induction and awakening. It has sedative/hypnotic, amnestic, and analgesic properties. It has been in clinical use as an anesthetic agent for more than 150 years and also has an extensive history of use in procedural sedation, primarily in emergency departments, burn units, and dental practices.

Nitrous oxide can be administered using either a demand-flow (face mask only) or free-flow (face mask or nasal cannula) gas system in concentrations of 30% to 70%. In the demand flow system, gas flow occurs only when the patient is sufficiently alert to hold the mask to his or her face and create a negative inspiratory pressure. Although this system effectively prevents inadvertent oversedation, it may preclude its use in the younger child (≤5 or 6 years) or the child with developmental delay. Safety features to prevent the delivery of a hypoxic gas mixture include an in-line FiO_2 monitor, a “fail-safe” device to cut off nitrous oxide flow if the oxygen supply fails, and a system to regulate the ratio of the flow rates of the oxygen and nitrous oxide so that more than 70% nitrous oxide cannot be delivered. Alternatively, commercially available tanks are manufactured that contain a 50/50 mixture of oxygen and nitrous oxide. A scavenger device attached to the delivery system is required to remove waste gases and prevent environmental pollution.

When administered at standard concentrations, nitrous oxide can cause mild hypotension. The solubility of nitrous oxide is such that it continues to diffuse into the alveoli from the blood after gas administration has been discontinued, thereby diluting the oxygen in the alveoli leading to the potential for diffusion hypoxemia. Therefore, 100% oxygen is routinely administered when nitrous oxide is discontinued. Nitrous oxide diffuses quickly into air-filled spaces, increasing the volume of the space, and is, therefore, contraindicated in bowel obstruction, with pneumocephalus, and intrathoracic injuries with the risk of pneumothorax. Nitrous oxide causes a mild increase in cerebral blood flow and ICP and is relatively contraindicated in patients with closed head injury and altered intracranial compliance. Repeated exposure of the patient or health care workers to nitrous oxide can lead to bone marrow suppression and peripheral neuropathy as a result of its effects on B_{12} metabolism and protein synthesis.

Combination of Agents

Lytic Cocktail

The lytic cocktail, or DPT, is a combination of meperidine (Demerol), promethazine (Phenergan), and chlorpromazine (Thorazine), which produces sedation and analgesia. The constituents usually are formulated in a 2:1:1 mixture, a combination developed from findings that opioid analgesia was potentiated by chlorpromazine, thus facilitating analgesia at lower opioid doses. The mixture initially was used for sedation for cardiac catheterization procedures more than 40 years ago[58] and remains in clinical use for such procedures.

Unfortunately, the DPT combination produces many undesirable side effects. All 3 agents are relatively long acting and sedation may be prolonged. Terndrup et al[59] reported that in 63 patients in the emergency department, the average time to discharge was 4.7 hours and a return to normal behavior was 19 hours. In addition, 29% of patients were inadequately sedated. The mixture may cause significant respiratory depression, which may occur long after the procedure is completed. Phenothiazines are vasodilators and may cause hypotension. Seizures have been reported and are related to the active metabolite of meperidine, normeperidine. The potential for seizures is increased by the concurrent administration of the phenothiazines.[60] Other adverse CNS effects include dystonic reactions, which also are related to the phenothiazines.

Due to these significant adverse effects and the development of safer and more effective sedative regimens, the lytic cocktail has become outdated. In 1995 the AAP Committee on Drugs issued a policy statement which, while not quite suggesting DPT be banned, recommended that alternative sedative and analgesic regimens be considered.[61]

Opioid and Benzodiazepine Reversal Agents

While careful monitoring of drug administration and vigilant patient monitoring should decrease the likelihood of adverse events, they still occur. Interpatient responses to sedative agents are not universal and human error never can be completely eliminated. The availability of specific antagonists for opioids and benzodiazepines has enhanced the safety of procedural sedation. However, these drugs should not take the place of appropriate monitoring and institution of airway management with assisted ventilation.

Opioid Antagonists

Two opioid receptor antagonists are available; naloxone is the most commonly used. It is a competitive antagonist of the μ- and κ-opioid receptors and reverses the effects of analgesia, respiratory depression, and sedation.[62] It may be administered via intravenous, intramuscular, or endotracheal routes, although intravenous administration is preferred. The mean duration of action with intravenous administration is 45 to 60 minutes, but ranges from 15 minutes to hours, and is dose-dependent. Because this is shorter than the duration of action of many opioids, monitoring must continue until the effects of the original drug are dissipated and there is no risk of recurrence of sedation and respiratory depression. Naloxone can precipitate full-blown withdrawal reactions, including seizures, when given to patients who are opioid-dependent, and may completely reverse the analgesia produced by the original opioid given. Therefore, naloxone should be administered in small doses and titrated to clinical effect. The starting dose is 1 to 2 μg/kg, repeated every 2 to 3 minutes until the desired effect is achieved. Slow injection and careful titration of the dose can maximize reversal of respiratory depression while minimizing analgesia reversal.

Nalmefene is a more recently developed opioid antagonist. It has the same receptor binding profile of naloxone, but its duration of action is 2 to 3 hours.[63] Intravenous dosing is 0.25 μg/kg every 2 minutes, up to 4 doses. Clinical benefit beyond a cumulative dose of 1 μg/kg has not been reported. Experience in pediatric patients is limited, but one study suggests that it is both effective and safe.[64]

Benzodiazepine Antagonists

Flumazenil is the only benzodiazepine antagonist currently available for clinical use. It competitively binds to central benzodiazepine receptors, thereby inhibiting GABA receptor activation.[65] Whereas naloxone and nalmefene reverse both sedation and respiratory depression, flumazenil primarily reverses sedation with less effect on respiratory depression. Flumazenil is only recommended for intravenous administration and for acute benzodiazepine intoxications. It is relatively lipophilic, so its onset of action is rapid (within 1-2 minutes). Similar to naloxone, its duration of activity (40-80 minutes) is shorter than that of most benzodiazepines, so there is a risk of resedation.[66] The standard dose is 0.01 to 0.02 mg/kg every 1 to 2 minutes to a maximum of 1.0 mg. Adverse effects occur in approximately 5% of patients. Common effects include agitation, crying, aggression, headache, nausea, and dizziness. Flumazenil is contraindicated in patients receiving chronic benzodiazepine therapy because it may precipitate seizures or withdrawal. Seizures also may occur if flumazenil is given to patients who have ingested medications that lower the seizure threshold (eg, tricyclic antidepressants, methylxanthines, cyclosporine). Flumazenil also can precipitate ventricular dysrhythmias when administered concomitantly with cocaine, methylxanthines, monoamine oxidase inhibitors, chloral hydrate, and tricyclic antidepressants.[65]

The reported pediatric experience is limited, particularly for procedural sedation. Shannon et al[66] administered flumazenil to 107 pediatric patients following sedation with midazolam with or without an opioid. Ninety-six percent of the patients responded to flumazenil at a mean dose of 0.017 mg/kg. Seven patients experienced resedation 19 to 50 minutes following flumazenil administration. There were no significant adverse events.

Despite the efficacy of both naloxone and flumazenil in reversing the sedative and respiratory depressant effects of opioids and benzodiazepines, their availability does not diminish the need for prompt detection of hypoventilation and the ability to intervene by establishing an airway and assisting ventilation.

Topical and Local Anesthetics

While systemic sedative agents play a vital role in relieving procedure-related anxiety and discomfort, appropriate topical preparation of the invasive procedure site is important and can significantly decrease or even eliminate the need for parenteral sedation. This may include the application of a topical anesthetic agent to the skin with or without subsequent infiltration with a local anesthetic agent. Additionally, when the sedation regimen uses an oral or rectal route, intravenous access still may be required. In such cases, a topical anesthetic cream can be applied at the same time the oral medication is given. After 20 to 30 minutes, an intravenous access generally can be established without causing pain.

The first of the topical anesthetic creams was eutectic mixture of local anesthetics (EMLA) cream (Astra-Zeneca Pharmaceutical, Wilmington, DE). It is a mixture of 2 local anesthetics, lidocaine and prilocaine, formulated into a cream for topical administration. A thick layer is applied to the skin, using 1 to 2 g/10 cm^2, and covered with an occlusive dressing.[67] Preformed discs also are available. The depth of analgesia penetration depends on the duration of contact with the skin. A 4 to 5 mm depth of penetration is achieved 45 to 60 minutes after application to intact skin.[68] Analgesia is maintained for up to 30 to 60 minutes following removal of the cream. EMLA cream may be sufficient for superficial procedures and also may facilitate painless deep infiltration of a local anesthetic for deeper procedures.

It has been used extensively in children for a variety of invasive procedures, including venipuncture, intravenous insertion, subcutaneous venous reservoir accessing, lumbar puncture, bone marrow aspiration, laser therapy of dermal lesions, joint aspiration, circumcision, cardiac catheterization, and central venous catheter placement.[67,69,70] It may be particularly useful in patients undergoing repeated procedures, such as those with oncologic diagnoses, in whom procedure-related anxiety and needle phobia can become severe. It is becoming common practice to have the parents apply the EMLA at home before coming to clinic, thereby avoiding delays while waiting for the cream to be effective.

Reported complications from EMLA are rare. The most serious is methemoglobinemia, which may be induced by the local anesthetic, prilocaine. This is most common in infants because methemoglobin reductase, which converts methemoglobin back to hemoglobin, may be deficient in this population.[71] Additionally, fetal hemoglobin is more susceptible to oxidant stresses and, therefore, is more likely to be converted to methemoglobin. Although demonstrated to be safe and effective during neonatal circumcision and heel stick, with no significant change in methemoglobin levels, EMLA cream should be used cautiously in infants younger than 1 month. Contraindications to use include patients with congential or idiopathic methemoglobinemia, or infants younger than 12 months who are receiving treatment with methemoglobin-inducing agents. Other reported complications have resulted from inadvertent ingestion, usually from young children picking at the dressing and licking the cream, resulting in airway anesthesia and loss of airway protective reflexes.[72] While serum drug concentrations should be low if the cream is properly applied, young children should be closely observed to prevent accidental ingestion, and prehospital application of EMLA should be avoided.

One of the major drawbacks of EMLA is the time required (60 minutes) for it to be effective. This limits its usefulness in procedures that must be performed semi-urgently. Newer topical anesthetic formulations that act more rapidly include a topical 2% lidocaine gel with epinephrine 1:100,000 using iontophoresis (Numby, Iomed Inc, Salt Lake City, UT), a 4% tetracaine gel (Ametop, Smith & Nephew, Hull, United Kingdom), and a 4% liposomal lidocaine mixture (ELA-Max, Ferndale Laboratories, Ferndale, MI). Bishai et al[73] performed a crossover comparison of 4% tetracaine gel with EMLA for Port-a-Cath puncture in 39 children and reported equivalent analgesia after only 30 minutes of tetracaine application compared with 60 minutes of EMLA. Similarly, Eichenfield et al[74] reported equivalent pain relief in 120 children 30 minutes after an application of a 4% liposomal lidocaine gel compared with a 60-minute application of EMLA. No significant adverse effects have been reported with either preparation.

A topically applied mixture of tetracaine, adrenaline, and cocaine (TAC) has been used for the control of pain associated with laceration suturing in the emergency department. Multiple reports have confirmed the safety and efficacy of TAC when used appropriately.[75,76] Dosages should be based on the patient's weight and the concentrations of cocaine and tetracaine in the solution calculated because considerable inter-institutional variation exists among the formulations of TAC. Because both cocaine and epinephrine are vasoconstrictors, TAC should not be applied to areas with limited circulation, such as the pinna of the ear, penis, or digits.

Significant toxicity related to the absorption of cocaine can occur, especially when TAC is inappropriately applied to mucosal surfaces. Complications include seizures, respiratory distress, and death.[77] While these events were reported as resulting from direct application to mucosal surfaces, inadvertent mucosal absorption from solution dripping or running off of a non-mucosal wound also must be avoided. Newer formulations with a lower cocaine content seem to be efficacious, as do non-cocaine containing solutions.[78]

Superficial and deep infiltration with local anesthetic solutions also can provide effective analgesia during invasive procedures. Because systemic toxicity can occur with all agents, limiting the total dose of the drug (based on the patient's weight and the concentration of the solution used) on a mg/kg basis is necessary. This is especially important in smaller patients or if the area to be infiltrated is large. See Chapter 2 for a full discussion of the various local anesthetic agents and their pharmacology.

Most practitioners are familiar with the use of lidocaine for topical anesthesia. Use of the 0.5% preparation is suggested because toxic doses are reached more quickly with higher concentrations. The total dose should not exceed 5 mg/kg or 1 mL/kg of the 0.5% solution. The injection of lidocaine can be painful due to its acidity (pH = 5.0). Ways to decrease discomfort include using a topical anesthetic cream first (see previous text), slow injection, using small-gauge (27 or 30 gauge) needles, and buffering with the addition of 0.1 mEq of sodium bicarbonate per each milliliter of lidocaine.[79] Alternatively, chloroprocaine, a local anesthetic of the ester class, can be used. Vials of chloroprocaine have a pH close to 7.0, thereby obviating the need of adding sodium bicarbonate. Additionally, given its rapid metabolism by serum esterases with a half-life of less than 60 seconds, the risk of toxicity with chloroprocaine is less than with other local anesthetic agents.

Non-pharmacologic Methods

Non-pharmacologic methods may be used either alone or as an adjunct to pharmacologic treatment. Distraction techniques, along with appropriate preparation, can significantly influence the amount of sedation required. Preparation can be as simple as informing the child of the intended procedure and the steps involved. This may be done by the treating physician or with the aid of child life specialists. See Chapter 11 for a full discussion of non-pharmacologic methods of alleviating procedure-related pain and anxiety.

Summary

With increasing recognition of the importance of adequate procedural comfort and the availability of safe and effective agents with which to provide these effects, there are no longer excuses for subjecting children to painful procedures without adequate sedation and analgesia. Conversely, with growing recognition of the factors associated with adverse sedation outcomes, it is incumbent on all practitioners to ensure that children be sedated in the safest environment possible with conformance to the guidelines outlined by the AAP and ASA. Despite extensive experience with procedural sedation, pediatric literature regarding various regimens remains limited. Future directions in pediatric procedural sedation should include the development of multicenter collaborative groups to better document the effectiveness of specific agents/regimens and the components of safe practices.

References

1. American Academy of Pediatrics Committee on Drugs, Section on Anesthesiology. Guidelines for the elective use of conscious sedation, deep sedation, and general anesthesia in pediatric patients. *Pediatrics.* 1985;76:317-321
2. American Academy of Pediatrics Committee on Drugs. Guidelines for monitoring and management of pediatric patients during and after sedation for diagnostic and therapeutic procedures. *Pediatrics.* 1992;89:1110-1115

3. American Academy of Pediatrics Committee on Drugs. Guidelines for monitoring and management of pediatric patients during and after sedation for diagnostic and therapeutic procedures: addendum. *Pediatrics.* 2002;110:836-838
4. Cote CJ. Sedation for the pediatric patient. *Pediatr Clin North Am.* 1994;41:31-58
5. Practice guidelines for sedation and analgesia by non-anesthesiologists: an updated report by the American Society of Anesthesiologists Task Force on Sedation and Analgesia by Non-anesthesiologists. *Anesthesiology.* 2002:96:1004-1017
6. Tinker JH, Dull DH, Caplan RA, Ward RJ, Cheney PW. Role of monitoring devices in prevention of anesthetic mishaps: a closed claims analysis. *Anesthesiology.* 1989;71:541-546
7. Malviya S, Voepel-Lewis T, Tait AR. Adverse events and risk factors associated with the sedation of children by nonanesthesiologists. *Anesth Analg.* 1997;85:1207-1213
8. Cote CJ, Notterman DA, Karl HW, Weinberg JA, McCloskey C. Adverse sedation events in pediatrics: a critical incident analysis of contributing factors. *Pediatrics.* 2000;105:805-814
9. Sinex JE. Pulse oximetry: principles and limitations. *Am J Emerg Med.* 1999;17:59-67
10. Moyle JTB. Uses and abuses of pulse oximetry. *Arch Dis Child.* 1996;74:77-80
11. Malviya S, Reynolds PI, Voepel-Lewis T, et al. False alarms and sensitivity of conventional pulse oximetry versus the Masimo SET™ technology in the pediatric postanesthetic care unit. *Anesth Analg.* 2000;90:1336-1340
12. Bebout DE, Mannheimer PD. The OxiMax system: Nellcor's new platform for oximetry. *Minerva Anestesiol.* 2002;68:236-239
13. Hart LS, Berns SD, Houck CS, Boenning DA. The value of end-tidal CO_2 monitoring when comparing three methods of conscious sedation for children undergoing painful procedures in the emergency department. *Pediatr Emerg Care.* 1997;13:189-193
14. Tobias JD. End-tidal carbon dioxide monitoring during sedation with a combination of midazolam and ketamine for children undergoing painful, invasive procedures. *Pediatr Emerg Care.* 1999;15:173-175
15. Chernik DA, Gillings D, Laine H, et al. Validity and reliability of the Observer's Assessment of Alertness/Sedation Scale: study with intravenous midazolam. *J Clin Psychopharmacol.* 1990;10:244-251

16. Macnab AJ, Levine M, Glick N, Susak L, Baker-Brown G. A research tool for measurement of recovery from sedation: the Vancouver Sedative Recovery Scale. *J Pediatr Surg.* 1991;26:1263-1267
17. Malviya S, Voepel-Lewis T, Tait AR, Merkel S, Trempers K, Naughton M. Depth of sedation in children undergoing computed tomography: validity and reliability of the University of Michigan Sedation Scale (UMSS). *Br J Anaesth.* 2002;88:241-245
18. Sebel PS, Lang E, Rampil IJ, et al. A multicenter study of bispectral electroencephalogram analysis for monitoring anesthetic effect. *Anesth Analg.* 1997;84:891-899
19. Denman WT, Swanson EL, Rosow D, Ezbicki K, Connors PD, Rosow CE. Pediatric evaluation of the bispectral index (BIS) monitor and correlation of BIS with end-tidal sevoflurane concentration in infants and children. *Anesth Analg.* 2000;90:872-878
20. Berkenbosch JW, Fichter CR, Tobias JD. The correlation of the bispectral index monitor with clinical sedation scores during mechanical ventilation in the pediatric intensive care unit. *Anesth Analg.* 2002;94:506-511
21. Aneja R, Heard AM, Fletcher JE, Heard CM. Sedation monitoring of children by the Bispectral Index in the pediatric intensive care unit. *Pediatr Crit Care Med.* 2003;4:60-64
22. Gill M, Green SM, Krauss B. A study of the Bispectral Index Monitor during procedural sedation and analgesia in the Emergency Department. *Ann Emerg Med.* 2003;41:234-241
23. McDermott NB, VanSickle T, Motas D, Friesen RH. Validation of the bispectral Index monitor during conscious and deep sedation in children. *Anesth Analg.* 2003;97:39-43
24. Ronchera-Oms CL, Casillas C, Marti-Bonmati L, et al. Oral chloral hydrate provides effective and safe sedation in paediatric magnetic resonance imaging. *J Clin Pharm Therap.* 1994;19:239-243
25. Lipschitz M, Marino BL, Sanders ST. Chloral hydrate side effects in young children: causes and management. *Heart Lung.* 1993;22:408-414
26. Jastak JT, Pallasch T. Death after chloral hydrate sedation: report of a case. *J Am Dent Assoc.* 1988;116:345-348
27. Cote CJ, Karl HW, Notterman DA, Weinberg JA, McCloskey C. Adverse sedation events in pediatrics: analysis of medications used for sedation. *Pediatrics.* 2000;106:633-644
28. Klein EJ, Diekema DS, Paris CA, Quan L, Cohen M, Seidel KD. A randomized, clinical trial of oral midazolam plus placebo versus oral midazolam plus oral transmucosal fentanyl for sedation during laceration repair. *Pediatrics.* 2002;109:894-897

29. Cote CJ, Cohen IT, Suresh S. A comparison of three doses of a commercially prepared oral midazolam syrup in children. *Anesth Analg.* 2002;94:37-43
30. Kennedy RM, Porter FL, Miller J, Jaffe DM. Comparison of fentanyl/midazolam with ketamine/midazolam for pediatric orthopedic emergencies. *Pediatrics.* 1998;102:956-963
31. Litman RS. Conscious sedation with remifentanil and midazolam during brief painful procedures in children. *Arch Pediatr Adolesc Med.* 1999;153:1085-1088
32. Venn RM, Bradshaw CJ, Spencer R, et al. Preliminary UK experience of dexmedetomidine, a novel agent for postoperative sedation in the intensive care unit. *Anaesthesia.* 1999;54:1136-1142
33. Tobias JD, Berkenbosch JW. Initial experience with dexmedetomidine in pediatric-aged patients. *Paediatr Anaesth.* 2002;12:171-175
34. Venn RM, Hell J, Grounds RM. Respiratory effects of dexmedetomidine in the surgical patient requiring intensive care. *Crit Care.* 2000;4:302-308
35. Dyck JB, Maze M, Haack C, Vuorilehto L, Shafer SL. The pharmacokinetics and hemodynamic effects of intravenous and intramuscular dexmedetomidine hydrochloride in adult human volunteers. *Anesthesiology.* 1993;78:813-820
36. Berkenbosch JW, Tobias JD. Development of bradycardia during sedation with dexmedetomidine in an infant concurrently receiving digoxin. *Pediatr Crit Care Med.* 2003;4:203-205
37. Dahlstrom B, Bovine P, Feychting H, Noack G, Paalzow L. Morphine kinetics in children. *Clin Pharmacol Ther.* 1979;26:354-365
38. Schechter NL, Weisman SJ, Rosenblum M, Bernstein B, Conard PL. The use of transmucosal fentanyl citrate for painful procedures in children. *Pediatrics.* 1995;95:335-339
39. Klein EJ, Diekema DS, Paris CA, Quan L, Cohen M, Seidel KD. A randomized, clinical trial of oral midazolam plus placebo versus oral midazolam plus oral transmucosal fentanyl for sedation during laceration repair. *Pediatrics.* 2002;109:894-897
40. Reyle-Hahn M, Niggemann B, Max M, Streich M, Rossaint R. Remifentanil and propofol for sedation in children and young adolescents undergoing diagnostic flexible bronchoscopy. *Paediatr Anaesth.* 2000;10:59-63
41. Keidan I, Berkenstadt H, Sidi A, Perel A. Propofol/remifentanil versus propofol alone for bone marrow aspiration in paediatric haemato-oncologic patients. *Paediatr Anaesth.* 2001;11:297-301
42. White PF, Way WL, Trevor AJ. Ketamine — its pharmacology and therapeutic uses. *Anesthesiology.* 1982;56:119-136

43. McCarty EC, Mencio GA, Walker LA, Green NE. Ketamine sedation for the reduction of children's fractures in the emergency department. *J Bone Joint Surg.* 2000:82:912-918
44. Parker RI, Mahan RA, Giugliano D, Parker MM. Efficacy and safety of intravenous midazolam and ketamine as sedation for therapeutic and diagnostic procedures in children. *Pediatrics.* 1997;99:427-431
45. Green SM, Klooster M, Harris T, Lynch EL, Rothrock SG. Ketamine sedation for pediatric gastroenterology procedures. *J Pediatr Gastroenterol Nutr.* 2001;32:26-33
46. Tobias JD, Phipps S, Smith B, Mulhern RK. Oral ketamine premedication to alleviate the distress of invasive procedures in pediatric oncology patients. *Pediatrics.* 1992;90:537-541
47. Green SM, Rothrock SG, Lynch EL, et al. Intramuscular ketamine for pediatric sedation in the emergency department: safety profile in 1,022 cases. *Ann Emerg Med.* 1998;31:688-697
48. Berkenbosch JW, Graff GR, Stark JM. Safety and efficacy of ketamine sedation for infant flexible fiberoptic bronchoscopy. *Chest.* 2004;125:1132-1137
49. Thorsen T, Gran L. Ketamine/diazepam infusion anaesthesia with special attention to the effect on cerebrospinal fluid pressure and arterial blood pressure. *Acta Anaesth Scand.* 1980;24:1-4
50. Audenaert SM, Montgomery CL, Thompson DE, Sutherland S. A prospective study of rectal methohexital: efficacy and side effects in 648 cases. *Anesth Analg.* 1995;81:957-961
51. Nguyen MT, Greenberg SB, Fitzhugh KR, Glasier CM. Pediatric imaging: sedation with an injection formulation modified for rectal administration. *Radiology.* 2001;221:760-762
52. Alp H, Orbak Z, Guler I, Altinkaynak S. Efficacy and safety of rectal thiopental, intramuscular cocktail and rectal midazolam for sedation in children undergoing neuroimaging. *Pediatr Int.* 2002;44:628-634
53. Strain JD, Campbell JB, Harvey LA, Foley LC. IV Nembutal: safe sedation for children undergoing CT. *Am J Roentgen.* 1988;151:975-979
54. Short SM, Aun CST. Haemodynamics of propofol in children. *Anaesthesia.* 1991;46:783-785
55. Stecker MM, Kramer TH, Raps EC, O'Meeghan R, Dulaney E, Skaar DJ. Treatment of refractory status epilepticus with propofol: clinical and pharmacokinetic findings. *Epilepsia.* 1998;39:18-26
56. Klement W, Arndt JO. Pain on injection of propofol: effects of concentration and delivery. *Br J Anaesth.* 1991;67:281-284

57. Lowrie L, Weiss AH, Lacombe C. The pediatric sedation unit: a mechanism for pediatric sedation. *Pediatrics.* 1998;102:e30
58. Smith C, Rowe RD, Vlad P. Sedation of children for cardiac catheterization with an ataractic mixture. *Can Anaesth Soc J.* 1958;5:35-40
59. Terndrup TE, Dire DJ, Madden CM, Davis H, Cantor RM, Gavula DP. A prospective analysis of intramuscular meperidine, promethazine, and chlorpromazine in pediatric emergency department patients. *Ann Emerg Med.* 1991;20:31-35
60. Hassan H, Bastani B, Gellens M. Successful treatment of normeperidine neurotoxicity by hemodialysis. *Am J Kid Dis.* 2000;35:146-149
61. American Academy of Pediatrics Committee on Drugs. Reappraisal of Lytic Cocktail/Demerol, Phenergan, Thorazine (DPT) for the sedation of children. *Pediatrics.* 1995;95:598-602
62. Chamberlain JM, Klein BL. A comprehensive review of naloxone for emergency physician. *Am J Emerg Med.* 1994;12:650-660
63. Barsan WG, Seger D, Danzl DF, et al. Duration of antagonistic effects of nalmefene and naloxone in opiate-induced sedation for emergency department procedures. *Am J Emerg Med.* 1989;7:155-161
64. Chumpa A, Kaplan RL, Burns MM, Shannon MW. Nalmefene for elective reversal of procedural sedation in children. *Am J Emerg Med.* 2001;19:545-548
65. Hunkeler W, Mohler H, Pieri L, et al. Selective antagonists of benzodiazepines. *Nature.* 1981;290:514-516
66. Shannon M, Albers G, Burkhart K, et al. Safety and efficacy of flumazenil in the reversal of benzodiazepine-induced conscious sedation. *J Pediatr.* 1997;131:582-586
67. Gajraj NM, Pennant JH, Watcha MF. Eutectic mixture of local anesthetics (EMLA) cream. *Anesth Analg.* 1994;78:574-583
68. Hallen B, Olsson GL, Uppfeld TA. Pain-free venipuncture: effect of timing of application of local anesthetic cream. *Anaesthesia.* 1984;39:969-972
69. Halperin DL, Koren G, Attias D, Pellegrini E, Greenberg ML, Wyss M. Topical skin anesthesia for venous, subcutaneous drug reservoir and lumbar punctures in children. *Pediatrics.* 1989;84:281-284
70. Benini F, Johnston C, Faucher D, Aranda J. Topical anesthesia during circumcision in newborn infants. *J Am Med Assoc.* 1993;270:850-853
71. Frayling IM, Addison GM, Chattergee K, Meakin G. Methaemoglobinemia in children treated with prilocaine-lidocaine cream. *Br Med J.* 1990;301:153-154

72. Norman J, Jones PL. Complications of the use of EMLA [letter]. *Anaesthesia.* 1990;64:403
73. Bishai R, Taddio A, Bar-Oz B, Freedman MH, Koren G. Relative efficacy of amethocaine gel and lidocaine-prilocaine cream for Port-a-Cath puncture in children. *Pediatrics.* 1999;104:e31
74. Eichenfield LF, Funk A, Fallon-Frielander S, Cunningham BB. A clinical study to evaluate the efficacy of ELA-Max (4% liposomal lidocaine) as compared with eutectic mixture of local anesthetics cream for pain reduction of venipuncture in children. *Pediatrics.* 2002;109:1093-1099
75. Hegenbarth MA, Altieri MF, Hawk WH, Greene A, Ochsenschlager DW, O'Donnell R. Comparison of topical tetracaine, adrenaline and cocaine anesthesia with lidocaine anesthesia for repair of lacerations in children. *Ann Emerg Med.* 1990;19:63-67
76. Anderson AB, Colecchi C, Baronoski R, Dewitt TG. Local anesthesia in pediatric patients: topical TAC versus lidocaine. *Ann Emerg Med.* 1990;19:519-522
77. Grant SAD, Hoffman RS. Use of tetracaine, epinephrine, and cocaine as a topical anesthetic in the emergency department. *Ann Emerg Med.* 1992;21:987-997
78. Smith GA, Strausbaugh SD, Harbeck-Weber C, Cohen DM, Shields BJ, Powers JD. New non-cocaine-containing topical anesthetics compared with tetracaine-adrenaline-cocaine during repair of lacerations. *Pediatrics.* 1997;100:825-830
79. Palmon SC, Lloyd AT, Kirsch JR. The effect of needle gauge and lidocaine pH on pain during intradermal injection. *Anesth Analg.*1998;86:379-381

Chapter 6

Sedation in the Pediatric Intensive Care Unit

Joseph D. Tobias, MD, FAAP

The Decision Points: Agent, Route, and Mode of Administration
Tools for Assessing Depth of Sedation in the Pediatric Intensive Care Unit
Agents for Sedation
- Inhalational Anesthetic Agents
- Benzodiazepines
- Ketamine
- Propofol
- Barbiturates
- Opioids
- Miscellaneous Agents
  - Phenothiazines and Butyrophenones
  - Choral Hydrate
  - α_2-adrenergic Agonists

Introduction

Several factors may cause pain and anxiety in infants and children in the pediatric intensive care unit (PICU), and the importance of appropriate sedation and pain control for the PICU patient cannot be overemphasized. Acute pain can be directly related to the underlying medical illness, surgical procedure, or traumatic event. Emotional distress may be caused by separation from parents, disruption of the day-night cycle, the presence of unfamiliar people, the noise of imposing machines and monitoring devices, fear of death, and loss of self-control. Dressing changes for burns, the presence of an endotracheal tube, placement of central venous or arterial cannula, and other invasive procedures are other causes of pain. Although open communication, reassurance, and parental presence may lessen the effect of some of these problems, pharmacologic intervention frequently is necessary to control pain and prevent emotional distress. To avoid potential complications, the administration of sedative and analgesic agents in the PICU should proceed only with appropriate planning, preparation, and caution (Table 6-1).[1]

Few studies have evaluated the pharmacokinetics and pharmacodynamic properties of analgesic and sedative drugs in critically ill patients in general and children in particular.[2-6] Pharmacokinetic studies generally are performed in healthy adult volunteers or postoperative patients and then extrapolated to the critical care population. Unstable patients present significant differences with regard to end-organ function, cardiorespiratory stability, volume of distribution, and metabolic processes. The variability in the PICU patient includes drug-drug interactions, end-organ (hepatic, renal) failure, malnutrition, low plasma proteins with altered drug binding, and alterations in uptake (of particular concern when using non-intravenous routes), delivery (due to alterations in cardiac output), and volume of distribution. While there are no clear guidelines to identify each of these variables and their eventual effects on the specific analgesic or sedative agent used, all should be considered when selecting a specific drug, its dose, and route of administration.

Despite the potential difficulties and risk of adverse effects of providing sedation and analgesia to the PICU patient, the benefits of such care are significant. Aside from the obvious humanitarian concerns, clinical studies have demonstrated improvements in morbidity and mortality with effective analgesic regimens following cardiovascular surgery for congenital heart disease in neonates and infants.[7,8] Although it may not be possible to extrapolate these benefits to the entire PICU population, effective sedation may provide benefits under other circumstances. Sedation during mechanical ventilation has become increasingly important with newer modalities of mechanical ventilation, such as permissive hypercapnia, reverse inspiratory-expiratory ratio ventilation, and high-frequency techniques. Without effective tech-

Table 6-1. Preparation for Pediatric Intensive Care Unit Sedation

1. Rule out treatable causes of agitation.
   - Hypoxia
   - Hypercarbia
   - Cerebral hypoperfusion
   - Bladder distention
   - Surgical lesion—necrotic bowel
2. Identify etiology of pain or agitation to guide appropriate selection of agent or agents.
3. Monitor patient according to standards outlined by the American Academy of Pediatrics.
4. Identify
   - Agent to be used.
   - Route of administration (intravenous, inhalation, subcutaneous, oral, neuraxial).
   - Mode of administration (intermittent bolus, continuous infusion, or patient-controlled delivery).
5. Titrate the dose based on the patient's clinical response.
6. Observe for adverse effects.
7. Monitor response using formalized pain/sedation scale.
8. Observe for signs of tolerance and continue to increase dose as needed.

niques for sedation, there may be a need for neuromuscular blocking agents and their associated risks.[9] Additionally, sedation may serve as a therapeutic tool in the treatment of intracranial hypertension or to modulate pulmonary vascular resistance in patients at risk for pulmonary hypertension.

The Decision Points: Agent, Route, and Mode of Administration

The 3 primary decision points for sedation and analgesia in the PICU include the following: 1) the agent to be used, 2) the route of administration, and 3) the mode of administration. Although several different agents have been used for sedation in the PICU setting (Table 6-2), no single agent can be expected to be effective in all patients or fulfill the criteria of the ideal agent (Table 6-3). Therefore, health care providers should attempt to become facile with several agents to allow a switch from one agent to another when the first-line drug is either ineffective or leads to adverse effects.

When initiating a sedation/analgesia regimen, monitoring the response to the therapy is important. The importance of titrating the

Table 6-2. Agents for Pediatric Intensive Care Unit Sedation

Agents
Inhalational anesthetic agents
Benzodiazepines
Opioids
Phenothiazines
Butyrophenones
Antihistamines
Chloral hydrate
Etomidate
Ketamine
Barbiturates
Propofol
α_2-adrenergic agonists

dose of the sedative/analgesic agent to the desired effect is illustrated by the study of Katz and Kelly.[5] When evaluating the infusion rate of fentanyl required to provide sedation during mechanical ventilation in neonates and infants, they noted variability ranging from 0.47 to 10.3 μg/kg/h to achieve a similar effect. This variability is magnified in the PICU patient who may have alterations in volume of distribution, protein binding, hepatic blood flow, or renal/hepatic function, thereby further altering the pharmacokinetics of sedative/analgesic agents.[6] Given this diversity, it is not possible to formulate a "cookbook" with strict guidelines about the medications to be used and especially the doses required for sedation and analgesia. These medications are not dosed on a per kilogram basis like antibiotics, but must be titrated up and down to achieve the desired level of sedation. The dosing recommendations given later in the chapter are only meant to be starting doses. The actual amount should be titrated up or down to achieve the desired level of sedation or analgesia, while avoiding the occurrence of

Table 6-3. Properties of the Ideal Agent for Pediatric Intensive Care Unit Sedation

Rapid onset
Easy to titrate by intravenous infusion
Predictable duration of effect
Lack of active metabolites
Effects dissipate rapidly when agent discontinued
Non-parenteral options for route of delivery
Limited effects on cardiorespiratory function
Limited adverse effect profile
Effects and duration not altered by renal or hepatic disease
No interference with effect or metabolism by other medications
Wide therapeutic index
Cost-effective
Slow development of tolerance

adverse effects. (See page 214 for a discussion regarding tools for the assessment of the depth of sedation.)

Options for route of delivery in the PICU patient have expanded. In most patients, the intravenous route is chosen; however, in certain situations, alternative, non-intravenous routes may become necessary. Drug incompatibilities may preclude intravenous administration in patients with limited intravenous access. With specific drugs, alternative routes of delivery may be available (Table 6-4). For example, chloral hydrate may be administered orally or rectally, isoflurane may be administered by inhalation, while propofol requires intravenous administration. Other agents, such as midazolam, may be administered via several routes (intravenous, intramuscular, subcutaneous, oral, nasal, sublingual). However, the non-intravenous route may not be optimal for repeated administration and also negates a rapid titration to the desired level of sedation, which is easily achieved with intravenous administration.

The third of the 3 primary decision points is the mode of administration. Options include continuous administration, intermittent dosing, or patient-controlled techniques. Although longer-acting agents

Table 6-4. Potential Routes of Delivery for Sedative/Analgesic Agents

Route
Intravenous
Intramuscular
Subcutaneous
Oral
Transmucosal
Buccal
Nasal
Rectal
Sublingual
Transdermal
Inhalation

(lorazepam, pentobarbital, morphine) may be used by intermittent, bolus administration, when the need for sedation/analgesia is prolonged, short-acting agents (midazolam, fentanyl) usually are best administered by a continuous infusion to maintain a steady state serum concentration, thereby providing an ongoing effect. An alternative mode, used most commonly in the postoperative period for the delivery of analgesic agents, is a patient-activated device otherwise known as patient-controlled analgesia (PCA). Although not in widespread use in the PICU population, PCA devices also may be considered for the delivery of sedative and anxiolytic agents to allow patients some control over their level of sedation. The initial clinical studies in adults in the operating room setting, where PCA has been used during brief surgical procedures, have demonstrated similar results as studies using PCA for postoperative analgesia. Patients report an increased level of satisfaction with a decreased requirement for sedative or analgesic agents. When used in this manner, it has been suggested that the technique be called "patient-controlled anxiolysis." An additional advantage of this technique is that the device is continuously attached to the intravenous infusion and, therefore, repeated entering of the line is not required to administer bolus doses. When central venous access is in place, limitations of "breaks" into the line may theoretically decrease the overall incidence of central line sepsis.

Tools for Assessing Depth of Sedation in the Pediatric Intensive Care Unit

Assessing depth of sedation should be an ongoing process, and the infusion rates of sedatives and analgesics should be increased or decreased as needed. In many cases, a subjective measure is used to evaluate the dose of sedative. For example, the amount of sedative agent administered is titrated to allow the patient to tolerate mechanical ventilation. Although the amount of sedative necessary for tolerating an endotracheal tube and mechanical ventilation are frequently used end points, monitoring also may involve the use of formal pain/sedation scoring systems by the nursing staff. These sedation scores can be assessed with other routine vital signs at specific intervals. The most commonly used PICU sedation scores take into account 2 basic parameters: physiologic variables and an objective assessment of the patient's depth of sedation. The latter frequently includes the patient's response to a tactile stimulus. The COMFORT scale combines a patient's response/movement with physiologic parameters.[10] It relies on the measurement of alertness, respiration, blood pressure, muscle tone, agitation, movement, heart rate, and facial tension. This scoring system has been validated in the pediatric patient and may have utility in assessing mechanically ventilated pediatric patients.[10,11] Alternatively, other scoring systems, such as the Agitation-Sedation Scale, do not rely on physiologic parameters such as heart rate and blood pressure, but rather visually assess the level of the patient's comfort, grading it from 1 (unarousable) to 7 (dangerous agitation, such as pulling at the endotracheal tube).[12] Similarly, the Ramsay score assigns a value ranging from 1 (awake, anxious, and agitated) to 6 (no response to a glabellar tap) based on observing the patient.[13] Both the Ramsay score and the Agitation-Sedation Scale use a physical or noxious stimulus to evaluate deeper levels of sedation. Although many of these scales have been validated for the intensive care unit (ICU) population, there are significant problems with their use. Scales that rely on physiologic parameters can be misleading in an ICU setting, where significant alterations in vital signs can occur unrelated to the level of sedation. Patients with severe cardiovascular dysfunction requiring vasoactive medications may not develop tachycardia and hypertension despite severe degrees of agitation. Scales that assess the response to a tactile stimulus require disturbing a sleeping or resting patient to differentiate between the deeper levels of sedation. Obviously, scales that evaluate a patient's response to a stimulus or observe their behavior are not valid in patients receiving neuromuscular blocking agents that prevent patient movement. Additionally, because many factors may need to be assessed to derive a score, use of these scales can be time consuming.

The Bispectral Index (BIS) (Aspect Medical, Newton, MA) is a processed electroencephalographic (EEG) parameter, expressed as a numeric value ranging from 0 (isoelectric) to 100 (awake with eyes open), which is used clinically as a measure of hypnosis and awareness. Routinely it has been used to monitor the effects of anesthetic and sedative agents intraoperatively. Lower numeric values indicate deeper hypnosis, while higher values indicate a lightly sedated or awake patient. Bispectral Index values of 60 or less have been shown to indicate a low probability of intraoperative awareness.[14,15] More recently, the BIS monitor has been used in ICU settings where assessment of sedation is critical to interventions such as mechanical ventilation or invasive procedures.[16-19] Clinical experience suggests that it may be particularly efficacious in situations that preclude the use of conventional ICU scoring systems, such as patients receiving neuromuscular blocking agents or medications that may alter heart rate and blood pressure responses. An additional advantage is that it provides a continuous numerical readout, thereby providing a simplistic scale that is immediately available at the bedside, eliminating the need to assess and add various parameters.

Agents for Sedation

Although opioids and benzodiazepines remain the most frequently used agents for sedation,[9] several alternatives are available, including inhalational anesthetic agents, ketamine, propofol, phenothiazines, butyrophenones, α_2-adrenergic agonists, and barbiturates (Table 6-2). These alternative agents are most commonly chosen when opioids and benzodiazepines, either alone or in combination, are ineffective or associated with significant adverse physiologic effects.

Before widespread application and administration to the PICU population, a thorough evaluation of new agents is required. Lessons learned from the past with agents such as etomidate emphasize the importance of this practice. After its introduction into clinical practice, etomidate seemed to be a beneficial agent for ICU sedation due to its lack of adverse effects on cardiovascular function. However, when used by continuous infusion for prolonged periods in the ICU population, increased mortality occurred related to its depressant effects on adrenocortical function and the inhibition of cortisol production.[20] Because of such problems, etomidate is no longer used by continuous infusion in the ICU setting; however, given its lack of effects on cardiovascular function and its beneficial effects on the cerebral metabolic rate for oxygen resulting in a lowering of intracranial pressure (ICP), it remains a useful agent during endotracheal intubation in the patient with increased ICP or altered cardiovascular function. In this setting, etomidate is used as a single bolus dose of 0.2 to 0.3 mg/kg with a neuromuscular blocking agent.[21,22] Other associated adverse effects of etomidate include pain on injection, myoclonic movements, and nausea and vomiting.

Inhalational Anesthetic Agents

The inhalational anesthetic agents (halothane, isoflurane, desflurane, enflurane, sevoflurane) are used routinely to provide intraoperative amnesia during surgical procedures. Clinical experience with inhalational anesthetic agents in the operating room setting has revealed characteristics that may be beneficial for ICU sedation, including a rapid onset, rapid awakening on discontinuation, and ease of control of the depth of sedation. Additionally, these agents are administered through the respiratory system, eliminating the need for mixing infusions and intravenous administration. Although they have seen limited use in the United States, certain centers in Europe have reported favorable experiences when these agents are used for sedation during mechanical ventilation in adult ICU patients.[23]

To date there are no reports on the administration of sevoflurane for ICU sedation. The 4 other inhalational anesthetic agents, halothane, enflurane, isoflurane and, most recently, desflurane,[24] have been used in the ICU setting; however, isoflurane remains the agent most commonly used for ICU sedation. Problems with halothane include a direct negative inotropic and chronotropic effect on myocardial function; the potential for a pro-arrhythmogenic effect, especially in the presence of increased catecholamines or when used in conjunction with other medications (aminophylline); and the occurrence of hepatitis, which is related to an immunologic reaction to trifluoroacetic acid.[25,26] Although the latter problem has been reported with other inhalational agents, including isoflurane, its incidence is less with isoflurane due to its limited metabolism (0.2%) compared with halothane (15%-20%). The risk of developing hepatitis exists not only for the patient, but also health care providers who work in the area, which may be contaminated with inhalational agents. Enflurane has a similar negative inotropic effect and releases fluoride during metabolism. Although only 2% of enflurane is metabolized, its content of fluoride is high enough that, with a 2% metabolism rate, serum fluoride concentrations can increase with prolonged administration. Fluoride concentrations greater than 50 µmol/L can result in nephrotoxicity with a decreased glomerular filtration rate and renal tubular resistance to vasopressin with nephrogenic diabetes insipidus. Sevoflurane also undergoes significant metabolism (3%-5%), and prolonged administration also can result in elevated serum fluoride concentrations.

Given the potential problems with the other agents, isoflurane remains the agent of choice for prolonged use in the ICU setting. Its primary hemodynamic effect is peripheral vasodilatation. This decreases afterload, thereby increasing cardiac output, as opposed to the decrease in cardiac output that occurs with halothane or enflurane. With peripheral vasodilatation, there may be a reflex tachycardia, which can increase myocardial oxygen demand. This effect could lead to an imbalance in the myocardial oxygen delivery/demand ratio in susceptible patients. Isoflurane should be used cautiously in patients at risk for myocardial ischemia or in those who are unable to tolerate tachycardia and a decrease in systemic vascular resistance.

The use of inhalational anesthetic agents poses additional concerns. In addition to the cost of the specialized equipment for delivery and monitoring of the agent, the daily cost for isoflurane can range from $50 to $150 per day, depending on the inspired concentration, the size of the patient, and the minute flow through the ventilator. All inhalational agents are nonspecific vasodilators and can cause cerebral vasodilatation, resulting in an increase in ICP. The degree of cerebral vasodilatation is least with isoflurane and can be partially prevented by hyperventilation to a $PaCO_2$ of 25 to 30 torr.[27,28] With the availability of other agents, which have beneficial effects on the cerebral metabolic rate for oxygen and ICP, the inhalational anesthetic agents are not recommended for continuous sedation in patients with altered intracranial compliance. The inhalational agents alter the metabolism of several other medications, including lidocaine, β-adrenergic antagonists, benzodiazepines, local anesthetics, and other agents that may be administered in the PICU setting.[29] They also may trigger malignant hyperthermia.

Logistic problems may limit the use of inhalational anesthetic agents outside the operating room. These agents are considered general anesthetics, and hospital and state regulations may restrict those who are allowed to adjust the inspired concentration. Changes in concentration may need to be made by physicians or even members of the anesthesiology staff and not the nursing staff, thereby affecting the cost and convenience of this form of sedation. When administered in the operating room, exhaled gases are collected or scavenged and vented from the operating room. Because ICU ventilators do not routinely scavenge exhaled gases, effective scavenging devices must be connected to them to prevent environmental pollution. Delivery of these agents requires specialized equipment, including a vaporizer that converts the liquid to a gas and a monitor to measure the end-tidal (exhaled) concentration of the drug. Although all this equipment is readily available in the operating room, it may be possible to move an anesthesia machine into the ICU. Additionally, anesthesia machine ventilators do not have the diverse functions available on ICU ventilators, which makes their use difficult or impossible in patients with poor pulmonary resistance and compliance. Intensive care units that rely on inhalational sedation may use an ICU ventilator with a vaporizer attached to it. Alternatively, the output from the vaporizer can be added to the ventilator gas through the auxiliary gas inlet.

There remains limited reported clinical experience with the administration of the inhalational anesthetic agents for prolonged sedation in the PICU population. Arnold et al[30] reported their experience with isoflurane for sedation during mechanical ventilation in 10 patients, ranging in age from 3 weeks to 19 years. Effective sedation was achieved in all patients without adverse effects on end-organ function. The highest fluoride concentration was 26.1 μmol/L, and no evidence of renal toxicity was noted. Given the previously mentioned issues, this group of agents will have a limited role for the provision of sedation in the PICU patient; however, they still may have a role in treating refractory status asthmaticus and status epilepticus.

Benzodiazepines

Benzodiazepines remain the most commonly used agents for sedation in the PICU. Benzodiazepines act through the inhibitory neurotransmitter γ-aminobutyric acid (GABA). Binding of the benzodiazepine molecule to the α subunit of the GABA receptor facilitates binding of the GABA molecule to the β subunit, resulting in increased chloride conduction across the neuronal membrane and neuronal hyperpolarization. The benzodiazepines provide amnesia and anxiolysis, but have no intrinsic analgesic properties. Therefore, concomitant administration of an opioid is necessary in situations requiring analgesia.

The benzodiazepines in common clinical use in the United States include diazepam, midazolam, and lorazepam. Previously diazepam was the agent of choice for sedation in both pediatric and adult ICUs. Diazepam's high lipid solubility results in a rapid onset of action; however, its low solubility in water requires administration in a solution of propylene glycol, which can cause pain and thrombophlebitis when administered through a peripheral vein. A new formulation of diazepam eliminates the propylene glycol diluent and delivers diazepam in a lipid base, thereby alleviating the discomfort associated with intravenous administration. Use of diazepam in the PICU setting is limited because of the presence of active metabolites, including oxazepam and N-desmethyldiazepam, which have elimination half-lifes that far exceed that of the parent compound. With repeated administration, the metabolites may accumulate and cause prolonged sedation and delayed awakening once the drug is discontinued.

Midazolam is an imidazobenzodiazepine with a rapid onset of action and a short elimination half-life.[31] Given its short half-life, midazolam is frequently administered by a continuous infusion, except for brief procedures. Clinical experience has demonstrated the efficacy of continuous midazolam infusions for sedation in the PICU patient in starting doses ranging from 0.05 to 0.2 mg/kg/h.[32-34] Midazolam has been approved by the US Food and Drug Administration (FDA) for use by continuous infusion for ICU sedation. Although price had been a concern, with costs ranging from $50 to $100 per day for a patient weighing 20 kg who requires an infusion of 0.1 to 0.2 mg/kg/h, the introduction of generic forms has made midazolam a more cost-effective agent.

Rosen and Rosen[34] reported their retrospective experience with midazolam infusions for sedation during mechanical ventilation in 55 pediatric patients. Dosing included a bolus dose of 0.25 mg/kg followed by a continuous infusion of 0.4 to 4 μg/kg/min (0.02-0.2 mg/kg/h). Midazolam was effective in all patients without significant hemodynamic effects. The authors noted that midazolam became ineffective in one patient following the institution of extracorporeal membrane oxygenation (ECMO) and attributed that to midazolam binding to the surface of the membrane oxygenator.

Although intravenous administration is preferable in the PICU patient, several investigators have described novel routes of delivery for midazolam including oral, rectal, transmucosal (nasal, rectal, sublingual) and subcutaneous.[35-39] Due to the decreased bioavailability in these routes, except for subcutaneous administration, increased doses are required. These alternative routes, although rarely indicated and generally not practical for ongoing sedation in the PICU, may have some role for one-time sedation for brief diagnostic/invasive procedures. (See Chapter 5 for a full discussion of procedural sedation.)

Midazolam is metabolized by isoforms of the cytochrome P_{450} 3A enzyme system to the major hydroxylated metabolite 1-OH midazolam, which has similar potency to the parent compound. It undergoes further hepatic metabolism via the glucuronyl transferase system to 1-OH midazolam-glucuronide. The latter compound also has sedative properties and subsequently undergoes renal excretion because it is water-soluble. In the presence of renal failure, 1-OH midazolam-glucuronide can accumulate and potentiate the effects of midazolam.[40] Several factors, including age and underlying illness, may alter midazolam pharmacokinetics. As mentioned previously, it should be anticipated that similar alterations can occur with any of the agents used in the PICU setting and, therefore, dosing of these medications must be titrated up and down based on the patient's response and, potentially, the BIS number. de Wildt et al[41] evaluated midazolam pharmacokinetics in 21 PICU patients ranging in age from 2 days to 17 years. Because metabolism depends on the hepatic P_{450} system, clearance increases and half-life decreases with age. de Wildt et al[41] also noted in their PICU cohort that midazolam clearance in patients aged 3 to 10 years was significantly longer (5.5 ± 3.5 hours) than that reported in healthy children (1.2 ± 0.3 hours).[42] They concluded that midazolam cannot be considered a drug with a short-elimination half-life in PICU patients and, given that a steady-state serum concentration is not achieved for approximately 20 hours after initiating an infusion (4-5 half-lifes of the medication), sedation should be initiated with a bolus dose prior to the start of the continuous infusion. From this study, they also concluded that renal insufficiency, hepatic failure, and the concomitant administration of medications that affect the P_{450} system significantly affect midazolam pharmacokinetics. Alterations in protein binding with increases in the free fraction also may occur with heparin administration and hepatic/renal dysfunction.[43-45]

Lorazepam is a water-soluble benzodiazepine that has been used for sedation in the PICU. Lorazepam's duration of action is longer and it can be administered effectively by either a continuous infusion or by intermittent, on-demand dosing. Unlike midazolam, lorazepam is metabolized by glucuronyl transferase and not the P_{450} system. Medications known to alter the P_{450} system (anticonvulsants, rifampin, cimetidine) have no effect on the pharmacokinetics of lorazepam. Phase II reactions (glucuronyl transferase) tend to be better preserved in patients with hepatic dysfunction than phase I reactions (P_{450} system), so that the pharmacokinetics of lorazepam remain unchanged. Lorazepam has no active metabolites.

Reported clinical experience with lorazepam in the PICU patient is somewhat limited, especially when compared with midazolam. Pohlman et al[46] compared lorazepam with midazolam for sedation in 20 adult ICU patients. The mean infusion rate for achieving adequate sedation was 0.06 and 0.15 mg/kg/h, respectively, for lorazepam and midazolam. The maximum and mean infusion rates (mg/kg/h) for the entire study period were 0.1/0.06 for lorazepam and 0.29/0.24 for midazolam. The mean number of infusion rate adjustments per day was 1.9 for lorazepam and 3.6 for midazolam. The mean time to return to baseline mental status was 261 minutes with lorazepam and 1,815 minutes with midazolam. Three of 6 surviving patients in the midazolam group required more than 24 hours to return to their baseline mental status, while all 7 in the lorazepam group returned in less than 12 hours. The investigators reported a potency ratio of lorazepam to midazolam of 2.5:1 to achieve the initial sedation, 2.9:1 at the point of maximum infusion rate, and 4:1 overall during the study.

Dundee et al[47] performed a prospective, open-label investigation evaluating lorazepam in 25 adult ICU patients. Lorazepam in a dose of 4 mg was administered at 4- to 6-hour intervals. Lorazepam provided effective sedation without significant adverse effects. No significant change in the hemodynamic profile was noted in 9 patients who had cardiac output measurements following lorazepam administration.

There are limited published data concerning lorazepam for sedation of the PICU patient. Lugo et al[48] described the use of enteral lorazepam to decrease the need for intravenous midazolam, thereby decreasing costs during mechanical ventilation in 30 infants and children. The midazolam infusion was continued until the requirements were stable for 24 hours. The enteral lorazepam dose, administered every 4 to 6 hours, was started at one sixth the total daily intravenous midazolam dose. The midazolam infusion was then titrated to provide the desired level of sedation. The dose of midazolam was significantly reduced on day 1. By day 3, the midazolam infusion was discontinued in 24 of 30 patients. In the remaining 6 patients, although the midazolam could not be discontinued, the daily infusion requirements were reduced by 52%. The projected cost savings was more than $40,000 for the 30 patients. Oral administration of lorazepam also has been reported by Tobias et al[49] for the treatment/prevention of withdrawal following prolonged administration of intravenous benzodiazepines in the PICU patient. (See Chapter 7.)

Each 2 mg/mL of the lorazepam solution is diluted with 0.8 mL (800 mg) of propylene glycol. Several case reports have described propylene glycol toxicity with high-dose or prolonged infusions of lorazepam manifested by metabolic acidosis, renal failure/insufficiency, and an elevated osmolar gap.[50,51] Propylene glycol is metabolized in the liver to lactic acid and pyruvic acid accounting, in part, for the lactic acidosis that occurs. Propylene glycol also is excreted unchanged in the urine, which makes toxicity more likely in patients with renal insufficiency. Because of such concerns, calculation of the propylene glycol infusion rate as well as periodic measurement of the osmolar gap (measured minus calculated serum osmolarity) should be considered during high-dose or prolonged lorazepam infusions. An increasing osmolar gap is suggestive of increasing serum propylene glycol levels. Alternatively, serum propylene glycol levels can be measured by some reference laboratories (concentrations >18 mg/dL can be associated with toxicity). These problems highlight the importance of considering not only the compound itself, but also the carrier vehicle and diluents when considering potential toxicities (see following text for a discussion of problems related to the intralipid carrier for propofol).

The benzodiazepines generally are well tolerated, with limited effects on cardiorespiratory function, especially when used as monotherapy. However, specific situations may arise that necessitate a reversal agent. Flumazenil is a GABA antagonist, or reversal agent, for the benzodiazepines. Breheny[52] demonstrated reversal of midazolam sedation in 14 of 15 ICU patients following administration of flumazenil. However, because the half-life of flumazenil is less than that of midazolam and its metabolites, resedation occurred in 7 of the patients. Given these findings, continued observation of patients is necessary when flumazenil is used to reverse life-threatening adverse effects. With increased clinical use, adverse effects have been reported following flumazenil administration. Seizures may occur, especially in patients chronically receiving benzodiazepines or those exposed to other medications that lower the seizure threshold.[53] Therefore, flumazenil is not recommended for use in the PICU patient who has been chronically receiving benzodiazepines.

Ketamine

Ketamine is an intravenous anesthetic agent chemically related to phencyclidine that was introduced in 1965.[54] Unlike many of the other agents discussed in this chapter that possess only analgesic or sedative effects, a unique attribute of ketamine is that it provides amnesia and analgesia. Ketamine is a racemic mixture of the 2 optical (+,-) isomers; however, preliminary trials are underway to develop an isolated isomer form, which may limit the adverse effects of ketamine. Metabolism of ketamine occurs primarily by hepatic N-methylation to norketamine, which is further metabolized via hydroxylation pathways with subsequent urinary excretion. Norketamine retains approximately one third of the analgesic and sedative properties of the parent compound. Hepatic metabolism suggests that doses should be reduced in patients with hepatic dysfunction. Additionally, due to the renal excretion of norketamine, dose adjustments also may be required in patients with renal dysfunction.

Beneficial properties of ketamine include preserved cardiovascular function, limited effects on respiratory mechanics, and maintenance of central control of ventilation in most patients. These properties make it an effective agent for providing amnesia and analgesia during brief, painful, invasive procedures in the spontaneously breathing patient.[55] Although some centers have switched to shorter-acting agents to allow for a more rapid recovery, ketamine remains a frequently used agent for procedures such as central line placement, bone marrow biopsy, or burn dressing changes. For such purposes, it is administered in incremental, intermittent bolus doses (0.5-1 mg/kg every 1-2 minutes) and titrated to effect. It often is combined with or preceded by an antisialagogue, such as glycopyrrolate, to prevent salivation and a benzodiazepine to limit emergence phenomena.

In most clinical situations, ketamine is associated with the release of endogenous catecholamines, resulting in increased heart rate and blood pressure.[56] Ketamine also acts as a bronchodilator and is a useful agent for patients with status asthmaticus during spontaneous or controlled ventilation. The indirect sympathomimetic effects from endogenous catecholamine release generally overshadow ketamine's direct negative inotropic properties, acting to maintain blood pressure and heart rate. However, hypotension may occur in patients with diminished myocardial contractility.[57,58] In these patients, ketamine's direct negative inotropic properties may predominate when endogenous catecholamine stores have been depleted by stress or chronic illness.

A controversial issue with the use of ketamine, especially in patients with congenital heart disease, is its potential effect on pulmonary vascular resistance (PVR). Conflicting results have been reported in the literature.[59] However, because many of the studies were performed during spontaneous ventilation, the alterations in PVR may have been related to alterations in the $PaCO_2$ and not a direct effect of ketamine on the pulmonary vasculature. Following ketamine administration to spontaneously breathing infants with congenital heart disease, Morray et al[60] noted statistically significant increases in pulmonary artery pressure (from a mean of 20.6-22.8 mmHg) and increases in PVR. Although the PVR change met statistical significance, it is unlikely that there is clinical significance of an average PVR increase of 2.2 mmHg. Hickey et al[61] noted no change in PVR in infants receiving minimal ventilatory support (4 breaths/min and an F_iO_2 of 0.4) in a study that included 14 patients (7 with normal and 7 with elevated baseline PVR). Given the current clinical knowledge, ketamine should be used cautiously in patients with pulmonary hypertension, especially during spontaneous ventilation.

Many respiratory parameters remain unchanged following ketamine administration. Mankikian et al[62] demonstrated no change in functional residual capacity, minute ventilation, and tidal volume following ketamine administration, while other investigators have demonstrated improved pulmonary compliance, decreased resistance, and prevention of bronchospasm.[63] The effects on respiratory mechanics have been at least partially attributed to the release of endogenous catecholamines. Although minute ventilation is generally maintained, elevations of

$PaCO_2$ and a rightward shift of the carbon dioxide response curve have been reported.[64] The potential alterations in $PaCO_2$ should be taken into consideration when administering ketamine to spontaneously breathing patients with increased PVR or alterations in intracranial compliance.

Various reports provide conflicting information about ketamine's effects on protective airway reflexes.[65] Although clinical use and experimental studies suggest that airway reflexes and respiratory function are maintained, aspiration and laryngospasm have been reported following ketamine in spontaneously breathing patients without a protected airway.[66] Ketamine may cause increased oral secretions through stimulation of central cholinergic receptors. The concomitant administration of an antisialagogue, such as atropine or glycopyrrolate, is recommended. In higher doses or in compromised patients, ketamine can cause apnea, upper airway obstruction, laryngospasm, or respiratory compromise, thereby again emphasizing that all sedative/analgesic agents, especially when administered to critically ill patients, should be used only in a controlled environment with appropriate monitoring.

An additional area of controversy surrounding ketamine use is its effect on ICP. As with its effects on PVR, it has been postulated and subsequently demonstrated in laboratory animals that increased ICP associated with ketamine administration may relate more to changes in $PaCO_2$ rather than a direct effect on the cerebral vasculature. Early studies demonstrated that ketamine increased ICP, thereby suggesting that it should not be administered to patients with altered intracranial compliance.[67,68] Those clinical studies were supported by animal studies suggesting that ketamine's effects on ICP were the result of direct cerebral vasodilatation, mediated through central cholinergic receptors.[69,70] However, other animal studies demonstrated no change in ICP following ketamine administration to animals with altered intracranial compliance provided that mechanical ventilation was used to maintain a normal $PaCO_2$.[71,72] Furthermore, in adult patients with head trauma who were sedated with propofol and mechanically ventilated to maintain $PaCO_2$ at 35 to 38 mmHg, ketamine in doses of 1.5, 3, and 5 mg/kg have been shown to decrease ICP (mean decrease of 2 ± 0.5, 4 ± 1, and 5 ± 2 mmHg, respectively, from baseline with the 3 doses).[73] Additionally, the authors noted no change in cerebral perfusion pressure, jugular bulb venous oxygen saturation, and middle cerebral artery blood flow velocity.

Another issue related to the potential central nervous system (CNS) effects of ketamine is its use in patients at risk for or with an underlying seizure disorder. Electroencephalographic recordings in children and laboratory animals during ketamine administration demonstrate increased frequency and amplitude and occasional paroxysmal or seizure activity.[74,75] However, no clinical evidence of seizure activity has been reported with ketamine administration. Furthermore, ketamine has been shown to possess anticonvulsant activity in laboratory animals,[76,77] and at least one report outlines ketamine use for the treatment of refractory status epilepticus.[78]

The most concerning adverse effect of ketamine is emergence phenomena or hallucinations. Emergence phenomena are dose related and tend to occur more commonly in older patients. It is postulated that emergence phenomena result from the alteration of auditory and visual relays in the inferior colliculus and the medical geniculate nucleus, leading to the misinterpretation of visual and auditory stimuli.[79] The administration of a benzodiazepine (lorazepam or midazolam) before administration of ketamine generally is effective in preventing emergence phenomena. For years the ketamine solution available for clinical use was the racemic mixture of the 2 optical isomers. The single enantiomer form, [S or +] ketamine, has been released for clinical use outside of the United States.[80] The [S or +] enantiomer is more potent than the racemic mixture, and initial clinical studies have demonstrated fewer of the psychomimetic effects.[80]

There remains limited reported clinical experience with the use of a ketamine infusion for sedation of the PICU patient during mechanical ventilation. Tobias et al[81] reported anecdotal experience with the use of ketamine infusions for sedation in 5 PICU patients. Four of the 5 patients had experienced adverse cardiorespiratory effects following the administration of benzodiazepines and/or opioids. Ketamine provided effective sedation in all 5 patients without adverse effects. Hartvig et al[82] reported experience with a ketamine infusion to provide sedation and analgesia following cardiac surgery in 10 pediatric patients. The patients ranged in age from 1 week to 30 months. Ketamine was administered in a dose of 1 mg/kg/h to 5 of the patients and in a dose of 2 mg/kg/h to the other 5. Both groups received supplemental doses of midazolam as needed. The plasma clearance of ketamine was 0.94 ± 0.22 L/kg/h with an elimination half-life of 3.1 ± 1.6 hours. Norketamine demonstrated an elimination half-life of 6.0 ± 1.8 hours. The 2 groups had similar and acceptable levels of sedation. No adverse effects were noted.

Because of its favorable effects on cardiorespiratory function, ketamine may be useful in various PICU scenarios including 1) sedation during mechanical ventilation in patients who develop myocardial depression with opioids or benzodiazepines, 2) sedation with the preservation of spontaneous ventilation when using noninvasive ventilation techniques, and 3) sedation during mechanical ventilation in patients with status asthmaticus in whom the release of endogenous catecholamines following ketamine administration may be therapeutic. Dosing regimens for ketamine infusions include a bolus of 1 to 2 mg/kg followed by a continuous infusion starting at 1 mg/kg/h. The infusion can be supplemented with as-needed doses of midazolam to provide a steady baseline level of sedation as well as prevent emergence phenomena. Another option is to combine ketamine and midazolam in a single solution (ketamine 10 mg/mL and midazolam 1 mg/mL). An infusion starting at 0.1 mL/kg/h will provide ketamine 1 mg/kg/h and midazolam 0.1 mg/kg/h. Ketamine is also a useful agent to provide sedation and analgesia during painful invasive procedures, especially in spontaneously breathing patients. For this purpose, an anticholinergic agent (glycopyrrolate 5 µg/kg) and midazolam (0.03-0.05 mg/kg) are administered intravenously, followed by incremental boluses of ketamine (0.5 mg/kg up to a maximum of 25 mg) every 1 to 2 minutes as needed. As with midazolam, several alternative routes of delivery exist for ketamine. Oral, nasal, and rectal routes generally have been used for one-time dosing of the agent for sedation during a procedure. These options will have a limited role for ongoing sedation of the PICU patient.

Propofol

Propofol is an intravenous anesthetic agent of the alkyl phenol family. Given this classification, there may be debates in specific institutions (as there is with ketamine) as to who should be allowed to administer propofol—pediatricians, PICU physicians, or anesthesiologists. Currently, at the University of Missouri, the administration of ketamine and propofol by non-anesthesiologists is allowed, provided the person is accredited by the institution for procedural sedation. Such accreditation requires renewal every 2 years along with renewal of hospital privileges. Decisions such as these should be made by individual institutions.

Propofol is a sedative/amnestic agent with no analgesic properties. It should be combined with an opioid infusion in patients requiring analgesia. Propofol's chemical structure is distinct from that of other intravenous anesthetic agents, including the barbiturates.[83] However, it shares a similar mechanism of action with the benzodiazepines and the barbiturates via the GABA system. Propofol facilitates the binding of the inhibitory neurotransmitter, GABA, to specific membrane-bound receptors, which increase chloride conductance, resulting in neuronal hyperpolarization. Its binding site is distinctly different from that of the barbiturates or benzodiazepines.

Following its introduction into anesthesia practice, propofol's pharmacodynamic profile (rapid onset, rapid recovery time, and lack of active metabolites) made it a logical choice for evaluation as an agent for ICU sedation.[84,85] When compared with midazolam for sedation in adult patients, propofol provides shorter recovery times, improved titration efficiency, and reduced posthypnotic obtundation with faster weaning from mechanical ventilation.[86]

Propofol also has beneficial effects on CNS dynamics, including a decreased cerebral metabolic rate of oxygen ($CMRO_2$) with reflex cerebral vasoconstriction and lowering of ICP.[87] The latter effect is the same as that seen with the barbiturates and etomidate. Preliminary laboratory and clinical experience with propofol has demonstrated its potential as a therapeutic agent in regulating CNS dynamics and controlling ICP. Nimkoff et al[88] evaluated the effects of propofol, methohexital, and ketamine on cerebral perfusion pressure (CPP) and ICP in cytotoxic and vasogenic cerebral edema in felines. Vasogenic cerebral edema was induced by inflating an intracranial balloon, while cytotoxic cerebral edema was induced by an acute reduction of blood osmolarity using hemofiltration. Propofol administration lowered ICP and maintained CPP in vasogenic cerebral edema, but had no effect in cytotoxic cerebral edema. The authors postulated that the loss of autoregulatory function with diffuse cytotoxic edema uncouples $CMRO_2$ from cerebral blood flow (CBF), thereby eliminating propofol's efficacy.

Watts et al[89] evaluated the effects of propofol and hyperventilation on ICP and somatosensory-evoked potentials (SEPs) of intracranial hypertension in rabbits. An intracranial balloon was inflated to increase the ICP to 26 ± 2 mmHg and produce a 50% or greater reduction in SEPs. The animals were randomized to 2 groups: 1) propofol followed by hyperventilation or 2) hyperventilation followed by propofol. Mean arterial pressure (MAP) was maintained at baseline levels by a phenylephrine infusion. The ICP decrease was greater in group 1 (final ICP: 12 ± 2 mmHg vs 16 ± 5 mmHg, *P*=.008). When comparing propofol with hyperventilation, propofol resulted in a greater ICP decrease (final ICP: 16 ± 2 mmHg with propofol vs 21 ± 5 mmHg with hyperventilation, *P*=.007). When propofol was administered first, there was a significant increase in the amplitude of the SEPs. More phenylephrine (*P*<.02) was required to maintain the MAP with propofol than with hyperventilation.

The review of the literature on propofol in humans has provided conflicting results about efficacy in controlling ICP. Although several studies demonstrate a decrease in ICP, propofol's cardiovascular effects and lowering of the MAP generally result in a decrease in the CPP. With intact autoregulation of CBF, a decrease in CPP leads to reflex cerebral vasodilation to maintain CBF. The cerebral vasodilation can increase ICP in patients with altered intracranial compliance. This effect may negate the decrease in ICP related to the decrease in $CMRO_2$ induced by propofol.

Herregods et al[90] evaluated the effect of propofol (2 mg/kg) on ICP and MAP in 6 adults with an ICP greater than 25 mmHg. Mean ICP decreased from 25 ± 3 to 11 ± 4 mmHg (*P*<.05). However, there was a decrease in the MAP and consequently a decrease in the CPP from 92 ± 8 mmHg to a low of 50 ± 7 mmHg. The CPP was less than 50 mmHg in 4 of 6 patients. No vasoconstrictor agent was administered to maintain the MAP. Similar results were obtained by Pinaud et al[91] in adults with traumatic brain injury. Propofol administration resulted in a decreased ICP (11.3 ± 2.6-9.2 ± 2.5 mmHg, *P*<.001) and a decrease in MAP, which resulted in an overall decrease in CPP from 82 ± 14 to 59 ± 7 mmHg, *P*<.01. Other investigators have demonstrated similar results in patients with traumatic brain injury[92] and during cerebral aneurysm surgery.[93] In these studies, although propofol decreased ICP, the decrease in MAP was greater, resulting in an overall decrease in CPP.

If MAP is maintained, propofol can lower ICP and increase CPP. Farling et al[94] administered propofol (2-4 mg/kg/h) for sedation during mechanical ventilation in 10 adult patients with closed head injuries. Additional therapy for increased ICP included mannitol and hyperventilation. There was a statistically significant decrease in the mean ICP of 2.1 mmHg achieved at 2 hours following the start of the propofol infusion. No decrease in MAP was noted. The CPP increased during the 24-hour study period, and the difference was statistically significant at the 24-hour point (9.8 mmHg, P=.028). The authors concluded that propofol was a suitable agent for sedation in patients with head injury requiring mechanical ventilation.

Spitzfadden et al,[95] in their report on the use of propofol to provide sedation and control ICP in 2 adolescents, presented additional anecdotal experience about the therapeutic potential of propofol for the control of ICP. With dopamine used to maintain MAP and CPP, propofol resulted in adequate sedation and control of ICP. When compared with barbiturates, the usual therapy for pharmacologic control of ICP, the authors suggested that a significant advantage of propofol was a much more rapid awakening.

There is also increasing evidence demonstrating a potential beneficial effect of propofol in patients at risk for airway reactivity. In a prospective trial, 77 patients were randomized to receive propofol (2.5 mg/kg), etomidate (0.4 mg/kg), or thiopental (5 mg/kg) for anesthetic induction and tracheal intubation.[96] Following placement of the endotracheal tube, respiratory resistance was significantly lower with propofol when compared with etomidate and thiopental. Pizov et al[97] randomized asthmatic and non-asthmatic patients to anesthetic induction with either thiopental/thiamylal (5 mg/kg), methohexital (1.5 mg/kg), or propofol (2.5 mg). Following tracheal intubation, the presence of wheezing was noted by auscultation. In asthmatic patients, the incidence of wheezing was 45% with thiopental/thiamylal, 26% with methohexital, and 0% with propofol. In non-asthmatic patients, the incidence of wheezing was 16% with thiopental/thiamylal and 3% with propofol.

The potential beneficial effects of propofol on airway reactivity are further supported by animal studies. Propofol has been shown to attenuate carbachol-induced airway constriction in canine tracheal smooth muscle.[98] The reported mechanism involves a decrease of intracellular inositol phosphate, resulting in a decrease of intracellular calcium availability. Pedersen et al[99] demonstrated that propofol was effective in preventing bronchoconstriction following administration of several provocative agents in an isolated guinea pig trachea smooth-muscle model.

Despite these potential beneficial effects, clinical experience has demonstrated certain adverse effects with propofol (Table 6-5). Cardiovascular effects of propofol resemble those of the barbiturates and include the potential for hypotension from peripheral vasodilation and negative inotropic properties.[100] These effects occur most often following rapid bolus administration. Although tolerated by patients with adequate cardiovascular function, these effects may have detrimental

Table 6-5. Adverse Effects Described With Propofol

Adverse Effects
Hypotension
Negative inotropic effects
Vasodilation
Bradycardia
Neurologic sequelae
Opisthotonic posturing
Seizure-like activity
Myoclonus
Anaphylactoid reactions
Metabolic acidosis and cardiac failure
Pain on injection
Bacterial contamination of solution
Hyperlipidemia
Potential for depletion of trace elements (zinc)

physiologic effects in patients with compromised cardiovascular function. The administration of calcium chloride (10 mg/kg) has been shown to prevent the deleterious cardiovascular effects of propofol.[101]

In addition to the negative inotropic properties, central vagal tone may be affected, leading to bradycardia, conduction disturbances, and asystole.[102,103] Bradycardia may be more likely when propofol is combined with other medications known to alter cardiac chronotropic function (fentanyl or succinylcholine).[103] Although relative bradycardia generally is considered a beneficial effect in patients at risk for myocardial ischemia, it may be detrimental in patients with a fixed stroke volume in whom cardiac output is heart-rate–dependent.

Opisthotonic posturing, myoclonic movements (especially in children), and seizure-like activity may occur with propofol administration.[104-106] Movement disorders seen with propofol administration have been attributed to its antagonism at glycine receptors in subcortical structures. Although some of the initial reports attempted to link propofol with clinical seizure activity,[106] it seems that these concerns are unfounded. There is no EEG evidence of seizure activity with propofol administration. Hewitt et al[107] evaluated the effects of propofol and thiopental on the EEGs of 20 patients undergoing temporal lobe surgery. No difference in the rate of discharge or extension of the irritative zone was seen when comparing thiopental with propofol. Additionally, propofol has been used to treat status epilepticus and is included in suggested algorithms for treating patients with refractory status epilepticus.[108,109]

Despite the obvious benefits of using propofol for sedation in the PICU, routine use cannot be recommended because of reports of what has been termed the "propofol infusion syndrome" presenting as metabolic acidosis, bradydysrhythmias, and fatal cardiac failure.[110,111] Parke et al[110] were the first to describe propofol infusion syndrome in 5 children with respiratory infections and respiratory failure who were receiving relatively high doses of up to 13.6 mg/kg/h. Similar problems and their potential association with propofol have been reported by other investigators.[111-113] Bray[114] reviewed the medical records of 18 children with suspected propofol infusion syndrome. Risk factors for the syndrome included propofol administration for more than 48 hours or doses greater than 4 mg/kg/h. However, several children received doses greater than 4 mg/kg/h for longer than 48 hours without adverse effects, suggesting that factors other than dose and duration may be necessary for development of the syndrome. Other potential associated factors included age; 13 of the 18 patients were 4 years or younger and only 1 of 18 was older than 10 years. There also may be an association of respiratory tract infections in the etiology of the syndrome because a large percentage of the reported cases have been in children with upper respiratory tract infections. Since Bray's review,[114] the syndrome has been reported in a 17-year-old patient[112] and more recently in a cohort of adult patients with head injuries.[113] In addition to the cardiovascular manifestations, other clinical signs and symptoms include metabolic acidosis, lipemic serum, hepatomegaly, and muscle involvement with rhabdomyolysis and hyperkalemia. Treatment includes immediate discontinuation of the propofol infusion plus symptomatic treatment of cardiovascular dysfunction. In patients with rhabdomyolysis and renal failure, hemodialysis has been used.[112] Hemodialysis may play a role in the management of the renal dysfunction or as a therapeutic tool through the removal of a suspected toxic metabolite.

Recent investigations have provided some insight into the potential mechanisms responsible for the propofol infusion syndrome. In a guinea pig cardiomyocyte preparation, Schenkman and Yan[115] demonstrated that propofol impairs mitochondrial function either through an alteration in oxygen use or inhibition of electron flow along the electron transport chain. Wolf et al[116] provided further evidence for alteration of mitochondrial function as the etiology of the propofol infusion syndrome. Biochemical analysis of a 2-year-old boy who developed the propofol infusion syndrome revealed an increased concentration of malonyl-carnitine. This compound can inhibit the transport protein necessary for the movement of long-chain fatty acids into the mitochondria. They noted an increase in the concentration of C_5-acylcarnitine, indicative of inhibition of the respiratory chain at complex II. The authors began hemofiltration once the syndrome was detected and were able to reverse the clinical manifestations with effective recovery of their patient. As the evidence mounts that propofol may interfere with mitochondrial function and oxidative phosphorylation, there seems to be a similarity between propofol infusion syndrome and specific inborn errors of metabolism known as mitochondrial myopathies, which result in primary involvement of cardiac and skeletal muscle with lactic acidosis. Caution is recommended when propofol is administered by continuous infusion in the PICU patient in doses exceeding 4 mg/kg/h or for longer than 24 to 48 hours. Intermittent analysis of acid-base status and creatinine phosphokinase (evaluating for rhabdomyolysis) also is recommended. If a base deficit is noted with an increasing serum lactate, immediate discontinuation of the propofol is recommended. Immediate discontinuation of the propofol infusion with the first signs of developing lactic acidosis may allow for spontaneous resolution of the problem.[95] Hemodialysis[112] and hemofiltration[116] also have been suggested as potential therapeutic interventions.

The opinion that propofol should not be used for prolonged sedation of the PICU patient except potentially for the treatment of the head injured patient with increased ICP still is not unanimously embraced by the medical community. There remain reports in small cohorts of patients of the safe and successful use of propofol for sedation in the PICU setting.[117-120] In March 2001 AstraZeneca (Wilmington, DE), the manufacturers of Diprivan, one of the 2 commercially available propofol preparations,[121] reviewed the preliminary outcomes of a clinical trial in which propofol (either a 1% or 2% solution) was being compared with other agents used for PICU sedation. During the trial and the 28-day follow-up period, there were 12 (11%) deaths in the 2% propofol group, 9 (8%) in the 1% propofol group, and 4 (4%) in the standard sedation group. Although review failed to show a specific pattern to the causes of death, there was enough concern that the company issued the statement: "propofol is currently not approved for sedation in pediatric ICU patients in the United States and should not be used for this purpose."

Additional problems with propofol relate to its delivery in a lipid emulsion (the same lipid preparation that is used in parenteral hyperalimentation solutions otherwise known as intralipid). Problems include rare reports of anaphylactoid reactions (more likely in patients with a history of egg allergy[122]), pain on injection, and elevated triglyceride levels with prolonged infusions. Variable success in decreasing the incidence of injection pain has been reported with various maneuvers, including the preadministration of lidocaine, mixing lidocaine and propofol in a single solution, mixing the propofol with thiopental,[123] diluting the concentration of the propofol, or cooling it prior to bolus administration. Another alternative is the administration of a small dose of ketamine (0.5 mg/kg) prior to the administration of propofol.[124] Because propofol has limited analgesic properties, ketamine and propofol can be administered together, in separate or the same solution, to take advantage of the analgesia provided by ketamine and the rapid recovery of propofol. Ketamine can be added to the propofol solution to result in a mixture containing 3 to 5 mg/mL ketamine and 10 mg/mL propofol. For brief procedures, incremental doses of 0.1 mL/kg of the mixed solution can be administered, resulting in the delivery of 0.3 to 0.5 mg/kg of ketamine and 1 mg/kg of propofol.

Unlike most other medications used for continuous sedation, the initial production of propofol did not contain preservatives. Laboratory studies have demonstrated that the lipid emulsion can serve as a suitable culture media for bacteria.[125] Systemic bacteremia and postoperative wound infections have been linked to extrinsically contaminated propofol.[126] A modification of the initial preparation by AstraZeneca

Pharmaceuticals included the addition of disodium ethylenediaminetetraacetic acid (EDTA) as a preservative, which may limit the risk of bacterial contamination. Despite this modification, strict aseptic technique is still recommended when using propofol. Opened but unused vials should be disposed of promptly and not saved for later use. Current policy in some PICUs is to change the vial and tubing every 12 hours during continuous infusions. A theoretical problem with disodium EDTA is the potential for chelation and depletion of essential trace minerals such as zinc. Although there are no formal studies, this concern is outlined in the manufacturer's package insert.

Another preparation of propofol containing sodium metabisulfite as the preservative also is available from Baxter Pharmaceuticals (New Providence, NJ). Although there is some controversy over the possible association of sodium metabisulfite with allergic reactions, especially in patients with asthma and other atopic conditions, several other commonly used medications contain sodium metabisulfite. There have been no reports of problems with these medications, and evaluation by the FDA concluded that the 2 propofol preparations were equivalent, although Trissel[127] has provided preliminary data that the 2 formulations are different in their compatibility with other medications. This is an extremely important issue for pediatric patients in whom intravenous access may be limited, and future studies are needed to further define this issue. Furthermore, a retrospective analysis of dose requirements during sedation for magnetic resonance imaging suggests a decreased potency of the sodium metabisulfite propofol solution when compared to the EDTA soltuion.[128]

A problem related to the high lipid content of the propofol solution is hypertriglyceridemia.[129,130] A case report outlines the anecdotal association of a high-dose propofol infusion rate with an increasing $PaCO_2$ during mechanical ventilation.[130] The patient required up to 200 µg/kg/min of propofol to maintain an adequate level of sedation, which resulted in a total caloric intake of 4,500 cal/d (53% from the lipid in the propofol diluent). The $PaCO_2$ increased from 67 mmHg to a maximum value of 78 mmHg despite increasing the minute ventilation from 11 to 13 L/min. The lipid content of propofol should be taken into consideration when calculating the patient's daily caloric intake. A propofol infusion of 2 mg/kg/h provides approximately 0.5 g/kg/d of fat. In an attempt to eliminate or lessen such problems, a 2% solution of propofol (twice the amount of propofol with the same amount of lipid per milliliter as the 1% solution) is undergoing clinical evalua tions.[131,132] Although the issue of increased triglycerides may be eliminated with the 2% solution, there may be an alteration in propofol's bioavailability because there seems to be an increased dose requirement when the 2% solution is used compared with the 1% solution.[131,132]

Despite issues with the use of propofol for sedation, it remains an agent that has an important role in providing procedural sedation. (See also Chapter 5.) When used in the absence of airway control and mechanical ventilation, the respiratory depressant effects of propofol should not be overlooked because reports demonstrate a relatively high incidence of respiratory effects, including hypoventilation, upper airway obstruction, and apnea.[120] As with any sedative agent, some degree of hypoventilation is likely to occur in spontaneously breathing patients with the potential for hypercarbia and deleterious effects on ICP and CPP.

Barbiturates

The barbiturates can be classified according to their duration of activity. Short-acting agents such as methohexital, thiopental, and thiamylal have a duration of action of 5 to 10 minutes. These agents are used most commonly by intravenous, bolus administration for brief procedures such as endotracheal intubation. When a more prolonged effect is needed, a continuous infusion may be used to maintain constant plasma levels. However, when this is done, the offset time will also be markedly prolonged and dependent on the duration of the infusion.

Long-acting agents with half-lifes of 6 to 12 hours include pentobarbital and phenobarbital.

Beneficial physiologic effects of the barbiturates include a decreased $CMRO_2$ with a secondary reduction of CBF that is mediated through cerebral vasoconstriction, leading to a decrease in ICP.[133,134] The barbiturates are effective anticonvulsants and may be used to treat refractory status epilepticus.[135,136] Animal studies suggest that the barbiturates provide cerebral protection during periods of cerebral hypoxia or hypoperfusion.[137,138]

Although used most commonly for their therapeutic effects (as anticonvulsants or to decrease ICP), the barbiturates may be an effective alternative for providing sedation in the PICU patient when first-line agents, either alone or in combination, fail to provide adequate sedation or result in untoward side effects.[139] In a retrospective report, pentobarbital was administered to 50 children for sedation during mechanical ventilation.[140] The patients ranged in age from 1 month to 14 years and in weight from 3.1 to 56 kg. Pentobarbital was used when the level of sedation was inadequate despite midazolam doses of 0.4 mg/ kg/h, fentanyl doses of 10 µg/kg/h, and morphine doses of 100 µg/kg/h. The duration of pentobarbital infusion ranged from 2 to 37 days (median 4 days) in doses of 1 to 6 mg/kg/h (median 2 mg/kg/h). Twelve patients also received an ongoing opioid infusion for more than 48 hours after starting the pentobarbital infusion to control pain related to a surgical procedure or an acute medical illness. In the 14 patients who received pentobarbital for 5 days or more, the dose requirements increased from 1.2 mg/kg/h on day 1 to 3.4 mg/kg/h on day 5. No significant adverse effects related to pentobarbital were noted.

One particularly difficult situation is providing sedation during ECMO. While fentanyl is the most commonly used agent, clinical experience has demonstrated a rapid development of tolerance with dose escalations up to 30 to 50 µg/kg/h. Pentobarbital may be an effective alternative to the more conventional agents in sedating pediatric patients during ECMO.[139,140] The barbiturates also have been efficacious is providing sedation, anxiolysis, and comfort measures during the end stages of terminal cancer.[141]

The effect of barbiturates on cardiorespiratory function are dose-dependent. In healthy patients, sedative doses can be expected to have limited effects on cardiovascular function, respiratory drive, and airway protective reflexes. Larger doses, especially in patients with cardiorespiratory compromise, can produce respiratory depression, apnea, and hypotension. The cardiorespiratory effects intensify with other agents such as opioids. Hypotension results from peripheral vasodilation and a direct negative inotropic effect. Given the potential for adverse cardiovascular effects, barbiturates should be used cautiously in patients with cardiovascular dysfunction. The risks of adverse cardiovascular effects can be limited by slow administration (over 5 minutes) of the bolus doses.

Another problem that may limit barbiturate use is that the solution is alkaline, thereby making it incompatible with other medications and parenteral alimentation solutions. Therefore, the barbiturates should be administered separately from other medications. Local erythema and thrombophlebitis can occur with subcutaneous infiltration. Additionally, like propofol and midazolam, the barbiturates possess no analgesic properties and, therefore, should be used with an opioid in situations requiring analgesia.

Opioids

Although generally used for analgesia, opioids also possess sedative properties and are effective agents for providing sedation during mechanical ventilation in the PICU patient. Clinical experience suggests that the opioids are particularly efficacious, especially in neonates and infants, which may relate to the well-developed opioid receptor system of the neonate. Although these agents provide effective analgesia, even with high doses (fentanyl 50-75 µg/kg), the opioids do not provide amnesia. Use of additional agents is recommended when amnesia is desired (eg, in an older infant or child who is receiving a neuromuscular blocking agent).

Despite significant clinical experience, there is limited information about the most effective opioid for PICU sedation. In a patient with compromised cardiovascular status or at risk for pulmonary hypertension, such as an infant with a large preoperative systemic to pulmonary shunt, synthetic opioids (eg, fentanyl, sufentanil) provide cardiovascular stability, beneficial effects on pulmonary vascular resistance, and effective blunting of the sympathetic stress. Due to their prompt redistribution and resultant short plasma half-lifes following a bolus administration, synthetic opioids generally are administered by a continuous infusion to maintain plasma concentrations adequate to provide analgesia.

When comparing the synthetic opioids (fentanyl, sufentanil, alfentanil, remifentanil), there does not seem to be an inherent advantage to using any particular agent. However, fentanyl is the least expensive of the synthetic opioids. Fentanyl, sufentanil, and alfentanil, like other opioids, are dependent on hepatic metabolism. Although these agents are short acting when administered as a single bolus dose, they demonstrate a context-sensitive half-life, so the duration of their effect may be prolonged when administered over an extended period.

Remifentanil is metabolized by nonspecific esterases in the plasma with a clinical half-life of 5 to 10 minutes and a brief duration of effect even after 12 to 24 hours of continuous infusion.[142] Unlike other opioids, these pharmacokinetic parameters also hold true in the neonatal population.[143] Given these properties, remifentanil may be a useful agent for providing a deep level of sedation, and yet allow for a rapid dissipation of its effects when the infusion is discontinued. There is limited information about the use of remifentanil in the ICU population. Tobias[144] reported experience in 4 patients who required a deep level of sedation for tolerating endotracheal intubation for 12 to 24 hours. Remifentanil provided a deep level of sedation, yet allowed for rapid awakening when the infusion was discontinued. Cavaliere et al[145] reported similar anecdotal success with remifentanil infusions in 10 adult ICU patients. Potential problems with remifentanil use include the cost and rapid development of tolerance, thereby limiting its application to 24 hours or less.

Synthetic opioids may cause increased ICP and chest wall[146-149] rigidity. Sperry et al[146] noted a decrease in MAP and an increase in ICP, resulting in decreased CPP following the administration of synthetic opioids to adults with altered intracranial compliance. The mechanism underlying the effect on ICP is postulated to be reflex cerebral vasodilation in response to the decrease in MAP.[147] A similar effect has been described with propofol (see previous text). When MAP is maintained with a direct-acting vasoconstrictor, no change in ICP is noted.

Pokela et al[148] reported decreased respiratory compliance and oxygen saturation in 4 infants receiving alfentanil and concluded that these agents should not be used without concomitant neuromuscular blockade. The incidence of chest wall rigidity is related to the dose, rate of administration, and perhaps the age of patient. It is a centrally mediated, idiosyncratic reaction which, when severe, can interfere with effective respiratory function. Chest wall rigidity can be reversed with naloxone or interrupted with neuromuscular blocking agents. Chest wall rigidity does not occur in all patients receiving synthetic opioids. Irazuzta et al[150] demonstrated improved compliance of the respiratory system in neonates and infants receiving fentanyl for sedation during mechanical ventilation.

Other opioids also can be used to provide effective sedation during mechanical ventilation in the PICU setting. Morphine is a frequently used and cheaper alternative in patients with normal cardiovascular function. Morphine can cause venodilation and decrease blood pressure. The effect intensifies in hypovolemic patients. Lynn et al[151] demonstrated that morphine infusions of 10 to 30 μg/kg/h resulted in serum concentrations of 10 to 22 ng/mL and provided effective analgesia and sedation during mechanical ventilation after surgery for congenital heart disease without impairing the ability to wean mechanical ventilatory support. Morphine infusions have been shown to blunt the sympathetic response and reduce epinephrine levels in neonates who require endotracheal intubation and mechanical ventilation for hyaline membrane disease.[152] Follow-up of preterm infants 5 to 6 years after birth who received morphine analgesia during the neonatal period has demonstrated no adverse effects on intelligence, motor function, or behavior.[153] When compared with fentanyl, preliminary evidence suggests that while providing equivalent analgesia, morphine decreases the amount of supplemental analgesia required and has a lower prevalence of withdrawal.[154]

Potential alternative opioids include hydromorphone, meperidine, and methadone (Table 6-6). Although there is little or no information concerning the use of these agents for sedation in the PICU patient, there is ample information concerning use of these agents in the management of acute pain. Hydromorphone may be an effective alternative to morphine in patients who experience pruritis[155] or those with renal failure in whom metabolites of morphine may accumulate. Although there are no active metabolites of hydromorphone, morphine is metabolized in the liver to morphine-6-glucoronide (M6G), which is more potent than the parent compound. Because M6G is renally excreted,

Table 6-6. Potency and Half-life of Opioids

Agent	Potency	Half-life
Morphine	1	2-3 h
Meperidine	0.1	2-3 h
Hydromorphone	5	2-4 h
Fentanyl	100	0.3-0.5 h
Sufentanil	1000	0.2-0.4 h
Alfentanil	20	0.2-0.3 h
Remifentanil	100	0.1 h

accumulation may be an issue in patients with renal insufficiency. Hydromorphone is 5 to 7 times more potent than morphine (Table 6-6).

Problems that preclude meperdine use in the PICU patient are a relatively high incidence of adverse CNS effects, including dysphoria, agitation, and seizures.[156] Central nervous system toxicity (including seizures) results from the accumulation of normeperidine following hepatic N-methylation of the parent compound. Normeperidine has a long half-life (15-20 hours) and is dependent on renal excretion. High or toxic levels are more likely in patients with renal insufficiency, with the coadministration of drugs such as phenobarbital that stimulate hepatic microsomal enzymes, and with large doses (>2 g/d in an adult).

Although intravenous administration remains the optimal and most frequently used route in the PICU patient, certain situations, such as limited intravenous access and drug incompatibilities, may preclude intravenous administration. In such situations, the subcutaneous administration of several different opioids is possible. While most experience with subcutaneous opioid infusions has been in patients with terminal cancer,[157] Bruera et al[158] reported experience with subcutaneous opioid infusions in adult ICU patients. Thirteen patients received opioids by either intermittent subcutaneous dosing or continuous infusion for a total of 60 patient days. The infusions were delivered through a 25-gauge butterfly needle inserted subcutaneously in the subclavicular area or the anterior abdominal wall. No infectious complications were noted, and the insertion site was changed only 3 times because of conditions such as erythema. The authors expressed a theoretical concern over possible delays in onset of activity or decreased absorption in patients with decreased peripheral perfusion, although they noted no such problems in their patients.

The subcutaneous route also is a possible delivery alternative in the PICU patient.[159,160] A retrospective review demonstrated the utility of this technique in 24 PICU patients ranging in age from 2 weeks to 18 years.[160] Continuous subcutaneous fentanyl infusions were administered for 1.5 to 14 days in patients in whom intravenous administration was not feasible due to lack of intravenous access or drug incompatibilities. The indication for opioid administration included acute pain issues including postoperative pain, a gradual weaning regimen following prolonged opioid use, and the provision of comfort during the terminal stages of a disease.

Concentrated solutions of opioids/sedatives are used for subcutaneous infusion so that the total volume is limited to 3 mL/h or less and started at the same time that the intravenous infusion is discontinued. A standard 22-gauge intravenous catheter or a butterfly needle can be used. Prior to placement, the tubing and needle are flushed with the opioid solution and, after sterile preparation of the area, the needle is inserted subcutaneously and covered with a bio-occlusive dressing. The same infusion pumps that are used for intravenous drug administration can be used for subcutaneous administration. The pressure limit may need to be adjusted to allow for subcutaneous administration.

Miscellaneous Agents

Phenothiazines and Butyrophenones

Anecdotal experiences with PICU sedation have been reported with several other agents and combinations of agents (Table 6-7). The phenothiazines and butyrophenones are considered major tranquilizers. They have been used most commonly in treating psychiatric disturbances and severe nausea. Neither of these classes of agents have found great popularity as sedatives in the PICU, although haloperidol is the most frequently chosen butyrophenone for ICU sedation in adults. While not approved by the FDA for intravenous administration, there is significant clinical experience with its intravenous use. Riker et al[161] reported experience with haloperidol by continuous intravenous infusion (range: 3-25 mg/h) for sedation in 8 adult ICU patients. Suggested benefits of haloperidol include a rapid onset, minimal respiratory depression, and lack of active metabolites. Adverse effects associated with the butyrophenones and phenothiazines include hypotension related to α-adrenergic blockade and peripheral vasodilatation, dystonic and extrapyramidal effects, lowering of the seizure threshold and, in rare cases, neuroleptic malignant syndrome. Of even greater concern are the potential effects on the cardiovascular system, including cardiac arrest and torsades de pointes. In the study of Riker et al,[161] cardiac events included atrial dysrhythmias, prolongation of the QT interval, and ventricular tachycardia in one patient. Alterations in repolarization induced by this class of agent may be particularly dangerous in patients with altered sympathetic function related to fever, pain, or the stresses of an acute illness. Additionally, the FDA, through a black box warning, has focused on the potential association of another butyrophenone, droperidol and postoperative cardiac events, including torsades de pointes in adult patients.[162]

Health care providers may be more familiar with the use of phenothiazines in the pediatric population in combination with other agents in a formulation known as DPT (Demerol, Phenergan, and Thorazine) for invasive procedures. Although this formulation is effective, the combination of these agents may result in prolonged

Table 6-7. Miscellaneous Agents for Intensive Care Unit Sedation

Agents
Phenothiazines
Promethazine
Butyrophenones
Haloperidol
Droperidol
Chloral Hydrate
Antihistamines
Diphenhydramine
α_2-adrenergic agonists
Clonidine
Dexmedetomidine

sedation and the risk of respiratory depression and apnea.[163] These agents have no role in providing prolonged sedation in the PICU patient. If such combinations are used for invasive procedures, careful and prolonged post-procedure monitoring is recommended.

Chloral Hydrate

Chloral hydrate, a sedative-hypnotic agent, is metabolized in the liver to its active form, trichloroethanol, which has a half-life of 8 to 12 hours. Because there is no parenteral formulation, oral or rectal administration is necessary, which may result in a slow onset of action (up to 20 minutes), thereby limiting its use in controlling the acutely agitated PICU patient. Repeated administration can lead to the accumulation of active metabolites and prolonged sedation that may persist following its discontinuation. Additionally, the active metabolite trichloroethanol is related to the halogenated hydrocarbons and has been associated with ventricular arrhythmias, especially in patients at risk for such problems (tricyclic antidepressant ingestions).[164,165]

α_2-Adrenergic Agonists

Clonidine, a centrally acting α_2-adrenergic agonist that decreases central sympathetic outflow, was initially introduced for the treatment of hypertension. More recent clinical experience has demonstrated its efficacy as a surgery premedicant.[166,167] Beneficial physiologic effects of the α_2-adrenergic agonists include sedation, anxiolysis, decreased anesthetic requirements, cardiovascular stability, and the potentiation of opiate-induced analgesia.[166,168] In addition to its sedative properties, clonidine and the other α_2-adrenergic agonists provide analgesic effects that are mediated at the dorsal horn of the spinal cord. Activation of presynaptic receptors on first-order neurons decreases the release of the nociceptive transmitter substance P while post-synaptic activation decreases the rate of depolarization of second-order neurons. Data on the use of clonidine for ICU sedation have appeared only as anecdotal case reports.[169]

Dexmedetomidine was recently approved for clinical use. Like clonidine, it is a centrally acting, α_2-adrenergic agonist and has the same clinical properties as clonidine. However, it possesses an affinity of 8 times that of clonidine for the α_2-receptor, a differential α_1 to α_2 agonism of 1:1600, and a half-life of 2 hours, which is roughly 4-fold shorter than clonidine. The shorter half-life of dexmedetomidine allows for easy titration via a continuous intravenous infusion. Dexmedetomidine is currently approved by the FDA for short-term (≤24 hours) sedation of adult patients during mechanical ventilation. When compared with placebo in 119 adult patients who required mechanical ventilation following cardiac and general surgical procedures, patients who received dexmedetomidine required 80% less midazolam and 50% less morphine.[170] Dexmedetomidine dosing included an initial bolus dose of 1 µg/kg followed by an infusion of 0.2 to 0.7 µg/ kg/h. Eighteen of the 66 patients who received dexmedetomidine experienced hypotension (MAP <60 mmHg or >30% decrease from baseline) or bradycardia (heart rate <50 beats/min). The cardiovascular changes were noted during the administration of the bolus dose in 11 of the 18 patients. This resulted in the interruption of the infusion in 3 patients and a withdrawal from the study of 3 others.

Hall et al[171] evaluated the analgesic, sedative, and cardiovascular effects of 2 infusion rates of dexmedetomidine (0.2 and 0.6 µg/kg/h) in healthy, adult volunteers. Both of the dexmedetomidine infusion rates resulted in significant sedation, reduction of pain to the cold pressor test, and impairment of memory and psychometric performance. Small but clinically significant decreases in MAP and heart rate also were noted, although no patient developed bradycardia or hypotension. Respiratory effects included a decreased respiratory rate and increased end-tidal carbon dioxide concentrations.

There is only one prospective trial regarding dexmedetomidine in pediatric patients.[172] The efficacy of sedation during mechanical ventilation was evaluated using an objective scoring system (Ramsay score—see previous text) and by comparing the requirements for supplemental doses of morphine. At a dose of 0.25 µg/kg/h, dexmedetomidine was equivalent to midazolam at 0.22 mg/kg/h. At 0.5 µg/kg/h, dexmedetomidine was more effective than midazolam as demonstrated by a decreased need for supplemental morphine as well as a decrease in the number of Ramsay scores of 1 exhibited by the patients. Dexmedetomidine was less effective in infants; 5 of the 6 patients who exhibited a Ramsay score of 1 during dexmedetomidine were younger than 12 months. The only noted adverse effect was bradycardia in one patient receiving dexmedetomidine who was also receiving digoxin.[173] Similar slowing of sinus node function has been reported when dexmedetomidine is administered with propofol, another agent with known negative chronotropic effects.[174] Although the clinical experience with dexmedetomidine is limited in the pediatric population, the initial experience combined with the beneficial physiologic properties suggest a potential role as a sedative/analgesic in the PICU patient.

Summary

Due to the wide spectrum of patients, ages, and clinical scenarios in the PICU population, a "cookbook" approach to sedation and analgesia is not feasible. Health care providers of these patients should become facile with several different medications and routes of administration. A common choice for initiating amnesia/sedation frequently includes the continuous infusion of a benzodiazepine, such as midazolam or lorazepam. Lorazepam eliminates the concerns regarding metabolism by the P_{450} system and the presence of active metabolites. In situations requiring analgesia, an opioid administered by either a continuous infusion or a PCA device can be used. Although fentanyl is frequently chosen in the ICU setting, morphine is an acceptable and cost-effective alternative for patients with stable cardiovascular function. Preliminary data suggest that morphine may lead to a less rapid development of tolerance and decrease the incidence of withdrawal. Follow-up studies have demonstrated no adverse developmental effects from the administration of morphine in the neonatal population. The synthetic opioids are recommended in those patients at risk for pulmonary hypertension. In this setting, the use of the synthetic opioids may decrease postoperative morbidity and mortality and modulate the deleterious effects of pain and the stress response on the pulmonary vasculature.

Alternatives to opioids and benzodiazepines include ketamine and pentobarbital. Ketamine may be useful for the patient with hemodynamic instability or with increased airway reactivity as a result of their disease. Propofol has gained great favor in the adult population as a means of providing deep sedation while allowing for rapid awakening. Similar beneficial properties are achieved in the pediatric patient; however, concerns over the "propofol infusion syndrome" limit the use of this agent. As the pediatric experience increases, it seems there will be a role for newer agents such as dexmedetomidine. Starting guidelines for sedative and analgesic agents are listed in Table 6-8.

A stable level of sedation is generally best achieved with a continuous infusion. The continuous infusion should be supplemented with as-needed doses for breakthrough agitation. Patients requiring frequent bolus doses should have the baseline infusion rate increased. As the infusion rate is increased, the bolus doses should be increased to equal the hourly rate. The titration of the infusion and use of supplemental bolus doses should be adjusted using clinical sedation scales or newer devices, such as the BIS monitor, when objective assessment of the patient is not feasible. Following prolonged administration of sedative and analgesic agents, strategies should be implemented to prevent withdrawal syndromes. This may include a gradual tapering of the infusion rate or switching to oral or subcutaneous administration.

Table 6-8. Suggested Guidelines for Dosing of Sedative and Analgesic Agents

Agent	Dose	Comments
Fentanyl	2-3 μg/kg/h	Modulates stress response and pulmonary vascular resistance
Morphine	10-30 μg/kg/h	Inexpensive, venodilation
Midazolam	0.05-0.15 mg/kg/h	Abundant clinical experience, expensive, P_{450} metabolism
Lorazepam	0.025-0.05 mg/kg/h	Limited clinical experience, inexpensive, metabolism: glucuronyl transferase
Ketamine	1-2 mg/kg/h	Endogenous catecholamine release, bronchodilation, cardiovascular stability, can be mixed 10:1 with midazolam
Pentobarbital	1-2 mg/kg/h	Alternative to benzodiazepine/opioid, incompatible with other medications, vasodilation/negative inotropic effects
Propofol	1-3 mg/kg/h	Potential for propofol infusion syndrome, rapid awakening, high lipid content of solution
Remifentanil	0.1-0.2 μg/kg/min	Cardiorespiratory effects similar to other synthetic opioids, rapid development of tolerance and cost may limit application except for limited periods (<12-24 hours), rapid dissipation of effects when infusion is discontinued
Dexmedetomidine	0.25-0.7 μg/kg/h	FDA-approved for short-term (24 hours) sedation in adults; limited clinical data in pediatric population

The infusion rates are suggestions for starting doses. The infusion should be supplemented with bolus doses to provide the desired level of sedation. In patients requiring numerous bolus doses, the infusion should be increased by 10% to 20%. If the patient requires no supplemental doses or is excessively sedated, the infusion should be decreased by 10% to 20%.

References

1. American Academy of Pediatrics Committee on Drugs. Guidelines for monitoring and management of pediatric patients during and after sedation for diagnostic and therapeutic procedures. *Pediatrics.* 1992;89:1110-1115
2. Volles DF, McGory R. Pharmacokinetic considerations. *Crit Care Clin.* 1999;15:55-57
3. Buck ML, Blumer JL. Opioids and other analgesics: adverse effects in the intensive care unit. *Crit Care Clin.* 1991;7:615-637
4. Reed MD, Blumer JL. Therapeutic drug monitoring in the pediatric intensive care unit. *Pediatr Clin North Am.* 1994;41:1227-1243
5. Katz R, Kelly HW. Pharmacokinetics of continuous infusions of fentanyl in critically ill children. *Crit Care Med.* 1993;21:995-1000
6. de Wildt SN, de Hoog M, Vinks AA, van der Giesen E, van den Anker JN. Population pharmacokinetics and metabolism of midazolam in pediatric intensive care patients. *Crit Care Med.* 2003;31:1952-1958
7. Anand KJS, Hansen DD, Hickey PR. Hormonal-metabolic stress responses in neonates undergoing cardiac surgery. *Anesthesiology.* 1990;73:661-670
8. Anand KJS, Hickey PR. Halothane-morphine compared with high-dose sufentanil for anesthesia and postoperative analgesia in neonatal cardiac surgery. *N Engl J Med.* 1992;326:1-9
9. Hansen-Flaschen JH, Brazinsky S, Basile C, Lanken PN. Use of sedating drugs and neuromuscular blocking agents in patients requiring mechanical ventilation for respiratory failure. *JAMA.* 1991;266:2870-2875
10. Ambuel B, Hamlett KW, Marx CM, Blumer JL. Assessing distress in pediatric intensive care environments: the COMFORT scale. *J Pediatr Psychol.* 1992;17:95-109
11. Crain N, Slonim A, Pollack MM. Assessing sedation in the pediatric intensive care by using BIS and the COMFORT scale. *Pediatr Crit Care Med.* 2002;3:11-14
12. Simmons LE, Riker RR, Prato BS, Fraser GL. Assessing sedation during intensive care unit mechanical ventilation with the Bispectral Index and Sedation-Agitation Scale. *Crit Care Med.* 1999;27:1499-1504
13. Ramsay M, Savage TM, Simpson ER, et al. Controlled sedation with aphalaxone-alphadone. *BMJ.* 1974;2:656-659
14. Flaishon RI, Windsor A, Sigl J, Sebel PS. Recovery of consciousness after thiopental or propofol. Bispectral index and isolated forearm technique. *Anesthesiology.* 1997;86:613-619

15. Sebel PS, Lang E, Rampil IJ, et al. A multicenter study of bispectral elec troencephalogram analysis for monitoring anesthetic effect. *Anesth Analg.* 1997;84:891-899
16. Berkenbosch JW, Fichter CR, Tobias JD. The correlation of the bispectral index monitor with clinical sedation scores during mechanical ventilation in the pediatric intensive care unit. *Anesth Analg.* 2002;94:506-511
17. De Deyne C, Struys M, Decruyenaere J, Creupelandt J, Hoste E, Colardyn F. Use of continuous bispectral EEG monitoring to assess depth of sedation in ICU patients. *Intensive Care Med.* 1998;24:1294-1298
18. Aneja R, Heard AMB, Fletcher JE, Heard CMB. Sedation monitoring of children by the Bispectral Index in the pediatric intensive care unit. *Pediatr Crit Care Med.* 2003;4:60-64
19. Arbour RB. Using the bispectral index to assess arousal response in a patient with neuromuscular blockade. *Am J Crit Care.* 2000;9:383-387
20. Wagner RL, White PF, Kan PB, Rosenthal MH, Feldman D. Inhibition of adrenal steroidogenesis by the anesthetic etomidate. *N Engl J Med.* 1984;310:1415-1421
21. Tobias JD. Airway management in the pediatric trauma patient. *J Intensive Care Med.* 1998;13:1-14
22. Tobias JD. Etomidate: applications in pediatric anesthesia and critical care. *J Intensive Care Med.* 1997;12:324-326
23. Kong KL, Willatts SM, Prys-Roberts C. Isoflurane compared with midazolam for sedation in the intensive care unit. *BMJ.* 1989;298:1277-1280
24. Meiser A, Sirtl C, Bellgardt M, et al. Desflurane compared with propofol for postoperative sedation in the intensive care unit. *Br J Anaesth.* 2003;90:273-280
25. Satoh H, Gillette JR, Takemura T, et al. Investigation of the immunological basis of halothane-induced hepatotoxicity. *Adv Experiment Med Biol.* 1986;197:657-773
26. Kenna JG, Neuberger J, Williams R. Evidence for expression in human liver of halothane-induced neoantigens recognized by antibodies in sera from patients with halothane hepatitis. *Hepatology.* 1988;8:1635-1641
27. Adams RW, Cucchiara RF, Gronert GA, Messick JM, Michenfelder JD. Isoflurane and cerebrospinal fluid pressure in neurosurgical patients. *Anesthesiology.* 1981;54:97-99
28. Drummond JC, Todd MM, Scheller MS, Shapiro HM. A comparison of the direct cerebral vasodilating potencies of halothane and isoflurane in the New Zealand white rabbit. *Anesthesiology.* 1986;65:462-467

29. Reilly CS, Wood AJJ, Koshakji RP, Wood M. The effect of halothane on drug disposition: contribution of changes in intrinsic drug metabolizing capacity and hepatic blood flow. *Anesthesiology.* 1985;63:70-76
30. Arnold JH, Truog RD, Rice SA. Prolonged administration of isoflurane to pediatric patients during mechanical ventilation. *Anesth Analg.* 1993;76:520-526
31. Reves JG, Fragan RJ, Vinik HR, Greenblatt DJ. Midazolam: pharmacology and uses. *Anesthesiology.* 1985;62:310-324
32. Lloyd-Thomas AR, Booker PD. Infusion of midazolam in paediatric patients after cardiac surgery. *Br J Anaesth.* 1986;58:1109-1115
33. Silvasi DL, Rosen DA, Rosen KR. Continuous intravenous midazolam infusion for sedation in the pediatric intensive care unit. *Anesth Analg.* 1988;67:286-288
34. Rosen DA, Rosen KR. Midazolam for sedation in the paediatric intensive care unit. *Intensive Care Med.* 1991;17:S15-S19
35. Beebe DS, Belani KG, Chang PN, et al. Effectiveness of preoperative sedation with rectal midazolam, ketamine, or their combination in young children. *Anesth Analg.* 1992;75:880-884
36. McMillan CO, Spahr-Schopfer IA, Sikich, Hartley E, Lerman J. Premedication of children with oral midazolam. *Can J Anaesth.* 1992;39:545-550
37. Karl HW, Rosenberger JL, Larach MG, Ruffle JM. Transmucosal administration of midazolam for premedication of pediatric patients: comparison of the nasal and sublingual routes. *Anesthesiology.* 1993;78:885-891
38. Theroux MC, West DW, Corddry DH, et al. Efficacy of midazolam in facilitating suturing of lacerations in preschool children in the emergency department. *Pediatrics.* 1993;91:624-627
39. Tobias JD. Subcutaneous administration of fentanyl and midazolam to prevent withdrawal following prolonged sedation in children. *Crit Care Med.* 1999;27:2262-2265
40. Bauer TM, Ritz R, Haberthur C, et al. Prolonged sedation due to accumulation of conjugated metabolites of midazolam. *Lancet.* 1995;346:145-147
41. de Wildt SN, de Hoog M, Vinks AA, van der Giesen E, van den Anker JN. Population pharmacokinetics and metabolism of midazolam in pediatric intenisve care unit patients. *Crit Care Med.* 2003;31:1952-1958
42. Payne K, Mattheyse FJ, Liebenberg D, Dawes T. The pharmacokinetics of midazolam in paediatric patients. *Eur J Clin Pharmacol.* 1989;37:267-272
43. Trouvin JH, Farinotti R, Haberer JP, Servin F, Chauvin M, Duvaldestin P. Pharmacokinetics of midazolam in anesthetized cirrhotic patients. *Br J Anaesth.* 1988;60:762-767

44. Vinik HR, Reves JG, Greenblatt DJ, Abernathy DR, Smith LR. The pharmacokinetics of midazolam in chronic renal failure patients. *Anesthesiology.* 1983;59:390-394
45. Oldenhorf H, Jong M, Steenhock A, Janknegt RR. Clinical pharmacokinetics of midazolam in intensive care patients: a wide interpatient variability? *Clin Pharmacol Ther.* 1988;43:262-269
46. Pohlman AS, Simpson KP, Hall JCB. Continuous intravenous infusions of lorazepam versus midazolam for sedation during mechanical ventilatory support: a prospective, randomized study. *Crit Care Med.* 1994;22:1241-1247
47. Dundee JW, Johnston HM, Gray RC. Lorazepam as a sedative-amnestic in an intensive care unit. *Curr Med Res Opinion.* 1976;4:290-295
48. Lugo RA, Chester EA, Cash J, Grant MJ, Vernon DD. A cost analysis of enterally administered lorazepam in the pediatric intensive care unit. *Crit Care Med.* 1999;27:417-421
49. Tobias JD, Deshpande JK, Gregory DF. Outpatient therapy of iatrogenic drug dependency following prolonged sedation in the pediatric intensive care unit. *Intensive Care Med.* 1994;20:504-507
50. Arbour R, Esparis B. Osmolar gap acidosis in a 60 year old man treated for hypoxemic respiratory failure. *Chest.* 2000;118:545-546
51. Reynolds HN, Teiken P, Regan ME, et al. Hyperlactatemia, increased osmolar gap, renal dysfunction during continuous lorazepam infusion. *Crit Care Med.* 2000;28:1631-1634
52. Breheny FX. Reversal of midazolam sedation with flumazenil. *Crit Care Med.* 1992;20:736-739
53. McDuffee A, Tobias JD. Seizure following flumazenil administration in a child. *Pediatr Emerg Care.* 1995;11:186-187
54. Domino EF, Chodoff P, Corssen G. Pharmacologic effects of CI-581, a new dissociative anesthetic in man. *Clin Pharmacol Ther.* 1965;6:279-291
55. Tobias JD. End-tidal carbon dioxide monitoring during sedation with a combination of midazolam and ketamine for children undergoing painful, invasive procedures. *Pediatr Emerg Care.* 1999;15:173-175
56. Chernow B, Lake CR, Creuss D, et al. Plasma, urine, and cerebrospinal fluid catecholamine concentrations during and after ketamine sedation. *Crit Care Med.* 1982;10:600-603
57. Wayman K, Shoemaker WC, Lippmann M. Cardiovascular effects of anesthetic induction with ketamine. *Anesth Analg.* 1980;59:355-358
58. Spotoft H, Korshin JD, Sorensen MB, Skovsted P. The cardiovascular effects of ketamine used for induction of anesthesia in patients with valvular heart disease. *Can Anaesth Soc J.* 1979;26:463-467

59. Gooding JM, Dimick AR, Tavakoli M, Corssen G. A physiologic analysis of cardiopulmonary responses to ketamine anesthesia in non-cardiac patients. *Anesth Analg.* 1977;56:813-816
60. Morray JP, Lynn AM, Stamm SJ, Herndon PS, Kawabori I, Stevenson JG. Hemodynamic effects of ketamine in children with congenital heart disease. *Anesth Analg.* 1984;63:895-899
61. Hickey PR, Hansen DD, Cramolini GM, et al. Pulmonary and systemic hemodynamic responses to ketamine in infants with normal and elevated pulmonary vascular resistance. *Anesthesiology.* 1985;62:287-293
62. Mankikian B, Cantineau JP, Sartene R, Clergue F, Viars P. Ventilatory and chest wall mechanics during ketamine anesthesia in humans. *Anesthesiology.* 1986;65:492-499
63. Hirshman CA, Downes H, Farbood A, Bergman NA. Ketamine block of bronchospasm in experimental canine asthma. *Br J Anaesth.* 1979;51:713-718
64. Bourke DL, Malit LA, Smith TC. Respiratory interactions of ketamine and morphine. *Anesthesiology.* 1987;66:153-156
65. Lanning CF, Harmel MH. Ketamine anesthesia. *Annu Rev Med.* 1975;26:137-141
66. Taylor PA, Towey RM. Depression of laryngeal reflexes during ketamine administration. *Br Med J.* 1971;2:688-689
67. Shapiro HM, Wyte SR, Harris AB. Ketamine anesthesia in patients with intracranial pathology. *Br J Anaesth.* 1972;44:1200-1204
68. Gardner AE, Dannemiller FJ, Dean D. Intracranial cerebrospinal fluid pressure in man during ketamine anesthesia. *Anesth Analg.* 1972:51:741-745
69. Reicher D, Bhalla P, Rubinstein EH. Cholinergic cerebral vasodilator effects of ketamine in rabbits. *Stroke.* 1987;18:445-449
70. Oren RE, Rasool NA, Rubinstein EH. Effect of ketamine on cerebral cortical blood flow and metabolism in rabbits. *Stroke.* 1987;18:441-444
71. Pfenninger E, Dick W, Ahnefeld FW. The influence of ketamine on both the normal and raised intracranial pressure of artificially ventilated animals. *Eur J Anaesth.* 1985;2:297-307
72. Pfenninger E, Grunert A, Bowdler I, Kilian J. The effect of ketamine on intracranial pressure during haemorrhagic shock under the conditions of both spontaneous breathing and controlled ventilation. *Acta Neurochirurgica.* 1985;78:113-118
73. Albanese J, Arnaud S, Rey M, Thomachot L, Alliez B, Martin C. Ketamine decreases intracranial pressure and electroencephalographic activity in traumatic brain injury patients during propofol sedation. *Anesthesiology.* 1997;87:1328-1334

74. Rosen I, Hagerdal M. Electroencephalographic study of children during ketamine anesthesia. *Acta Anaesth Scand.* 1976;20:32-39
75. Manohar S, Maxwell D, Winters WD. Development of EEG seizure activity during and after chronic ketamine administration in the rat. *Neuropharmacology.* 1972;11:819-826
76. Bourn WM, Yang DJ, Davisson JN. Effect of ketamine enantiomers on sound-induced convulsions in epilepsy prone rats. *Pharm Res Commun.* 1983;15:815-824
77. Veliskova J, Velisek L, Mares P, Rokyta R. Ketamine suppresses both bicuculline and picrotoxin induced generalized tonic clonic seizures during ontogenesis. *Pharm Biochem Behav.* 1990;37:667-674
78. Sheth RD, Gidal BE. Refractory status epilepticus: response to ketamine. *Neurology.* 1998;51:1765-1766
79. White PR, Way WL, Trevor AJ. Ketamine—its pharmacology and therapeutic uses. *Anesthesiology.* 1982;56:119-136
80. Haeseler G, Zuzan O, Kohn G, Piepenbrock S, Leuwer M. Anaesthesia with midazolam and S (+) ketamine in spotanesouly breathing paediatric patients during magnetic resonance imaging. *Paediatr Anaesth.* 2000;10:513-519
81. Tobias JD, Martin LD, Wetzel RC. Ketamine by continuous infusion for sedation in the pediatric intensive care unit. *Crit Care Med.* 1990;18:819-821
82. Hartvig P, Larsson E, Joachimsson PO. Postoperative analgesia and sedation following pediatric cardiac surgery using a constant infusion of ketamine. *J Cardiothorac Vasc Anesth.* 1993;7:148-153
83. Sebel PS, Lowdon JD. Propofol: a new intravenous anesthetic. *Anesthesiology.* 1989;71:260-277
84. Harris CE, Grounds RM, Murray AM, Lumlay J, Royston D, Morgan M. Propofol for long-term sedation in the intensive care unit. A comparison with papaveretum and midazolam. *Anaesthesia.* 1990;45:366-372
85. Beller JP, Pottecher T, Lugnier A, Mangin P, Otteni JC. Prolonged sedation with propofol in ICU patients: recovery and blood concentration changes during periodic interruption in infusion. *Br J Anaesth.* 1988;61:583-588
86. Ronan KP, Gallagher TJ, George B, Hamby B. Comparison of propofol and midazolam for sedation in intensive care unit patients. *Crit Care Med.* 1995;23:286-293
87. Hemelrijck JV, Fitch W, Mattheussen M, Van Aken H, Plets C, Lauwers T. Effect of propofol on cerebral circulation and autoregulation in the baboon. *Anesth Analg.* 1990;71:49-54

88. Nimkoff L, Quinn C, Silver P, Sagy M. The effects of intravenous anesthetic agents on intracranial pressure and cerebral perfusion pressure in two feline models of brain edema. *J Crit Care.* 1997;12:132-136
89. Watts ADJ, Eliasziw M, Gelb AW. Propofol and hyperventilation for the treatment of increased intracranial pressure in rabbits. *Anesth Analg.* 1998;87:564-568
90. Herregods L, Verbeke J, Rolly G, Colardyn F. Effect of propofol on elevated intracranial pressure. Preliminary results. *Anaesthesia.* 1988;43(suppl):107-109
91. Pinaud M, Lelausque J, Chetanneau A, Fauchoux N, Menegalli D, Souron R. Effects of propofol on cerebral hemodynamics and metabolism in patients with brain trauma. *Anesthesiology.* 1990;73:404-409
92. Mangez JF, Menguy E, Roux P. Sedation par propofol a debit constant chez le traumatise cranien. Resultas preliminaires. *Ann Fr Anesth Reanim.* 1987;6:336-337
93. Ravussin P, Guinard JP, Ralley F, Thorin D. Effect of propofol on cerebrospinal fluid pressure and cerebral perfusion pressure in patients undergoing craniotomy. *Anaesthesia.* 1988;43(suppl):37-41
94. Farling PA, Johnston JR, Coppel DL. Propofol infusion for sedation of patients with head injury in intensive care. *Anaesthesia.* 1989;44:222-226
95. Spitzfadden AC, Jimenez DF, Tobias JD. Propofol for sedation and control of intracranial pressure in children. *Pediatr Neurosurg.* 1999;31:194-200
96. Eames WO, Rooke GA, Sai-Chuen R, Bishop M. Comparison of the effects of etomidate, propofol, and thiopental on respiratory resistance after tracheal intubation. *Anesthesiology.* 1996;84:1307-1311
97. Pizov R, Brown RH, Weiss YS, et al. Wheezing during induction of general anesthesia in patients with and without asthma. A randomized, blinded trial. *Anesthesiology.* 1995;82:1111-1116
98. Lin CC, Shyr MH, Tan PP, et al. Mechanisms underlying the inhibitory effect of propofol on the contraction of canine airway smooth muscle. *Anesthesiology.* 1999;91:750-759
99. Pedersen CM, Thirstrup S, Nielsen-Kudsk JE. Smooth muscle relaxant effects of propofol and ketamine in isolated guinea-pig tracheas. *Eur J Pharm.* 1993;238:75-80
100. Brussel T, Theissen JL, Vigfusson G, Lunkenheimer PP, Van Aken H, Lawin P. Hemodynamic and cardiodynamic effects of propofol and etomidate: negative inotropic properties of propofol. *Anesth Analg.* 1989;69:35-40

101. Tritapepe L, Voci P, Marino P, et al. Calcium chloride minimizes the hemodynamic effects of propofol in patients undergoing coronary artery bypass grafting. *J Cardiothorac Vasc Anesth.* 1999;13:150-153
102. Sochala C, Van Deenen D, De Ville A, Govaerts MJM. Heart block following propofol in a child. *Paediatr Anaesth.* 1999;9:349-351
103. Egan TD, Brock-Utne JG. Asystole and anesthesia induction with a fentanyl, propofol, and succinylcholine sequence. *Anesth Analg.* 1991;73:818-820
104. Trotter C, Serpell MG. Neurological sequelae in children after prolonged propofol infusions. *Anaesthesia.* 1992;47:340-342
105. Saunders PRI, Harris MNE. Opisthotonic posturing and other unusual neurological sequelae after outpatient anesthesia. *Anaesthesia.* 1992;47:552-557
106. Finley GA, MacManus B, Sampson SE, Fernandez CV, Retallick I. Delayed seizures following sedation with propofol. *Can J Anaesth.* 1993;40:863-865
107. Hewitt PB, Chu DL, Polkey CE, Binnie CD. Effect of propofol on the electrocorticogram in epileptic patients undergoing cortical resection. *Br J Anaesth.* 1999;82:199-202
108. McBurney JW, Teiken PJ, Moon MR. Propofol for treating status epilepticus. *J Epilepsy.* 1994;7:21-22
109. Lowenstein DH, Alldredge BK. Status epilepticus. *N Engl J Med.* 1998;338:970-976
110. Parke TJ, Stevens JE, Rice AS, et al. Metabolic acidosis and fatal myocardial failure after propofol infusion in children: five case reports. *Br Med J.* 1992;305:613-616
111. Strickland RA, Murray MJ. Fatal metabolic acidosis in a pediatric patient receiving an infusion of propofol in the intensive care unit: is there a relationship? *Crit Care Med.* 1995;23:405-409
112. Hanna JP, Ramundo ML. Rhabdomyolysis and hypoxia associated with prolonged propofol infusion. *Neurology.* 1998;50:301-303
113. Cremer OL, Moons KG, Bouman EA, Kruijswijk, de Smet AM, Kalkman CJ. Long-term propofol infusion and cardiac failure in adult head-injured patients. *Lancet.* 2000;357:117-118
114. Bray RJ. Propofol infusion syndrome in children. *Paediatr Anaesth.* 1998;8:491-499
115. Schenkman KA, Yan S. Propofol impairment of mitochondrial respiration in isolated perfused guinea pig hearts determined by reflectance spectroscopy. *Crit Care Med.* 2000;28:172-177

116. Wolf A, Weir P, Segar P, Stone J, Shields J. Impaired fatty acid oxidation in propofol infusion syndrome. *Lancet.* 2001;357:606-607
117. Rigby-Jones AE, Nolan JA, Priston MJ, Wright PM, Sneyd JR, Wolf AR. Pharmacokinetics of propofol infusions in critically ill noenates, infants, and children in an intensive care unit. *Anesthesiology.* 2002;97:1393-1400
118. Reed MD, Yamashita TS, Marx CM, Myers CM, Blumer IL. A pharmacokinetically based propofol dosing strategy for sedation of the critically ill, mechanically ventilated pediatric patient. *Crit Care Med.* 1996;24:1473-1481
119. Norreslet J, Wahlgreen C. Propofol infusion for sedation of children. *Crit Care Med.* 1990;18:890-892
120. Hertzog JH, Campbell JK, Dalton HJ, Hauser GJ. Propofol anesthesia for invasive procedures in ambulatory and hospitalized children: experience in the pediatric intensive care unit. *Pediatrics.* 1999;103:e30
121. Propofol (Diprivan) infusion: sedation in children aged 16 years or younger. *Curr Problems Pharmacovigilance.* 2001;27:10
122. Laxenaire MC, Mata-Bermejo E, Moneret-Vautrin DA, Gueant JL. Life-threatening anaphylactoid reactions to propofol. *Anesthesiology.* 1992;77:275-280
123. Griffin J, Ray T, Gray B, et al. Pain on injection of propofol: a thiopental/propofol mixture versus a lidocaine/propofol mixture. *Am J Pain Manage.* 2002;12:45-49
124. Tobias JD. Prevention of pain associated with the administration of propofol in children: lidocaine versus ketamine. *Am J Anesthesiol.* 1996;23:231-232
125. Sosis MB, Braverman B. Growth of *Staphylococcus aureus* in four intravenous anesthetics. *Anesth Analg.* 1993;77:766-768
126. Postsurgical infections associated with extrinsically contaminated intravenous anesthetic agent—California, Illinois, Maine, and Michigan, 1990. *MMWR Morb Mortal Wkly Rep.* 1990;39:426-427, 433
127. Trissel LA. Drug compatibility differences with propofol injectable emulsion products. *Crit Care Med.* 2001;46:466-468
128. Lewis TC, Janicki PK, Higgins MS, et al. Anesthetic potency of propofol with disodium edetate versus sulfite-containing propofol in patients undergoing magnetic resonance imaging: a retrospective analysis. *Am J Anesthesiol.* 200;27:30-32
129. Gottardis M, Khunl-Brady KS, Koller W, Sigl G, Hackl JM. Effect of prolonged sedation with propofol on serum triglyceride and cholesterol concentrations. *Br J Anaesth.* 1989;62:393-396

130. Valente JF, Anderson GL, Branson RD, Johnson DJ, Davis K Jr, Porembka DT. Disadvantages of prolonged propofol sedation in the critical care unit. *Crit Care Med.* 1994;22:710-712
131. Sandiumenge Camps A, Sanchez-Izquierdo Riera JA, Toral Vazquez D, et al. Midazolam and 2% propofol in long-term sedation of traumatized, critically ill patients: efficacy and safety comparison. *Crit Care Med.* 2000;28:3612-3619
132. Barrientos-Vega R, Sanchez-Soria M, Morales-Garcia C, Cuena-Boy R, Castellano-Hernandez M. Pharmacoeconomic assessment of propofol 2% used for prolonged sedation. *Crit Care Med.* 2001;29:317-322
133. Astrup J, Sorensen PM, Sorensen HR. Inhibition of cerebral oxygen and glucose consumption in the dog by hypothermia, pentobarbital and lidocaine. *Anesthesiology.* 1981;55:263-268
134. Cormio M, Gopinath SP, Valadka A, Robertson CS. Cerebral hemodynamic effects of pentobarbital coma in head-injured patients. *J Neurotrauma.* 1999;16:927-936
135. Krishnamurthy KB, Drislane FW. Depth of EEG suppression and out come in barbiturate anesthetic treatment for refractory status epilepticus. *Epilepsia.* 1999;40:759-762
136. Holmes GL, Riviello JJ Jr. Midazolam and pentobarbital for refractory status epilepticus. *Pediatr Neurol.* 1999;20:259-264
137. Ishimaru H, Takahashi A, Ikarashi Y, Maruyama Y. Effects of MK-801 and pentobarbital on cholinergic terminal damage and delayed neuronal death in the ischemic gerbil hippocampus. *Brain Res Bull.* 1997;43:81-85
138. Morimoto Y, Morimoto Y, Nishihira J, et al. Pentobarbital inhibits apoptosis in neuronal cells. *Crit Care Med.* 2000;28:1899-1904
139. Tobias JD, Deshpande JK, Pietsch JB, Wheeler TJ, Gregory DG. Pentobarbital sedation in the pediatric intensive care unit patient. *South Med J.* 1995;88:290-294
140. Tobias JD. Pentobarbital for sedation during mechanical ventilation in the pediatric ICU patient. *J Intensive Care Med.* 2000;15:115-120
141. Collins JJ, Grier HE, Kinney HC, Berde CB. Control of severe pain in children with terminal malignancy. *J Pediatr.* 1995;126:653-657
142. Burkle H, Dunbar S, Van Aken H. Remifentanil: a novel, short acting, mu opioid. *Anesth Analg.* 1996;83:646-651
143. Ross AK, Davis PJ, Dear Gd GL, et al. Pharmacokinetics of remifentanil in anesthetized pediatric patients undergoing elective surgery or diagnostic procedures. *Anesth Analg.* 2001;93:1393-1401
144. Tobias JD. Remifentanil: applications in the pediatric ICU population. *Am J Pain Manage.* 1998;8:114-117

145. Cavaliere F, Antonelli M, Arcangeli A, et al. A low-dose remifentanil infusion is well tolerated for sedation in mechanically ventilated, critically ill patients. *Can J Anesth.* 2002;49:1088-1094
146. Sperry RJ, Bailey PL, Reichman MV, Peterson JC, Peterson PB, Pace NL. Fentanyl and sufentanil increase intracranial pressure in head trauma patients. *Anesthesiology.* 1992;77:416-420
147. Milde LN, Milde JH, Gallagher WJ. Effects of sufentanil on cerebral circulation and metabolism in dogs. *Anesth Analg.* 1990;70:138-146
148. Pokela ML, Ryhanen PT, Koivisto ME, Olkkola KT, Saukkonen AL. Alfentanil-induced rigidity in newborn infants. *Anesth Analg.* 1992;75:252-257
149. Glick C, Evans OB, Parks BR. Muscle rigidity due to fentanyl infusion in the pediatric patient. *South Med J.* 1996;89:1119-1120
150. Irazuzta J, Pascucci R, Perlman N, Wessel D. Effects of fentanyl administration on respiratory system compliance in infants. *Crit Care Med.* 1993;21:1001-1004
151. Lynn AM, Opheim KE, Tyler DC. Morphine infusion after pediatric cardiac surgery. *Crit Care Med.* 1984;12:863-866
152. Quinn MW, Wild J, Dean HG, et al. Randomised double-blind controlled trial of effect of morphine on catecholamine concentrations in ventilated pre-term babies. *Lancet.* 1993;342:324-327
153. MacGregor R, Evans D, Sugden D, Gaussen T, Levene M. Outcome at 5-6 years of prematurely born children who received morphine as neonates. *Arch Dis Child Fetal Neonatal.* 1998;79:F40-43
154. Franck LS, Vilardi J, Durand D, Powers R. Opioid withdrawal in neonates after continuous infusions of morphine or fentanyl during extracorporeal membrane oxygenation. *Am J Crit Care.* 1998;7:364-369
155. Rosow CE, Moss J, Philbin DM, Savarese JJ. Histamine release during morphine and fentanyl anesthesia. *Anesthesiology.* 1982;56:93-96
156. Shochet RB, Murray GB. Neuropsychiatric toxicity of meperidine. *J Intensive Care Med.* 1988;3:246-252
157. Bruera E, Brenneis C, Michaud M, et al. Use of the subcutaneous route for the administration of narcotics in patients with cancer pain. *Cancer.* 1988;62:407-411
158. Bruera E, Gibney N, Stollery D, Marcushamer S. Use of the subcutaneous route of administration of morphine in the intensive care unit. *J Pain Symptom Manage.* 1991;6:263-265
159. Tobias JD, O'Connor TA. Subcutaneous administration of fentanyl for sedation during mechanical ventilation in an infant. *Am J Pain Manage.* 1996;6:115-117

160. Dietrich CC, Tobias JD. Subcutaneous fentanyl in the pediatric population. *Am J Pain Manage.* 2003;13:146-150
161. Riker RR, Fraser GL, Cox PM. Continuous infusions of haloperidol controls agitation in critically ill patients. *Crit Care Med.* 1994;22:433-440
162. US Food and Drug Administration. MedWatch. Available at: http://www.fda/gov/medwatch/SAFETY/2001/inapsine.htm. Accessed August 6, 2004
163. Nahata MC, Clotz MA, Krogg EA. Adverse effects of meperidine, promethazine, and chlorpromazine for sedation in pediatric patients. *Clin Pediatr.* 1985;24:558-560
164. Rokicki W. Cardiac arrhythmia in a child after the usual dose of chloral hydrate. *Pediatr Cardiol.* 1996;17:419-420
165. Seger D, Schwartz G. Chloral hydrate: a dangerous sedative for overdose patients? *Pediatr Emerg Care.* 1994;10:349-350
166. Maze MM, Tranquilli W. Alpha-2 agonists: defining the role in clinical anesthesia. *Anesthesiology.* 1991;74:581-591
167. Mikawa K, Maekawa N, Nishina K, Takao Y, Yaku H, Obara H. Efficacy of oral clonidine premedication in children. *Anesthesiology.* 1993;79:926-931
168. De Kock MF, Pichon G, Scholtes JL. Intraoperative clonidine enhances postoperative morphine patient-controlled analgesia. *Can J Anaesth.* 1992;39:537-544
169. Bohrer H, Bach A, Layer M, Werning P. Clonidine as a sedative adjunct in intensive care. *Intensive Care Med.* 1990;16:265-266
170. Venn RM, Bradshaw CJ, Spencer R, et al. Preliminary UK experience of dexmedetomidine, a novel agent for postoperative sedation in the intensive care unit. *Anaesthesia.* 1999;54:1136-1142
171. Hall JE, Uhrich TD, Barney JA, Arain SR, Ebert TJ. Sedative, amnestic, and analgesic properties of small-dose dexmedetomidine infusions. *Anesth Analg.* 2000;90:699-705
172. Tobias JD, Berkenbosch JW. Sedation during mechanical ventilation in infants and children: dexmedetomidine versus midazolam. *South Med J.* 2004;97:451-455
173. Berkenbosch JW, Tobias JD. Development of bradycardia during sedation with dexmedetomidine in an infant concurrently receiving digoxin. *Pediatr Crit Care Med.* 2003;4:203-205
174. Talke P, Chen R, Thomas B, et al. The hemodynamic and adrenergic effects of perioperative dexmedetomidine infusion after vascular surgery. *Anesth Analg.* 2000;90:834-839

Chapter 7

Tolerance, Physical Dependency, and Withdrawal

Joseph D. Tobias, MD, FAAP

Definitions
- Tolerance
- Withdrawal and Physical Dependency

Initial Clinical Reports—Opioids

Tolerance and Abstinence Syndromes With Other Agents
- Benzodiazepines
- Barbiturates
- Ketamine
- Propofol
- Inhalational Anesthetic Agents

Clinical Signs and Symptoms of Withdrawal

Factors Affecting the Development of Tolerance

Treatment Options

Introduction

As technology increases, so does the potential for patients surviving catastrophic illnesses. Patients may spend weeks or months in a pediatric intensive care unit (PICU), during which time aggressive analgesia and sedation may be required. Due to humanitarian issues, as well as the potential for adverse psychological and physiologic effects of inadequate pain management, there is a need to ensure adequate sedation and analgesia in critically ill patients, as described in formal policy statements concerning intensive care unit (ICU) sedation.[1] This heightened awareness, coupled with an appropriately increased use of sedative and analgesic agents, has led to physical dependency, tolerance, and withdrawal, which require definition and effective treatment strategies. Effective management schemes to treat these consequences, as well as methods to delay or prevent them, are needed so that they do not limit the appropriate use of sedative and analgesics in the PICU patient. This chapter reviews initial studies describing tolerance, physical dependency, and withdrawal following the prolonged use of sedative and analgesic agents; investigates the cellular mechanisms of tolerance and physical dependency to define techniques that may potentially limit their occurrence; and suggests treatment strategies. Although much of the focus of this chapter is on the PICU patient, the same problems and techniques apply to patients in any setting who require long-term administration of sedative/analgesic agents.

Definitions

Tolerance

Treating the patient who has tolerance and physical dependency begins with defining the terminology[2] so that communication among health care providers remains clear, eliminating misunderstanding that may hinder treatment. *Tolerance* is a decrease in the effect of a drug over time so that it is necessary to increase the dose to achieve the same effect. In most cases, tolerance is defined as alterations in a drug's effect related to changes at or distal to the receptor, usually at the cellular level. However, other authorities have grouped tolerance into various subcategories, including innate tolerance, which refers to a genetically predetermined lack of sensitivity to a drug (eg, lack of the enzyme system required for the metabolism of codeine to morphine); pharmacokinetic or dispositional tolerance referring to changes in a drug's effect because of alterations in distribution or metabolism (eg, when the hepatic microsomal enzymes are stimulated by another medication leading to enhanced metabolism of the sedative/analgesic medication); learned tolerance or a reduction in a drug's effect as a result of learned or compensatory mechanisms (eg, learning to walk a straight line after ethanol or cannabinoid use by repeated practice of the task); and pharmacodynamic tolerance (eg, alterations at or distal to the receptor).[3]

With pharmacodynamic tolerance, the plasma concentration of the drug remains constant, but a decreased effect (eg, sedation or analgesia) is noted. Pharmacodynamic tolerance occurs in the PICU patient who requires prolonged sedation/analgesia during a catastrophic illness. The potential magnitude of tolerance is illustrated by a case involving a 16-year-old adolescent weighing 52 kg who required mechanical ventilation for 5 weeks.[4] Tolerance resulted in the ultimate need to increase the fentanyl infusion to 3,500 μg/h (67.3 μg/kg/h, usual starting doses range from 1-3 μg/kg/h). Because administering such a large amount of fentanyl required infusing 70 mL/h of the fentanyl solution, which has a maximum concentration of 50 μg/mL, fentanyl was substituted with the more potent synthetic opioid sufentanil to limit fluid volume. The patient eventually made a full recovery and was discharged home on an oral methadone taper (see following text).

Tolerance also can be documented with newer ICU technology such as the Bispectral Index (BIS monitor, Aspect Medical, Newton, MA), which monitors the electroencephalographic pattern of the patient, providing a number from 0 (isoelectric) to 100 (awake). Using this monitor in the PICU patient has helped identify tolerance because the infusion rates of medications must be increased to maintain the same BIS number.[5] This effect is shown in a patient who required sedation over a 5- to 6-day period. The total daily doses of midazolam and fentanyl that were required to maintain the BIS number between 30 to 40 increased from 230 mg and 4,056 μg respectively on day 1 to 460.8 mg and 13,172 μg on day 5. Such monitoring not only provides a more objective measure of tolerance development, but also may be helpful in monitoring sedation level and thereby preventing oversedation (see following text).

Withdrawal and Physical Dependency

Withdrawal can be defined as the set of signs and symptoms that manifest following the abrupt discontinuation of a sedative or analgesic agent in a patient who is physically tolerant. Withdrawal symptoms vary and are affected by factors such as the specific agent and the patient's age, cognitive state, and associated medical conditions. Physical or physiologic dependence is the need to continue a sedative or analgesic agent to prevent withdrawal. Physical dependence must be distinguished from psychological dependence, or the need for a substance because of its euphoric effects. Addiction is a complex pattern of behaviors characterized by the repetitive, compulsive use of a substance; antisocial or criminal behavior to obtain the drug; and a high incidence of relapse after rehabilitative treatment. Psychological dependency and addiction are extremely rare following the appropriate use of sedative/analgesic agents, such as those used to treat pain or relieve anxiety in the PICU setting. The rare occurrence of psychological dependency and addiction, as well as concerns about tolerance, physical dependency, and withdrawal, should not limit the use of sedative/analgesic agents in the PICU population. These consequences can be effectively managed by using appropriate weaning schedules outlined in this chapter.

Initial Clinical Reports—Opioids

Opioid dependency and withdrawal in pediatric patients were first encountered in the 1970s and 1980s in infants of drug-addicted mothers.[6-8] Although there is an obvious difference in the cause, these studies can provide valuable information for treating today's PICU population, including potential pharmacologic treatment regimens and scoring systems to quantify the severity of withdrawal and evaluate the efficacy of treatment.

Awareness of opioid tolerance and withdrawal in the PICU population began in the late 1980s and early 1990s. Arnold and colleagues[9] were among the first to identify dependency and withdrawal following prolonged opioid administration. In a retrospective study of 37 neonates who had received fentanyl infusions for sedation during extracorporeal membrane oxygenation (ECMO) for respiratory failure, they identified the signs and symptoms and risk factors of the neonatal abstinence syndrome (NAS). There was an increase in the fentanyl infusion requirements to achieve the desired level of sedation from 11.6 ± 6.9 µg/kg/h on day 1 to 52.5 ± 19.4 µg/kg/h on day 8. There was an increase in the plasma fentanyl concentration required to achieve the same level of sedation, thereby demonstrating that the tolerance was pharmacodynamic and not pharmacokinetic. A follow-up study by the same investigators demonstrated tolerance in neonates and infants sedated with a continuous fentanyl infusion during mechanical ventilation, but not placed on ECMO.[10] Neonatal abstinence syndrome developed in 57% of neonates. Risk factors for the development of NAS included a cumulative fentanyl dose greater than 1.6 mg/kg, or the administration of the fentanyl infusion for more than 5 days (odds ratio 7 and 13.9, respectively).

These studies indicate: 1) NAS occurs following the prolonged administration of sedative/analgesic agents in the PICU population; 2) its incidence can be significant; and 3) over time, there is an increase in the plasma fentanyl concentration required to achieve the desired level of sedation, thereby demonstrating pharmacodynamic tolerance. Additionally, Arnold et al[9,10] used a standard scoring system described by Finnegan et al[6,7] to grade the severity of the NAS and assess the response to therapy (Table 7-1).

Table 7-1. Components of the Finnegan Score

Sign/Symptom	Score
Cry	
Excessive	2
Continuous	3
Sleep (h) after feeding	
<1 h	3
<2 h	2
<3 h	1
Moro reflex	
Hyperactive	2
Markedly hyperactive	3
Tremors	
Mild, disturbed	1
Mod-severe, disturbed	2
Mod-severe, undisturbed	3
Increased muscle tone	2
Frequent yawning	2
Excoriation	1
Seizures	5
Sweating	1
Fever	
100°F-101°F	1
>101°F	2
Mottling	1
Nasal congestion	1
Sneezing	1
Nasal flaring	2
Respiratory rate	
>60 breaths/min	1
>60 with retractions	2
Excessive sucking	1
Poor feeding	2
Regurgitation	2
Projectile vomiting	3
Stools	
Loose	2
Watery	3

A score of 0-7 indicates mild symptoms of withdrawal, 8-11 moderate withdrawal, and 12-15 severe withdrawal.

In 1990 the use of oral methadone to treat or prevent opioid withdrawal, following the prolonged administration of fentanyl in the PICU patient, was reported.[11] The 3 infants studied demonstrated opioid tolerance, dependency, and withdrawal in a PICU population that was older and had different medical/surgical problems (post-cardiovascular surgery patients) than those reported by Arnold et al.[9,10] Before this study and that of Arnold et al[9,10] there had been limited data on opioid tolerance, withdrawal, and physical dependency in the PICU population.

Tolerance and Abstinence Syndromes With Other Agents

In the PICU population, several classes of agents in addition to opioids are used for sedation, thereby raising additional questions. Do tolerance, physical dependency, and withdrawal occur with non-opioid agents? Are the signs and symptoms similar to opioid withdrawal? Are there specific risk factors that can be used to identify the at-risk population?

Benzodiazepines

Although less common than with opioids, benzodiazepine addiction and dependency occur in the drug-abuse population. Benzodiazepine withdrawal has been reported in the adult psychiatric and drug-addicted population[12,13] as well as the adult ICU population. Freda et al[14] reported a 72-year-old man, chronically medicated with alprazolam as an outpatient, who was admitted to the ICU following aortic aneurysm surgery. While in the ICU, 48 hours after the last dose of alprazolam, the patient developed agitation, delirium, and signs of sympathetic hyperactivity, including tachycardia, hypertension, and tachypnea. These symptoms resolved following intravenous administration of diazepam. Although the study deals with an adult ICU population, it describes signs and symptoms of benzodiazepine withdrawal in the ICU setting, as well as the importance of knowing what medications the patient had received before admission to the ICU. Although, in most cases, physical dependency and withdrawal result from drugs administered in the PICU, problems also may result from medications the patient received before admission. This may become more common as technology advances and more patients receive outpatient medications to treat chronic health conditions.

Sury et al[15] described benzodiazepine withdrawal in 3 children, ranging in age from 4 to 12 years, following prolonged sedation with a continuous infusion of midazolam. Midazolam was administered for 7, 14, and 17 days during mechanical ventilation at mean infusion rates of 0.17, 0.22, and 0.56 mg/kg/h in the 3 patients. The infusion was discontinued without tapering and within 24 hours. The patients manifested visual hallucinations, combative behavior, and seizures, which resolved once a benzodiazepine was reintroduced.

van Engelen et al[16] noted similar symptoms in 2 pediatric patients (aged 15 months and 14 days). The maximum midazolam infusion rates were 0.14 and 0.57 mg/kg/h with durations of 12 and 29 days. Following discontinuation of the medication, both patients demonstrated signs and symptoms of withdrawal manifested by agitation, tachycardia, hyperpyrexia, and gastrointestinal (GI) symptoms, which resolved with reinstitution of the midazolam infusion.

Fonsmark et al[17] studied sedative withdrawal in their retrospective review of 40 children who received sedation with midazolam, pentobarbital, or a combination of the 2 agents during mechanical ventilation. Withdrawal symptoms occurred in 14 of 40 patients (35%). Of those patients who manifested withdrawal symptoms, 8 received both midazolam and pentobarbital, 3 received only midazolam, and 3 received only pentobarbital. A cumulative midazolam dose of 60 mg/kg or greater was predictive of withdrawal, while the duration of the infusion was not. Sedation was gradually tapered in only 1 of 14 patients who experienced withdrawal.

Barbiturates

Withdrawal also has been reported following prolonged administration of pentobarbital in the PICU setting.[17-19] The previously mentioned report of Fonsmark et al[17] noted withdrawal in 11 children who received pentobarbital (8 received both pentobarbital and midazolam, while 3 received only pentobarbital). A cumulative pentobarbital dose of 25 mg/kg or greater was predictive of withdrawal.

A report by Tobias et al[18] also documented pentobarbital withdrawal in a 17-month-old infant. Pentobarbital was started at 2 mg/kg/h when sedation was inadequate, despite escalating doses of fentanyl and midazolam. The pentobarbital infusion was increased to 4 mg/kg/h after 8 days. The patient's trachea was extubated and, 6 to 8 hours after discontinuing the pentobarbital infusion, the child became irritable and developed tachycardia and hypertension. The symptoms resolved following the administration of pentobarbital (2 mg/kg bolus over 10 minutes) and restarting the infusion at 2 mg/kg/h. Oral pentobarbital was substituted for intravenous administration and a taper schedule started.

The relative rarity of reports of withdrawal following pentobarbital may relate to the infrequent use of barbiturates for ICU sedation.[19] However, with the use of pentobarbital in the author's practice as an alternative to the usual combination of opioids and benzodiazepines, additional cases have been noted. The potential for developing tolerance to barbiturates also is supported by animal studies.[20,21]

Ketamine

Because it remains an uncommonly used agent for PICU sedation, there are limited data concerning adverse effects of prolonged administration of ketamine, and no reports regarding withdrawal.[22] However, tolerance to the anesthetic effects of ketamine has been reported.[23-25] Ketamine remains a frequently used agent to provide sedation and analgesia in the nonsurgical environment (during radiation therapy or diagnostic imaging). Several reports have demonstrated tolerance to ketamine manifested as an increased dose requirement and/or decreased sleep time following repeated exposure to the medication.[23-25] To date, however, there are no reports regarding tolerance or withdrawal following ketamine administration in the PICU setting.

Propofol

Despite ongoing debates regarding its safety (see Chapter 6 for a full discussion of propofol use for sedation in the PICU patient), propofol continues to be used to sedate children and adults during mechanical ventilation. Cammarano et al[26] retrospectively reviewed the problem of acute withdrawal following prolonged propofol administration in the adult ICU population. The incidence of withdrawal behavior was higher in patients who received propofol for more than 1 day (P=.026) and more likely in patients who received prolonged infusions of propofol (P=.046). The authors were unable to definitively prove that the withdrawal was related to propofol because all of the patients received other agents, including opioids and benzodiazepines.

Au et al[27] reported a withdrawal syndrome following the administration of propofol for 5 days (dose unspecified) during mechanical ventilation following repair of an ascending aortic aneurysm in a 41-year-old man. The patient became increasingly confused, tremulous, and hallucinatory, and had a generalized tonic-clonic seizure when the the propofol infusion was discontinued after 5 days. Before extubation, the patient also was receiving an opioid infusion. Both the propofol and opioid infusions were restarted and gradually tapered over a 48-hour period. The patient had no other signs or symptoms of withdrawal.

Imray and Hay[28] reported propofol withdrawal in a 10-month-old girl who required mechanical ventilatory support for 2 weeks following an inhalation smoke injury. After discontinuing the propofol infusion, the authors reported "generalized twitching and jitteriness," which subsided in 3 days without additional therapy.

The limited reports of propofol withdrawal may be related to some unique property of the drug or, more likely, the fact that there remains limited clinical experience with prolonged propofol sedation in the ICU population. Although propofol has gained popularity for short-term sedation, clinical experience with prolonged use is limited, especially in children.

Inhalational Anesthetic Agents

An alternative approach for sedation during mechanical ventilation that has not gained widespread use in the United States is the administration of inhalational anesthetic agents such as isoflurane. Arnold and colleagues[29] reported their experience with 10 patients, ranging in age from 3 weeks to 19 years, who received isoflurane for sedation during mechanical ventilation after the usual combination of opioids and benzodiazepines proved to be ineffective. The duration of isoflurane administration varied from 29 to 769 hours (mean of 245 hours) while the minimum alveolar concentration (MAC) hours ranged from 13 to 497 (mean of 131 MAC hours). Agitation and non-purposeful movements occurred in 5 of the 10 patients within 2 hours of discontinuing isoflurane. The 5 patients who manifested withdrawal symptoms had received more than 70 MAC hours of isoflurane. The symptoms responded to the administration of benzodiazepines and/or opioids. These findings were somewhat surprising because studies in laboratory animals had suggested that tolerance and dependency did not occur following the prolonged administration of inhalational anesthetic agents.[30]

The same investigators subsequently reported tolerance and withdrawal phenomena following isoflurane administration to a 4-year-old boy for sedation during mechanical ventilation.[31] After 19 days of administration, despite end-tidal isoflurane concentrations of 0.8% to 1.2% (0.7-1 MAC), the patient was awake and able to follow commands. The MAC awake level of isoflurane is 0.3 to 0.4 MAC, so it was not expected that the patient would be awake and able to follow commands with an end-tidal concentration of 0.3% to 0.5% of isoflurane. After 32 days, the patient's trachea was extubated and the isoflurane was discontinued. The patient developed agitation, diaphoresis, tachycardia, hypertension, and profuse diarrhea. The symptoms were controlled with pentobarbital and midazolam infusions.

Another case of isoflurane withdrawal was reported by Hughes et al.[32] Isoflurane (unspecified concentration) was administered for 4 days. Following its discontinuation, the patient became agitated, experienced visual and auditory hallucinations, and had a generalized tonic-clonic seizure. The symptoms were treated with rectal diazepam and, within 5 days, the patient had returned to his baseline status.

Clinical Signs and Symptoms of Withdrawal

Developing strategies to provide effective treatment of physical dependency requires accurately identifying and recognizing withdrawal symptoms. Associated conditions that mimic the clinical signs and symptoms of withdrawal must be investigated and ruled out. In the PICU patient, associated conditions that mimic withdrawal include central nervous system (CNS) insults or infections, ICU psychosis, metabolic abnormalities, hypoxia, hypercarbia, and cerebral hypoperfusion from alterations in cardiac output or cerebral vascular disease. Given the potential effect of such conditions, a thorough search to rule out such problems is essential before treating what is assumed to be withdrawal.

Although many of the signs and symptoms of withdrawal are the same regardless of the agent, there may be subtle differences depending on the specific agent. The onset of withdrawal symptoms varies depending on the half-life of the agent and its active metabolites. The half-life of the latter may be several times longer than the parent compound. Clinical signs and symptoms may manifest shortly after discontinuation of the drug if the agent and its metabolites have a short half-life (propofol, fentanyl) or days later if the agent or its metabolites have long half-lives (diazepam). Delayed clearance of active metabolites or the parent compound in patients with underlying renal or hepatic dysfunction also may affect the onset time of withdrawal symptoms.

The signs and symptoms of sedative/analgesic agent withdrawal generally include 1) central and sympathetic nervous system activation and 2) GI disturbances. The CNS manifestations are excitatory and include irritability, increased wakefulness, tremulousness, hyperactive deep tendon reflexes, clonus, inability to concentrate, frequent yawning, sneezing, delirium, and hypertonicity. In the neonatal and infant population, a high-pitched cry and an exaggerated Moro reflex are additional signs of CNS excitability. Seizures have been reported with withdrawal from various substances including opioids, benzodiazepines, barbiturates, propofol, and the inhalational anesthetic agents. Opioid, benzodiazepine, barbiturate, and inhalational anesthetic withdrawal can provoke either visual or auditory hallucinations. Prolonged tinnitus, lasting 6 to 8 months, has been anecdotally associated with benzodiazepine withdrawal.[33]

Gastrointestinal manifestations of withdrawal may be especially prominent in neonates and infants. These include feeding intolerance with vomiting, diarrhea, uncoordinated suck and swallow, or persistent residuals with enteral tube feedings. In many cases, GI disturbances may be attributed to conditions other than withdrawal.

Sympathetic nervous system signs and symptoms include tachycardia, hypertension, tachypnea, nasal stuffiness, sweating, and fever. These clinical findings may be particularly troublesome in the PICU patient with multiple indwelling central lines in whom temperature instability requires immediate investigation and, at times, treatment with broad-spectrum antibiotics.

Although a complete withdrawal syndrome with multiple manifestations is easily recognized, patients may have subtle clinical findings that easily can be confused with other conditions in the PICU setting. The signs and symptoms vary in number, severity, and presentation. Equally important, especially in the PICU patient, withdrawal should not be overdiagnosed and it must remain a diagnosis of exclusion. Fever or vomiting should never be attributed to withdrawal until other etiologies are excluded.

In addition to the previously mentioned signs and symptoms, unique clinical scenarios that represent withdrawal phenomena have been reported in the literature. For example, 2 patients with upper airway obstruction with stridor, that was later thought to be a manifestation of opioid withdrawal, were reported.[34] In these 2 patients, upper airway obstruction with stridor developed shortly after tracheal extubation and discontinuation of the opioid infusion. Direct laryngoscopy and airway examination in the operating room revealed no anatomical etiology for the stridor. Upper airway obstruction and stridor resolved after reinstituting the opioid infusions. These 2 patients had associated closed head injuries and altered mental status with Glasgow Coma Scale scores of 10 to 11, which may have influenced the manifestations of opioid withdrawal. On retrospective analysis, both patients also demonstrated sympathetic hyperactivity with tachycardia and hypertension, which are signs of opioid withdrawal, but were initially attributed to the respiratory distress.

Lane et al[35] reported choreoathetoid movements and myoclonus in 5 children following discontinuation of fentanyl infusions. In addition to the usual manifestations of opioid withdrawal (tremor, irritability, and insomnia), the patients developed myoclonus, ataxia, and choreoathetosis. No treatment was instituted and the patients made a complete recovery without permanent neurologic sequelae. The authors concluded that this unusual movement disorder was a manifestation of opioid withdrawal.

Bergman et al[36] described a similar syndrome in infants sedated with a combination of fentanyl and midazolam. The symptom complex included choreoathetoid movements with poor social interactions, decreased visual attentiveness, and dystonic posturing. As in the previous report of Lane et al,[35] all patients eventually made a full recovery, although some were symptomatic for up to 4 weeks. Retrospective analysis revealed the following risk factors: the combination of a continuous infusion of midazolam and fentanyl, young age, female gender, low serum albumin, and concomitant administration of aminophylline.

The authors were unable to determine if this was a true withdrawal syndrome or a toxic adverse effect related to the sedative agents, perhaps in combination with other medications.

Factors Affecting the Development of Tolerance

Most of the information regarding cellular mechanisms of tolerance and dependence involves opioids and related compounds. Sedatives and analgesics exert their effects through agent-specific cell surface receptors. The 4 major opioid receptors are classified as μ, κ, δ, or σ receptor agonists. The μ receptor can be further subclassified into μ_1 and μ_2 subtypes. The μ, δ, and κ receptors produce analgesia through a similar mechanism, the end result of which involves the inhibition of synaptic transmission in the CNS. Binding of the opioid agonist to the receptor results in a conformational change of the receptor which, through interactions with the G-protein system, alters the intracellular concentrations of cyclic adenosine monophosphate (AMP), ions (K^+, CA^{++}, Na^+), and enzyme systems including phospholipases A_2 and C. These alterations result in a decrease in the release of excitatory neurotransmitters and the hyperpolarization of neural pathways involved in nociception.

The predominant factors that determine tolerance and dependence are occupancy of the receptor by an agonist and the specificity or avidity with which the agonist binds to the receptor. However, the exact cellular mechanisms responsible for tolerance and dependence remain poorly defined. The mechanism is likely not solely a decrease in receptor number or binding affinity, but rather alterations of the interactions between the receptor, the regulatory G proteins, and intracellular systems.[37] The abrupt discontinuation of the opioid agonist results in increased afferent activity to the CNS with activation of the reticular activating system as well as sympathetic centers. Sympathetic activation from areas such as the locus ceruleus result in increased efferent sympathetic activity and subsequent autonomic effects, including tachycardia and hypertension.

In the same manner as the opioids, benzodiazepines and barbiturates act through specific cell surface receptors. Although the receptors are specific for the individual agent, the activation of the receptor leads to a similar cascade of intracellular events with the resultant alteration of chloride conductance and hyperpolarization of the CNS. Benzodiazepines increase the affinity of the inhibitory neurotransmitter γ-amino butyric acid (GABA) at surface receptors located on postsynaptic neurons, leading to increased chloride conductance and hyperpolarization. During chronic benzodiazepine administration in laboratory animals, Miller et al[38] noted receptor down-regulation with decreased function as indicated by chloride uptake. Abrupt discontinuation of the benzodiazepine will lead to decreased pharmacologic efficacy of the same concentration of GABA with a resultant disinhibition of the CNS. Similar mechanisms of action have been suggested for propofol and the inhalation anesthetic agents.

To date most information about factors controlling tolerance, as well as ways to prevent or delay its development, are based on information obtained from laboratory and clinical studies with opioids. Duration of opioid receptor occupancy is the key factor in determining the development of tolerance.[39] Tolerance tends to develop more rapidly with the continuous versus the intermittent administration of sedative and analgesic agents.[39] Because of their increased affinity for the opioid receptor when compared with other opioids such as morphine, synthetic opioids (fentanyl, sufentanil, remifentanil) may lead to tolerance more rapidly.

In clinical practice, the amount of sedative/analgesic medication required for effective sedation or pain relief can be lessened (perhaps delaying tolerance) by the use of pain or sedation scales to allow for appropriate titration of the infusion. These scoring systems, which are discussed in more detail in Chapter 6, involve various combinations of the patient's self-reporting of the degree of pain, physiologic parameters such as alterations in heart rate or blood pressure, or objective observations made by the health care personnel of the patient's behavior or response to a stimulus. Based on a patient's score, the dose can be adjusted according to need so that the minimum necessary amount of medication is administered. The importance of dose titration is illustrated by the study of Katz and Kelly,[40] which demonstrated a 10-fold variability in the fentanyl infusion requirements to achieve the same degree of sedation in a population of PICU patients.

The potential effect of oversedation is illustrated by the study of Cammarano et al,[26] who noted that the concomitant use of neuromuscular blocking agents for more than 1 day was a risk factor for the development of tolerance. The authors speculated that, when caring for patients who are receiving neuromuscular blocking agents, many of the usual clues used to titrate the sedative and analgesic agents are lacking. Therefore, these patients may receive higher doses of sedative and analgesic agents. Because scoring systems that rely on the patient's self-reporting or response to stimuli are not feasible during the use of neuromuscular blocking agents, the use of physiologic monitors such as the BIS monitor may provide a guide for the titration of sedation.[41] The author has demonstrated that the BIS number correlates with clinical sedation scores and extrapolate from these data to suggest that the BIS monitor may be effectively used to guide the dosing of sedative agents in settings when objective or self-report pain scores are not feasible. Further studies are needed to determine if such strategies will allow more accurate titration of sedative agents and decrease the incidence of tolerance and dependence.

It is theoretically possible to delay tolerance related to receptor occupancy by rotating sedation regimens. This technique may be more feasible with the introduction of a novel agent for ICU sedation, the α_2-adrenergic agonist dexmedetomidine. (See Chapter 6.) There are now 3 different receptor systems that can be used to sedate PICU patients (benzodiazepine, opioid, and α_2-adrenergic systems). Rather than rotating regimens at fixed intervals, it also may be feasible to switch to another agent when an obvious dose escalation above specific predetermined doses is noted. Prospective evaluations are needed to determine the efficacy of these maneuvers to prevent or delay tolerance and physical dependency.

Basic science research has provided some insight into other ways to prevent or delay tolerance. Specific interactions between opioid receptor subtypes may be involved in the tolerance. In laboratory animals, blockade of δ receptors prevents acute and chronic tolerance to μ-receptor agonists.[42] The administration of μ antagonists increases the analgesic effects of κ agonists,[43] while the activation of spinal κ receptors attenuates tolerance to the μ agonist morphine.[44]

Non-opioid receptors such as the *N*-methyl-D-aspartate (NMDA) system also are involved in tolerance and physical dependency. Antagonism of central NMDA receptors slows the development of opioid tolerance[45] and attenuates certain withdrawal behaviors.[46] Although the current experience with NMDA-receptor antagonists is limited to laboratory studies with agents such as MK-801 and LY274614 (which are not available for clinical use), ketamine, dextromethorphan, and magnesium possess direct or indirect antagonistic properties at the NMDA receptor. The NMDA-receptor ion channels are blocked by magnesium in a voltage-dependent manner at a location deep within the ion channel. McCarthy et al[47] demonstrated that the coadministration of intrathecal magnesium with morphine delayed the development of tolerance to the antinociceptive effects of morphine. These properties, at least theoretically, suggest that these agents may delay tolerance in sedated PICU patients. Prospective studies are needed to better address the efficacy of rotating sedation regimens, intermittent versus continuous infusions of sedative/analgesic agents, and the role of other pharmacologic agents such as NMDA-receptor antagonists in preventing tolerance and dependence.

Treatment Options

The first phase of treating patients with dependence and tolerance is to identify risk factors and to develop a scoring system for identifying and quantifying withdrawal signs and symptoms. At-risk patients can then be identified and appropriate therapy initiated, such as slowly tapering infusions, thereby preventing, rather than treating, withdrawal. Katz et al[48] identified factors that placed patients at risk for opioid withdrawal in a cohort of 23 infants and children, aged 1 week to 22 months. All of the patients had received continuous infusions of fentanyl for sedation during mechanical ventilation. Once sedation was no longer required, the fentanyl infusion was rapidly decreased over a 48-hour period. Withdrawal was assessed using a neonatal scoring system originally described by Finnegan et al (Table 7-1).[49] Withdrawal was observed in 13 of 23 patients (57%). Risk factors for withdrawal included the total fentanyl dose and the duration of the infusion. A total fentanyl dose of 1.5 mg/kg or greater or a duration of infusion of 5 days or more was associated with a 50% incidence of withdrawal. A total fentanyl dose of 2.5 mg/kg or greater or a duration of infusion of 9 days or more was associated with a 100% incidence of withdrawal. Similar results were reported by the studies of Arnold et al,[9,10] who noted a correlation of both total dose (>1.6 mg/kg) and duration of administration (>5 days) with the incidence of withdrawal.

Arnold et al[31] also noted that the total dose administered was a risk factor for patients who received the inhalation anesthetic agent isoflurane. Withdrawal occurred only in patients who had received more than 70 MAC hours of isoflurane. In their retrospective review, Fonsmark et al[17] reported that an increased probability of withdrawal was noted with a total dose of midazolam of 60 mg/kg or greater or a total dose of pentobarbital of 25 mg/kg or greater.

Regardless of the agent(s) used for sedation, once the decision is made to start weaning the infusion, close observation of the patient using a formal scoring system is necessary to assess withdrawal. Kahn et al[8] were among the first to introduce a scoring system. The scoring system divided withdrawal into 3 grades: grade I included mild, but abnormal behavior; grade II included more severe symptoms that occurred when the infant was disturbed; and grade III included severe symptoms that occurred spontaneously. A more detailed scoring systems described later by Finnegan et al[49] assigned points to different types of abnormal behavior (Table 7-1). According to the Finnegan system, a total score greater than 6 to 8 was indicative of significant withdrawal and the need for treatment. Other scoring systems are outlined in the review of Anand and Arnold.[50] Such scoring symptoms were developed to determine the severity of withdrawal in infants of drug-addicted mothers by assessing neonatal behavior. However, they can provide useful information in the PICU patient as well.

The primary therapy to prevent withdrawal is a slow weaning of the sedative/analgesic infusions. Although this usually can be achieved rapidly (10%-15% every 6-8 hours) in patients who have been treated for brief periods (<3-5 days), following prolonged administration, the weaning process may take 2 to 4 weeks to prevent withdrawal symptoms.

Although the weaning process can be accomplished by slowly decreasing the intravenous infusion rate, this mandates the maintenance of intravenous access, ongoing hospitalization and, at times, continued monitoring in the PICU. In this setting, subcutaneous or oral administration may be considered to facilitate patient care and allow for discharge from the PICU setting. If it is decided that tapering the infusion can be accomplished within a reasonable period that will not delay hospital discharge, the patient may be considered a candidate for subcutaneous therapy.[51] These patients generally are those who require moderate doses of fentanyl (5-10 μg/kg/h) and/or midazolam (0.1-0.3 mg/kg/h) to provide effective sedation. Subcutaneous administration is not feasible for the barbiturates or propofol. Concentrated solutions of fentanyl (25-50 μg/mL) and midazolam

(2.5-5 mg/mL) are used so that the maximum infusion rate does not exceed 3 mL/h. The subcutaneous infusions are started at the dose currently used for intravenous administration. Several sites are suitable for subcutaneous administration, including the subclavicular region, abdomen, deltoid, or anterior aspect of the thigh. Eutectic mixture of local anesthetics (Astra Zeneca Pharmaceuticals, Westborough, MA) is placed over the site of anticipated subcutaneous cannulation. After 2 hours the site is cleaned with an iodine solution followed by alcohol. Either a standard 22-gauge intravenous cannula or a 23-gauge butterfly needle is inserted into the subcutaneous tissue. Prior to placement, the tubing and needle are flushed with the opioid/benzodiazepine solution. The insertion site is covered with a transparent, bio-occlusive dressing. The site should be changed every 7 days, or more frequently if erythema develops. The same infusion pumps that are used for intravenous administration can be used for subcutaneous administration. The pressure limit may need to be adjusted to allow for subcutaneous administration. Alternatively, a syringe pump can be used. If symptoms of withdrawal develop, additional boluses can be administered subcutaneously if necessary. See Chapter 8 for a full discussion regarding the use of subcutaneous opioids.

When prolonged administration of opioids or other sedative agents is necessary, switching to oral administration of long-acting agents such as methadone may allow for earlier hospital discharge.[52] Patients who meet the criteria of Katz et al[48] for a 50% incidence of withdrawal should be considered for oral methadone therapy. Although the initial report by Tobias et al[11] on methadone use in the inpatient setting suggested a starting dose of 0.1 mg/kg every 12 hours, the 3 patients in the study had received relatively low opioid doses and, therefore, higher doses of methadone were not needed. Subsequent clinical experience has shown that higher methadone doses may be needed depending on the dose of fentanyl.[52]

Although several authors have recommended methadone to wean patients from intravenous opioids, dosing regimens and weaning times vary.[52-54] Additionally, some of these protocols recommend intravenous methadone, which may not be widely available. The protocol by Tobias[52] suggests that the switch from intravenous fentanyl to oral methadone should account for the difference of the potency of the 2 drugs (fentanyl:methadone = 100:1), the difference in the half-life (fentanyl:methadone = 1:75-100), and the oral bioavailability of methadone (75%-80%). The conversion is relatively straightforward because the difference in potency (100:1) is offset by the difference in half-life (1:100) and, therefore, the total daily dose of methadone should equal the total daily dose of fentanyl. Alteration in the dose to compensate for the decreased oral bioavailability of methadone (75%-80%) is generally not needed to prevent withdrawal symptoms and, therefore, left out to simplify the equation. For example, a patient weighing 10 kg who receives 10 µg/kg/h of fentanyl receives 2.4 mg/d of fentanyl and should, therefore, receive 2.4 mg/d of oral methadone. Because cross-tolerance of opioids is not 100%, switching from one opioid to another may result in a decrease in the total dose required when calculated on a standard potency ratio.

The oral methadone regimen begins with a dose every 8 to 12 hours. Following the second oral dose of methadone, the fentanyl infusion is decreased by 50%, by 50% following the third dose, and then discontinued after the fourth dose. Symptoms of opioid withdrawal are graded according to the system proposed by Finnegan et al[6,49] (Table 7-1) and treated with "rescue" doses of morphine (0.05-0.1 mg/kg/dose). One third to one fourth of the total morphine required in 24 hours is added to the next day's methadone dose. Further rescue doses of morphine are used as needed during the next 72-hour period, but no change is made in the subsequent methadone dose until 72 hours have elapsed to allow for a new steady state serum concentration following the change in the methadone dose. If excessive sedation occurs, one methadone dose is held and the dose decreased by 10% to 20%. Once an appropriate dose is achieved, the patient is discharged to the inpatient ward and then discharged home once the physician staff is comfortable with the family's ability to administer the medication at home. The oral methadone dose is then tapered once a week after a follow-up phone call to ensure that the infant or child is doing well. The dose is decreased by 20% of the initial dose so that the oral dose is gradually decreased and then discontinued after 5 to 6 weeks. A once-a-week taper is somewhat arbitrary and will result in a prolonged time for the administration of methadone (5-6 weeks in the author's experience), so other authors have suggested that a more rapid weaning of the methadone is feasible (10-20 days).[53,54] These authors also describe a different approach for calculating the methadone dose from the fentanyl or morphine requirements.

Given its use in drug-rehabilitation centers, the author's experience suggests there remain stigmata about the use of methadone. Therefore, a thorough discussion with the parents is necessary regarding why methadone is being used and to explain the differences between addiction and physical dependence. Long-acting morphine preparations (MS Contin), which are used to treat children with chronic pain problems, have been used instead of methadone. Based on potency and half-life, the dosing of methadone and MS Contin are similar. MS Contin is available only in tablets that cannot be crushed, so administration may be more difficult in younger patients compared with methadone, which is available in a liquid formulation.

Several other agents, both opioid and non-opioid, have been used for the treatment and prevention of opioid withdrawal.[55] Mixtures of opioid alkaloids (paregoric and tincture of opium) were among the first medications used to treat withdrawal in infants of drug-addicted mothers. However, because of the potential toxicity of its other components (CNS effects from camphor and cardiovascular manifestations of benzoic acid), paregoric is no longer recommended in neonates and infants. Tincture of opium is still used to treat opioid withdrawal in neonates of drug-addicted mothers. Frequent administration at 4-hour intervals is necessary due to its short half-life.

Non-opioid agents also have been used to treat opioid withdrawal. This approach may be theoretically less than optimal because it makes physiologic sense to treat withdrawal by replacing the missing agent, rather than treating the symptoms. Although diazepam has been used to treat opioid withdrawal in neonates and infants,[56] when compared with opioids such as paregoric, data from clinical studies have shown adverse effects on behavior, including increased sedation and poor sucking, as well as poor control of the autonomic hyperactivity that occurs with opioid withdrawal.[57] Because there is no cross-tolerance between opioids and benzodiazepines, the use of benzodiazepines should be limited to the treatment of seizures and extreme irritability and not as a replacement for opioid therapy.

Similar results have been reported when using phenobarbital in the treatment of infants of drug-addicted mothers.[58,59] Phenobarbital therapy leads to a greater degree of sedation with adverse effects on sucking behavior while inadequately controlling the GI effects (vomiting and diarrhea) of opioid withdrawal. Although the phenothiazines (chlorpromazine) also have been used to treat infants of drug-addicted mothers,[60] adverse effects including α-adrenergic blockade with hypotension and a lowering of the seizure threshold have limited widespread use.[61]

More recently, the centrally acting α_2-adrenergic agonist, clonidine, has been used to treat opioid withdrawal in both neonates and adults.[62,63] α_2-adrenergic receptors mediate part of their pharmacologic actions through the activation of the same potassium channel as opioid receptors. Due to its prolonged duration of action (12-18 hours), once- or twice-a-day dosing is possible. Adverse effects from clonidine include sedation, bradycardia, and hypotension. Although the use of clonidine is becoming more widespread in pediatric anesthesia as a premedicant for the operating room, as well as for caudal/epidural anesthesia, to date there are limited clinical data with its use in the treatment of opioid withdrawal. Further information is needed to more clearly define the efficacy and safety of this agent, as well as its role in treating opioid withdrawal in the PICU patient. The introduction of the intravenously administered α_2-adrenergic agonist, dexmedetomidine, may increase the use of this class of drug for the treatment of substance withdrawal. Animal data and anecdotal human data support its efficacy in treating or preventing substance withdrawal.[64,65]

As with many of the other aspects of tolerance and dependency, most of the treatment strategy information relates to opioids and less information and clinical experience discusses other agents such as benzodiazepines and barbiturates. Although subcutaneous administration of midazolam is a viable option for long-term weaning, the technique requires ongoing hospitalization and, perhaps, continued ICU admission. Substituting a longer-acting agent that can be administered orally is an option to transition from the continuous intravenous administration of midazolam. Lorazepam may be preferred over diazepam to avoid problems with active metabolites with variable half-lifes and durations of action that may occur with repeated diazepam administration. The conversion from midazolam to lorazepam should account for differences in potency (1:3-4) and half-life (1:2-3), as well as the decrease in bioavailability (60%-70%) with oral administration. Lugo et al[66] recommended starting lorazepam at a dose equivalent to one sixth of the total daily dose of midazolam and administering it every 4 to 6 hours. Although other agents have been evaluated in the adult population for treating benzodiazepine withdrawal, including propranolol, carbamazepime, phenobarbital, and clonidine,[67] there is no information concerning their use for benzodiazepine withdrawal in children to date.

Barbiturate tolerance presents similar problems as benzodiazepine tolerance in that there is limited information to suggest and evaluate treatment options. With the increased use of opioids and benzodiazepines, the use of barbiturates for prolonged sedation in the PICU patient has declined. Based on the author's initial experience, a switch to oral pentobarbital to replace intravenous administration was recommended. However, due to pentobarbital's short half-life, dosing every 6 hours may be necessary. More recently, it has been found that phenobarbital can be used instead of pentobarbital (unpublished data). This not only provides for easy oral administration because phenobarbital is available as an elixir and as tablets, but allows for 12-hour dosing intervals.[68]

Summary

Heightened awareness of the need for aggressive sedation and pain management for the PICU patient has resulted in sequelae, including tolerance, physical dependency, and withdrawal phenomena, that must be recognized and treated by PICU health care providers. Prevention, recognition, and treatment strategies are needed so that our ability to provide the appropriate level of sedation and analgesia to our patients is not limited. Laboratory investigations are beginning to elucidate the cellular mechanisms of tolerance and dependency with insight into ways of delaying their development. Although the initial work is promising, clinical application is not yet practical. Managing these patients includes careful observation for signs/symptoms of withdrawal and the use of formal scoring systems to document withdrawal symptoms. When sedative and analgesic agents have been administered for less than 5 days, the infusions can generally be weaned rapidly (10%-15% every 6-8 hours). When prolonged weaning is necessary, options include switching to longer-acting oral agents or subcutaneous administration, which may eliminate the need for intravenous access. During the initial switch from intravenous to oral medications, cardiorespiratory status monitoring is suggested because information is limited regarding these techniques. The initial switch is probably best accomplished in the PICU setting. Ongoing education for parents, patients, and health care providers about the differences between tolerance, physical dependency, and addiction is essential.

References

1. Shapiro BA, Warren J, Egol AB, et al. Practice parameters for intravenous analgesia and sedation for adult patients in the intensive care unit: an executive summary. *Crit Care Med.* 1995;23:1596-1600
2. Newman RG. The need to redefine "addiction." *N Engl J Med.* 1983;308:1096-1098
3. Collett BJ. Opioid tolerance: the clinical perspective. *Br J Anaesth.* 1998;81:58-68
4. Tobias JD. Fentanyl for sedation in the pediatric intensive care unit: dealing with the problems. *J Pharm Care Pain Symptom Control.* 1996;4:21-32
5. Tobias JD, Berkenbosch JW. Tolerance during sedation in a pediatric ICU patient: effects on the BIS monitor. *J Clin Anesth.* 2001;13:122-124
6. Finnegan LP. Effects of maternal opiate abuse on the newborn. *Fed Proc.* 1985;44:2314-2317
7. Finnegan LP, Connaughton JF Jr, Kron RE, et al. Neonatal abstinence syndrome: assessment and management. *Addict Dis.* 1975;2:141-158
8. Kahn EJ, Neumann LL, Polk GA. The course of the heroin withdrawal syndrome in newborn infants treated with phenobarbital or chlorpromazine. *J Pediatr.* 1969;75:495-500
9. Arnold JH, Truog RD, Orav EJ, et al. Tolerance and dependence in neonates sedated with fentanyl during extracorporeal membrane oxygenation. *Anesthesiology.* 1990;73:1136-1140
10. Arnold JH, Truog RD, Scavone JM, Fenton T. Changes in the pharmacodynamic response to fentanyl in neonates during continuous infusion. *J Pediatr.* 1991;119:639-643
11. Tobias JD, Schleien CL, Haun SE. Methadone as treatment for iatrogenic opioid dependency in pediatric intensive care unit patients. *Crit Care Med.* 1990;18:1292-1293
12. Levy AB. Delirium and seizures due to abrupt alprazolam withdrawal: case report. *J Clin Psychiatry.* 1984;45:38-39
13. Mellman TA, Uhde TW. Withdrawal syndrome with gradual tapering of alprazolam. *Am J Psychiatry.* 1986;143:1464-1466
14. Freda JJ, Bush HL, Barie PS. Alprazolam withdrawal in a critically ill patient. *Crit Care Med.* 1992;20:545-546
15. Sury MRJ, Billingham I, Russell GN, Hopkins CS, Thornington R. Acute benzodiazepine withdrawal syndrome after midazolam infusions in children. *Crit Care Med.* 1989;17:301-302

16. van Engelen BG, Gimbrere JS, Booy LH. Benzodiazepine withdrawal reaction in two children following discontinuation of sedation with midazolam. *Ann Pharmacother.* 1993;27:579-581
17. Fonsmark L, Rasmussen YH, Carl P. Occurrence of withdrawal in critically ill sedated children. *Crit Care Med.* 1999;27:196-199
18. Tobias JD, Deshpande JK, Gregory DF. Outpatient therapy of iatrogenic drug dependency following prolonged sedation in the pediatric intensive care unit. *Intensive Care Med.* 1994;20:504-507
19. Tobias JD, Deshpande JK, Pietsch JB, Wheeler TS, Gregory DF. Pentobarbital sedation for patients in the pediatric intensive care unit. *South Med J.* 1995;88:290-294
20. Ho IK, Yamamoto I, Loh HH. A model for the rapid development of dispositional and functional tolerance to barbiturates. *Eur J Pharmacol.* 1975;30:164-171
21. Jaffe JH, Sharpless SK. The rapid development of physical dependence on barbiturates. *J Pharmacol Exp Ther.* 1965;150:140-145
22. Tobias JD, Martin LD, Wetzel RC. Ketamine by continuous infusion for sedation in the pediatric intensive care unit. *Crit Care Med.* 1990;18:819-821
23. Bennett JA, Bullimore JA. The use of ketamine hydrochloride anaesthesia for radiotherapy in young children. *Br J Anaesth.* 1973;45:197-201
24. Cronin MM, Bousfield JD, Hewett EB, et al. Ketamine anaesthesia for radiotherapy in small children. *Anaesthesia.* 1972;27:135-142
25. Byer DE, Gould AB Jr. Development of tolerance to ketamine in an infant undergoing repeated anesthesia. *Anesthesiology.* 1981;54:255-256
26. Cammarano WB, Pittet JF, Weitz S, Schlobohm RM, Marks JD. Acute withdrawal syndrome related to the administration of analgesic and sedative medications in adult intensive care unit patients. *Crit Care Med.* 1998;26:676-684
27. Au J, Walker S, Scott DHT. Withdrawal syndrome after propofol infusion. *Anaesthesia.* 1991;46:238-239
28. Imray JM, Hay A. Withdrawal syndrome after propofol [letter]. *Anaesthesia.* 1991;46:704
29. Arnold JH, Truog RD, Rice SA. Prolonged administration of isoflurane to pediatric patients during mechanical ventilation. *Anesth Analg.* 1993;76:520-526
30. Smith RA, Winter PM, Smith M, et al. Tolerance to and dependence on inhalational anesthetics. *Anesthesiology.* 1979;50:505-509

31. Arnold JH, Truog RD, Molengraft JA. Tolerance to isoflurane during prolonged administration. *Anesthesiology.* 1993;78:985-988
32. Hughes J, Leach HJ, Choonara I. Hallucinations on withdrawal of isoflurane used as sedation. *Acta Paediatr.* 1993;82:885-886
33. Busto U, Sellers EM, Naranjo CA, et al. Withdrawal reaction after long-term therapeutic use of benzodiazepines. *N Engl J Med.* 1986;315:854-859
34. Tobias JD. Opioid withdrawal presenting as stridor. *J Intensive Care Med.* 1997;112:104-106
35. Lane JC, Tennison MB, Lawless ST, et al. Movement disorder after the withdrawal of fentanyl infusion. *J Pediatr.* 1991;119:649-651
36. Bergman I, Steeves M, Burckart G, Thompson A. Reversible neurologic abnormalities associated with prolonged intravenous midazolam and fentanyl administration. *J Pediatr.* 1991;119:644-649
37. Lutfy K, Yoburn BC. The role of opioid receptor density in morphine tolerance. *J Pharmacol Exp Ther.* 1991;256:575-580
38. Miller LG, Greenblatt DJ, Roy RB, Summer WR, Shader RI. Chronic benzodiazepine administration. II. Discontinuation syndrome is associated with upregulation of gamma-aminobutyric acid A receptor complex binding and function. *J Pharmacol Exp Ther.* 1988;246:177-182
39. Hovav E, Weinstock M. Temporal factors influencing the development of acute tolerance to opiates. *J Pharmacol Exp Ther.* 1987;242:251-256
40. Katz R, Kelly HW. Pharmacokinetics of continuous infusions of fentanyl in critically ill children. *Crit Care Med.* 1993;21:995-1000
41. Berkenbosch JW, Fichter CR, Tobias JD. The correlation of the bispectral index monitor with clinical sedation scores during mechanical ventilation in the pediatric intensive care unit. *Anesth Analg.* 2002;94:506-511
42. Abdelhamid EE, Sultana M, Portoghese PS, Takemori AE. Selective blockage of delta opioid receptors prevents the development of morphine tolerance and dependence in mice. *J Pharmacol Exp Ther.* 1991;258:299-303
43. Walker MJ, Le AD, Poulos CX, Cappell H. Chronic selective blockade of mu opioid receptors produces analgesia and augmentation of the effects of a kappa agonist. *Brain Res.* 1991;538:181-186
44. Takahashi M, Senda T, Kaneto H. Role of spinal kappa opioid receptors in the blockade of the development of antinociceptive tolerance to morphine. *Eur J Pharmacol.* 1991;200:293-297
45. Trujillo KA, Akil H. Inhibition of morphine tolerance and dependence by the NMDA receptor antagonist MK-801. *Science.* 1991;251:85-87

46. Rasmussen K, Fuller RW, Stockton ME, Perry KW, Swinford RM. NMDA receptor antagonists suppress behaviors, but not norepinephrine turnover or locus coeruleus unit activity induced by opiate withdrawal. *Eur J Pharmacol.* 1991;197:9-16
47. McCarthy RJ, Kroin JS, Tuman KJ, Penn RD, Ivankovich AD. Antinociceptive potentiation and attenuation of tolerance by intrathecal co-infusion of magnesium sulfate and morphine in rats. *Anesth Analg.* 1998;86:830-836
48. Katz R, Kelly HW, Hsi A. Prospective study on the occurrence of withdrawal in critically ill children who receive fentanyl by continuous infusion. *Crit Care Med.* 1994;22:763-767
49. Finnegan LP, Kron RE, Connaughton JF Jr, et al. A scoring system for evaluation and treatment of the neonatal abstinence syndrome: a new clinical and research tool. In: Morselli PL, Garattini S, Sereni F, eds. *Basic and Therapeutic Aspects of Perinatal Pharmacology.* New York, NY: Raven Press; 1975:139-152
50. Anand KJS, Arnold JH. Opioid tolerance and dependence in infants and children. *Crit Care Med.* 1994;22:334-342
51. Tobias JD. Subcutaneous administration of fentanyl and midazolam to prevent withdrawal following prolonged sedation in children. *Crit Care Med.* 1999;27:2262-2265
52. Tobias JD. Outpatient therapy of iatrogenic opioid dependency following prolonged sedation in the pediatric intensive care unit. *J Intensive Care Med.* 1996;11:284-287
53. Robertson RC, Darsey E, Fortenberry JD, Pettignano R, Hartley G. Evaluation of an opiate-weaning protocol using methadone in pediatric intensive care unit patients. *Crit Care Med.* 2000;1:119-123
54. Meyer MT, Berens RJ. Efficacy of an enteral 10-day methadone wean to prevent opioid withdrawal in fentanyl-tolerant pediatric intensive care unit patients. *Crit Care Med.* 2001;2:329-333
55. American Academy of Pediatrics. Neonatal drug withdrawal statement. *Pediatrics.* 1983;72:895-897
56. Nathenson G, Golden GS, Litt IF. Diazepam in the management of the neonatal narcotic withdrawal syndrome. *Pediatrics.* 1971;48:523-527
57. Kaltenbach K, Finnegan LP. Neonatal abstinence syndrome, pharmacotherapy, and developmental outcome. *Neurobehav Toxicol Teratol.* 1986;8:353-355
58. Kron RE, Litt M, Eng D, Phoenix MD, Finnegan LP. Neonatal narcotic abstinence: effects of pharmacotherapeutic agents and maternal drug usage on nutritive sucking behavior. *J Pediatr.* 1976;88:637-641

59. Madden JD, Chappel JN, Zuspan F, Gumpel J, Mejia A, Davis R. Observation and treatment of neonatal narcotic withdrawal. *Am J Obstet Gynecol.* 1989;127:199-201
60. Kandall SR. Managing neonatal withdrawal. *Drug Ther.* 1976;6:47-59
61. Cobrinik RW, Hood RT Jr, Chusid E. The effect of maternal narcotic addiction on the newborn infant. *Pediatrics.* 1959;24:288-293
62. Gold MS, Redmond DE Jr, Kleber HD. Clonidine blocks acute opiate-withdrawal symptoms. *Lancet.* 1978;2:599-602
63. Hoder EL, Leckman JF, Ehrenkranz R, Kleber H, Cohen DJ, Poulsen JA. Clonidine in neonatal narcotic-abstinence syndrome. *N Engl J Med.* 1981;305:1284-1285
64. Riihioja P, Jaatinen P, Oksanen H, et al. Dexmedetomidine alleviates ethanol withdrawal symptoms in the rat. *Alcohol.* 1997;14:537-544
65. Maccioli GA. Dexmedetomidine to facilitate drug withdrawal. *Anesthesiology.* 2003;98:575-577
66. Lugo RA, Chester EA, Cash J, et al. A cost analysis of enterally administered lorazepam in the pediatric intensive care unit. *Crit Care Med.* 1999;27:417-421
67. Roy-Byrne PP, Hommer D. Benzodiazepine withdrawal: overview and implications for the treatment of anxiety. *Am J Med.* 1988;84:1041-1052
68. Tobias JD. Tolerance, withdrawal and physical dependency after long-term sedation and analgesia of children in the pediatric intensive care unit. *Crit Care Med.* 2000;28:2122-2132

Chapter 8

Acute and Postoperative Pain Management

Joseph D. Tobias, MD, FAAP

Management of Acute Pain

Mild to Moderate Pain, Outpatient Setting—Prostaglandin Synthesis Inhibitors and Weak Opioids

- Agent and Route of Administration

Moderate to Severe Pain, Inpatient Setting—Prostaglandin Synthesis Inhibitors

Moderate to Severe Pain, Inpatient Setting—Opioids

- Agent, Mode, and Route of Administration

The Non-intravenous Administration of Opioids

Adverse Effects of Opioids

Measurement of Pain

Introduction

The belief that neonates, infants, and children do not feel or react to pain like adults was based on the misconception that the immaturity of the central nervous system (CNS) of infants made them less likely to perceive and respond to painful stimuli. This theory, compounded by fears of addiction and adverse effects from analgesic agents, led to the undertreatment of pain in the outpatient and hospital setting. More recently, clinical studies have demonstrated that infants and children experience a similar severity of postoperative pain as adults[1] and that even premature infants demonstrate alterations in heart rate, blood pressure, and oxygen saturation in response to painful stimuli. These findings have led to fundamental changes and advancement in understanding and treating pain in pediatric patients.

Etiologies of acute pain in the pediatric patient include trauma, acute medical illnesses, postoperative pain, and invasive procedures. Pain treatment may occur in the outpatient or the inpatient setting, in a tertiary care center, or in a community hospital. Patient variables that may affect the pain process and treatment include age, ranging from the neonatal period through adolescence, and the patient's underlying status, ranging from a healthy patient who has no systemic disease to one who is compromised. Despite ongoing emphasis on the control of acute pain, several recent studies demonstrate that there remains significant room for improving the treatment of pain and the need for ongoing education and scientific evaluation to determine optimal methods for acute pain management.

Management of Acute Pain

A 3-step analgesic "ladder" (Table 8-1), initially described by the World Health Organization for the treatment of cancer-related pain, may be used in treating acute pain.[2] The 3-step ladder can be used in outpatient and inpatient settings. Non-intravenous routes, including oral administration, are needed for outpatient management, while the inpatient setting provides an appropriate scenario for administering parenteral opioids. Mild pain, such as that following a soft-tissue surgical procedure or due to a mild illness, initially can be treated with a non-opioid analgesic agent, such as a prostaglandin synthesis inhibitor (acetaminophen, acetylsalicylic acid), or a nonsteroidal anti-inflammatory drug (NSAID), such as ibuprofen. Moderate pain such as that following a bony orthopedic procedure or a fracture usually can be controlled with a combination of a prostaglandin synthesis inhibitor and a weak opioid for the outpatient (eg, an acetaminophen with codeine preparation), or intravenous opioids or a regional anesthetic technique for the inpatient. More severe pain, such as that related to sickle cell vaso-occlusive crisis, major burn, or following a major surgical procedure (thoracotomy or an exploratory laparotomy), generally requires either a regional anesthetic or parenteral opioids.

Table 8-1. The World Health Organization Ladder for Pain Treatment

Mild Pain
NSAIDs, acetaminophen ± adjuvants*
Moderate Pain
NSAIDs or acetaminophen ± weak opioid (oxycodone, hydrocodone, codeine) ± adjuvants
Intravenous opioids (with addition of fixed interval NSAID or acetaminophen) ± adjuvants
Intravenous opioid by PCA
Continuous infusion of opioid with PRN rescue doses of opioid
Fixed, interval dosing of opioid
Regional anesthetic techniques ± adjuvants
Severe Pain (continue NSAID or acetaminophen)
Intravenous opioid by PCA ± adjuvants
Regional anesthetic techniques ± adjuvants

*Adjuvants include tricyclic antidepressants, anticonvulsants, and other agents with similar clinical effect. These agents generally are used only for prolonged acute problems.

Mild to Moderate Pain, Outpatient Setting—Prostaglandin Synthesis Inhibitors and Weak Opioids

Nonsteroidal anti-inflammatory drugs, acetaminophen, and salicylates inhibit the enzyme cyclooxygenase, thereby blocking the synthesis of prostaglandins that stimulate the free nerve endings of the peripheral nervous system. Unlike opioids, these agents demonstrate a ceiling effect, so that once a specific plasma concentration is achieved, increasing the dose provides no further analgesia. Although available as over-the-counter medications, these agents represent an effective means to control mild to moderate pain. They are classified according to their chemical structure as 1) para-amino phenol derivatives (acetaminophen), 2) NSAIDs (ibuprofen), and 3) salicylates (acetylsalicylic acid, choline magnesium trisalicylate) (Table 8-2).[3] Among the para-amino phenol derivatives, acetaminophen has a significant role in the management of acute pain, whereas phenacetin is no longer used given its potential toxicity profile (renal papillary necrosis). The use of salicylates in pediatric patients has decreased markedly due to concerns about Reye syndrome. However, choline magnesium trisalicylate offers the analgesic advantages of an aspirin product while having limited effects on platelet function, making it a commonly used salicylate in patients with qualitative and quantitative platelet issues. Refer to Reference 3 for a full discussion of the prostaglandin synthesis inhibitors. Those that are used most commonly in children and their various preparations are listed in Table 8-3.

Table 8-2. Prostaglandin Synthesis Inhibitors

1. Para-amino Phenol Derivatives
   Acetaminophen, phenacetin
2. Nonsteroidal Anti-inflammatory Agents
   Ibuprofen, indomethacin, tolmetin, fenoprofen, naproxen, mefenamic acid, ketorolac, sulindac
3. Salicylates
   Acetylsalicylic acid, choline magnesium trisalicylate

Table 8-3. Salicylate and NSAID Preparations

Medication	Preparation	Dosage Forms
Ibuprofen	Oral suspension Infant drops Chewable tablets Children's caplets Tablets	100 mg/5 mL 50 mg/1.25 mL 50 & 100 mg 100 mg 200, 400, 600 & 800 mg
Choline magnesium Trisalicylate	Liquid Tablets	500 mg/5 mL 500, 750 & 1,000 mg
Naproxen	Suspension Delayed release tablets Tablets	125 mg/5 mL 275 & 500 mg 250, 275, 375, 500 & 550 mg
Tolmetin	Tablets Capsules	200 & 600 mg 400 mg
Acetylsalicylic acid	Several different preparations available	

Prostaglandin synthesis inhibitors can be used alone to treat minor pain and combined with weak opioids for oral administration to control moderate pain. They can be added to parenteral opioids and regional anesthetic techniques for severe pain, thereby lowering the total amount of opioid required. Most opioid-related adverse effects are dose-related, and modalities that decrease total opioid consumption play a significant role in decreasing or preventing opioid-associated adverse effects.

Agent and Route of Administration

In most cases, oral administration of prostaglandin synthesis inhibitors is used, thereby providing obstacles to effective analgesia that must be considered, including a delay in the onset of relief, decreased bioavailability when compared with parenteral administration, patient refusal to take the medication, vomiting, and an inability to receive enteral medications due to ileus or abdominal complaints. For the pediatric patient, acetaminophen and ibuprofen are the most commonly prescribed agents. Both are available in several preparations, including chewable tablets, elixirs, and drops. Acetaminophen also is available in suppository form and sustained release tablets. An intravenous acetaminophen product is available in Europe and is undergoing trials in the United States.

A technique used frequently in the perioperative setting is the combination of the oral premedication (midazolam) with either acetaminophen (15 mg/kg) or ibuprofen elixir (10 mg/kg).[4] Following minor outpatient procedures, this technique allows the patient to have some analgesia on board on awakening and also masks the taste of the midazolam premedication. If preoperative administration is not chosen, an acetaminophen suppository (40 mg/kg) can be placed following anesthetic induction. A larger dose of acetaminophen is required to achieve effective plasma levels with rectal administration because absorption is decreased and at times erratic. To achieve serum concentrations of 10 to 20 µg/mL, an initial dose of 40 mg/kg *per rectum* currently is recommended.[5] The third option is the postoperative administration of either ibuprofen or acetaminophen when the child complains of pain in the recovery room. This latter option is less desirable because the onset of activity of these agents following oral or rectal administration is 20 to 30 minutes. The administration of a small dose of an intravenous opioid (fentanyl 0.5 µg/kg, morphine 0.02 mg/kg, or nalbuphine 0.02-0.04 mg/kg) can be used to provide immediate analgesia while waiting for the onset of the oral/rectal acetaminophen or ibuprofen. When the patient is ready for discharge home, ongoing analgesia can be provided with either acetaminophen or ibuprofen. While it is most common to administer these agents on a PRN or "as needed" basis, fixed interval dosing may provide more effective analgesia. This entails administering the medication around the clock for the first 24 to 48 hours and not waiting for the child to complain of pain. For this purpose, acetaminophen (10-15 mg/kg) every 4 hours or ibuprofen

(10 mg/kg) every 6 hours can be used. If the patient is receiving acetaminophen as a fixed interval dose and complains of pain, an as needed or supplemental dose of ibuprofen can be administered and vice versa.

When acetaminophen is used around the clock or at fixed intervals, it is important to ensure that the child is not receiving acetaminophen in other forms (eg, cold medicines). Additionally, given the various acetaminophen preparations that are available, it is equally as important to ensure that the parents and the health care provider are certain of the exact concentration of acetaminophen or ibuprofen in the elixir. Rivera-Peneera et al[6] reported the most common cause of acetaminophen toxicity in patients younger than 10 years was inadvertent overdosing by parents. Unfortunately, when inadvertent overdosing occurs, medical attention is not sought until signs of hepatic dysfunction or gastrointestinal (GI) distress have already started, thereby making treatment less effective and increasing the chances of hepatic failure and the need for transplantation.

When moderate pain needs to be treated on an outpatient basis, or when the first step of the ladder fails in what was thought to be mild pain, an NSAID, aspirin, or acetaminophen can be combined with a weak opioid such as codeine, oxycodone, or hydrocodone. Several preparations are available in both tablet and liquid formulations, depending on the patient's age and preference. For younger patients, acetaminophen with codeine elixir containing 120 mg of acetaminophen and 12 mg of codeine per 5 mL generally is effective. Dosing is based on the codeine component and ranges from 0.5 to 1.0 mg/kg every 4 to 6 hours. Tablet preparations contain 325 mg of acetaminophen with 15 mg of codeine (Tylenol #2, Ortho-McNeil Pharmaceutical, Raritan, NJ), 30 mg of codeine (Tylenol #3, Ortho-McNeil Pharmaceutical, Raritan, NJ), or 60 mg of codeine (Tylenol #4, Ortho-McNeil Pharmaceutical, Raritan, NJ). Although generally effective, codeine must be metabolized by hepatic microsomal enzymes to morphine for a significant part of its analgesic effect. In a cohort of 96 children, Williams et al[7] reported that 47% of patients had genotypes associated with a reduction of the activity of the enzymes necessary for the conversion of codeine to morphine and that no morphine or metabolites were detected in 36% of the patients given codeine. The authors concluded that reduced ability to metabolize codeine may be more common than previously reported and that codeine analgesia was less reliable than morphine. Although used most commonly and perhaps exclusively in pediatric patients via the oral route, codeine also is available as a parenteral formulation for subcutaneous administration. Although there are reports of intravenous administration, this is not recommended because of the potential for allergic and anaphylactoid reactions. It also should be remembered that there is no inherent safety feature of codeine. All opioids when used in equipotent doses result in equivalent degrees of sedation and respiratory depression.

Alternatives to codeine for oral administration include oxycodone or hydrocodone preparations. These "weak opioids" also are available in both liquid and tablet forms with either acetaminophen or acetylsalicylic acid. Hydrocodone (7.5 mg) also is available as a tablet combined with 200 mg of ibuprofen (Vicoprofen, Abbott Laboratories, Abbott Park, IL). The dose should be based on the oxycodone or hydrocodone component, starting at 0.1 to 0.15 mg/kg every 4 to 6 hours. Regardless of the preparation used, it should be noted that with dose escalations, the amount of acetaminophen may exceed the recommended dose of 15 mg/kg/dose or 60 to 90 mg/kg/d. When higher doses of the opioid component are needed, it is best to switch to preparations that contain codeine, oxycodone, or hydrocodone without acetaminophen or aspirin to avoid the possibility of toxicity. A sustained release formulation of oxycodone also is available (Oxycontin, Purdue Pharma LP, Stamford, CT). Its sustained release action provides an analgesic plasma concentration that can be maintained with a dosing interval of every 8 to 12 hours. Given reports of its abuse potential, illegal use, and a lack of data regarding pharmacokinetics in pediatric patients, the author does not recommend its use.

Another potential option to control mild to moderate pain in the outpatient setting is tramadol (Ultram, Ortho-McNeil Pharmaceutical, Raritan, NJ).[8] Introduced into clinical practice in Europe in 1977, tramadol is an analgesic agent with a dual mechanism of action that includes agonistic effects at the μ-opioid receptor and inhibition of the reuptake of the neurotransmitters norepinephrine and serotonin in the CNS. These 2 mechanisms interact synergistically to produce analgesia. Tramadol's potency is roughly equivalent to that of meperidine. It is available in several formulations, including an injectable solution, suppository, liquid, and tablet. A tablet containing 50 mg of tramadol and a combination of 37.5 mg of tramadol with 325 mg of acetaminophen in a tablet (Ultracet) are the only 2 preparations available in the United States. Although there is no liquid preparation available, the 50-mg tablet is scored and can be cut in half, allowing it to be administered to smaller pediatric patients. Dosing recommendations include 0.5 to 1.0 mg/kg of tramadol every 3 to 4 hours. Although initially thought to have limited abuse potential, clinical experience has demonstrated an abuse potential at least equivalent to codeine and oxycodone.

There are limited reports regarding tramadol use in the pediatric population.[8-10] Viitanen and Annila[9] compared the analgesic efficacy of an intravenous intraoperative dose of tramadol (2 mg/kg) with placebo in 80 children following outpatient surgery (adenoidectomy). The authors noted a decrease in the need for supplemental opioid analgesia in the recovery room in patients receiving tramadol. Forty-five percent of children receiving tramadol required no supplemental postoperative analgesia compared with 15% of children receiving placebo (P=.003). There was no difference in adverse effects and recovery times. Rose et al[10] evaluated the efficacy of oral tramadol in a group of 113 children. The patients ranged in age from 7 to 16 years, weighed at least 20 kg, and were expected to require analgesia for 7 to 30 days. Dosing started with 1 mg/kg and was increased up to 2 mg/kg as needed. The authors concluded that tramadol was well tolerated and provided effective pain relief. Adverse events generally were mild and similar in incidence to that seen with other oral opioids.

Tramadol has a longer half-life (6-7 hours) than other oral agents as well as an active metabolite with a half-life of 10 to 11 hours. The active metabolite is renally excreted and can accumulate in patients with renal insufficiency or failure, thereby making it a poor choice in that setting. Despite its longer half-life, the study of Viitanen and Annila[9] failed to demonstrate a decrease in analgesic needs after discharge when compared with placebo. The adverse effect profile of tramadol is similar to that of other opioids (see following text); however, like meperidine, seizure activity is a unique adverse effect generally seen only with large doses or in patients with renal failure.[11] Preliminary data suggest that there is less respiratory depression with equipotent doses of tramadol when compared with other opioids.[12] This fact is supported by a case report of a 12.4-kg girl who inadvertently received a 50-mg intravenous dose of tramadol.[11] Although the patient developed seizure activity, no respiratory depression was noted.

Moderate to Severe Pain, Inpatient Setting—Prostaglandin Synthesis Inhibitors

In patients receiving opioids, either by continuous infusion or a patient-controlled analgesia (PCA) device, the addition of ibuprofen (10 mg/kg PO every 6 hours) or acetaminophen (15 mg/kg PO/PR every 4 hours), on a fixed interval, not PRN schedule, is recommended. Several studies have demonstrated the opioid sparing effects of ibuprofen and acetaminophen. Maunuksela et al[13] evaluated the efficacy of rectal ibuprofen (40 mg/kg/d) following inpatient surgery in children. The children who received ibuprofen had lower pain scores and decreased opioid requirements in the recovery room, during the day of operation, and during the first 72 hours following the procedure. Additionally, the incidence of opioid-related adverse effects was lower in the patients receiving ibuprofen. Although rectal preparations of ibuprofen are not available in the United States, similar results have been reported in both children and adults with the use of rectal indomethacin or acetaminophen.[14]

In patients who cannot tolerate or will not accept oral or rectal medications, intravenous administration is possible with the parenteral NSAID ketorolac (Toradol, Roche Pharmaceuticals, Nutley, NJ). When first released, the initial clinical trails suggested that ketorolac was as effective as opioids in treating acute pain. However, its more realistic role is similar to that of other NSAIDs as an adjunct to opioid analgesia. Vetter and Heiner[15] evaluated the efficacy of intravenous ketorolac as a supplement to morphine PCA in children during the postoperative period. Ketorolac (0.8 mg/kg, up to a maximum of 60 mg) was administered intravenously before the completion of the surgical procedure. Patients who received ketorolac had decreased morphine requirements, lower pain scores, and a decreased incidence of adverse effects during the study period that included the first 12 postoperative hours.

Ketorolac also may be effective in treating acute pain of other etiologies, including inflammatory and musculoskeletal pain such as in patients with pleuritic pain or vaso-occlusive crisis due to sickle cell disease. Because ketorolac is relatively more expensive than non-parenteral NSAIDs, future studies are needed to determine its advantages over more inexpensive agents and routes of delivery (oral or rectal) in various acute pain situations. The author's current practice includes fixed interval administration of ketorolac for the initial post-operative period or immediately following the onset of acute pain, switching to either acetaminophen or ibuprofen once the patient is able to tolerate oral or rectal medications. Dsida et al[16] evaluated the pharmacokinetics of a single dose of ketorolac (0.5 mg/kg) in 36 children ranging in age from 1 to 16 years. The patients were grouped according to their age (1-3 years, 4-7 years, 8-11 years, and 12-16 years). No difference in the pharmacokinetic variables (volume of distribution, elimination clearance) was noted among the 4 age groups. The authors concluded that, in patients ranging in age from 1 to 16 years, ketorolac in a dose of 0.5 mg/kg demonstrated similar pharmacokinetic properties as that reported in adults and will provide a plasma concentration in the adult therapeutic range for 6 hours in most patients.

There are limited data regarding the use of ketorolac in patients younger than 1 year. Burd and Tobias[17] reported a retrospective evaluation of ketorolac use following surgical procedures in infants younger than 6 months. The 10 infants who received ketorolac (1-1.5 mg/kg/d for up to 48 hours) required significantly less morphine than the 8 control patients who did not receive ketorolac (0.04 ± 0.05 versus 0.15 ± 0.06 mg/kg/d, P<.01). No difference in pain scores was noted between the 2 groups. In this limited cohort of patients, no adverse effects related to ketorolac were noted.

In the adult population, a ceiling effect has been reported so that no further analgesia was noted with doses of ketorolac higher than 7.5 to 10 mg.[18] Although there are no comparable studies in pediatric patients, our current practice includes dosing at 0.5 mg/kg up to a maximum of 10 mg every 6 hours. Once the patient is able to tolerate oral medications, the switch is made to an oral NSAID or acetaminophen.

Ketorolac is contraindicated in patients with bleeding dyscrasias or in settings where acute hemorrhage is a concern (ie, patients with abnormal coagulation function, the trauma patient, or following intracranial or otolaryngologic surgery). Foster and Williams[19] reported 2 patients who developed bradycardia that was temporally related to the administration of ketorolac. Given their experience, the authors recommended considering the use of an anticholinergic agent concurrently or before the administration of ketorolac. Additionally, they recommended that ketorolac be given to children by slow intravenous administration and only with continuous electrocardiogram monitoring.* Most of the adverse effects of NSAIDs and acetylsalicylic acid (Table 8-4) are the result of the inhibition of prostaglandins distant from the site of inflammation. Adverse effects include decreased platelet function, peptic ulcer formation with GI bleeding, decreased glomerular filtration rate, and bronchospasm. Acetaminophen or the NSAID magnesium choline trisalicylate should be used in patients with qualitative or quantitative platelet disorders because neither agent alters platelet function. Alterations in glomerular filtration rate with NSAIDs are uncommon except in patients with preexisting renal dysfunction, with the concomitant administration of other nephrotoxic agents, in the presence of hypovolemia, or with prolonged administration. Clinical experience suggests that the risk of nephrotoxicity may be greater with certain NSAIDs, including ketorolac and, therefore, use of this agent is limited to 72 hours or less. An additional concern with NSAIDs is the inhibition of new bone formation and, in some centers, use of these agents is restricted in patients undergoing spinal fusion and other procedures in which bone grafts are used.[20]

Recent efforts to maintain analgesia while diminishing the incidence of adverse effects of NSAIDs have focused on 2 fronts 1) agents that

Table 8-4. Adverse Effects of NSAIDs

Adverse Effects of NSAIDs
Headache/dizziness/drowsiness
Nausea/vomiting
Peptic ulcer formation
Gastrointestinal bleeding
Decreased glomerular filtration rate, renal insufficiency/failure
Platelet dysfunction
Bronchospasm
Interaction with other medications (This effect varies from one NSAID to another.)

*The author has noted no such problems.

selectively inhibit cyclooxygenase (COX) type 2 versus type 1 and 2) the use of specific isomers of the NSAIDs. The use of specific NSAID isomers is still in the investigational phase. However, experience with other medications has demonstrated the potential for decreasing adverse effects while maintaining efficacy by separating the 2 enantiomers of a chiral compound. Ibuprofen is a chiral mixture of its 2 optical isomers. Preliminary animal data suggest that the S (+) isomer can be used alone to provide analgesia while having limited effects on the homeostatic COX (see following text), thereby limiting its adverse effect profile.[21]

Cyclooxygenase type 1, referred to as the homeostatic COX, is responsible for controlling renal blood flow, protecting the gastric mucosa, and normal platelet function. Cyclooxygenase type 2, referred to as inducible COX, is responsible for the inflammatory process. Three COX-2 inhibitors are available for clinical use: celecoxib (Celebrex, Pfizer, New York, NY), valdecoxib (Bextra, Pfizer, New York, NY), and rofecoxib (Vioxx, Merck, Whitehouse Station, NJ). Rofecoxib (Vioxx, Merck, Whitehouse, NY) is available in a liquid formulation (12.5 and 25 mg/5 mL). Additionally, a parenteral COX-2 inhibitor (parecoxib, which is metabolized to valdecoxib) will be released soon. There currently are limited data regarding the efficacy and safety of the COX-2 agents in the pediatric population. Joshi et al[22] demonstrated that a single 1 mg/kg preoperative dose of rofecoxib resulted in a decreased incidence of vomiting and lower 24-hour pain scores following tonsillectomy in children ranging in age from 3 to 11 years. The selectivity of these drugs for the different isoforms of COX is not 100% accurate. Although the incidence of adverse effects is less than with nonspecific prostaglandin synthesis inhibitors, there have been reports of nephrotoxicity and GI bleeding with the COX-2 agents. As with many other medications, a formal evaluation for efficacy, adverse effect profile, and pharmacokinetics is needed in pediatric patients.

Moderate to Severe Pain, Inpatient Setting—Opioids

Opioids can be grouped into 3 classes, including the naturally occurring, semi-synthetic, and synthetic agents (Table 8-5). Although chemical structure can be used to distinguish the various opioids, the more clinically relevant differences are their potency, duration of action, and the presence or absence of active metabolites (See Table 8-6). The opioids interact with specific opioid receptors (μ or κ) in the peripheral and central nervous system. Opioids may act as either pure agonists (bind and activate both μ and κ receptors) or agonist-antagonists (bind and activate κ receptors while binding to, but not activating μ receptors). The agonist-antagonists, including nalbuphine (Nubain, Endo Pharmaceuticals, Chadds Ford, PA), butorphanol (Stadol, Bristol-Meyers-Squibb, Princeton, NJ), and pentazocine (Talwin, Sanofi-Synthelabo, New York, NY) should not be administered to patients who have been receiving opioids long term because they may precipitate withdrawal symptoms and/or reverse analgesia. Although these agents have a decreased potential to cause repression depression, there also is an analgesic ceiling effect. With dose escalation for increasing or persistent pain, there is a limit to the amount of analgesia achieved. Their potency and efficacy for severe pain is less than that of pure agonists. They may be useful for mild to moderate pain when oral administration of other agents, such as acetaminophen with codeine, is not feasible or when a more rapid onset of action is desired. The author's practice frequently includes the intravenous administration of a single dose of these agents to treat moderate pain after anesthesia followed by a switch to oral agents when the patient is discharged home. An additional benefit of a drug such as nalbuphine is that it clinically provides more sedation than other opioids and, therefore, in addition to providing analgesia, may provide sedation for the agitated postoperative patient.

The agonist-antagonists also should be considered when supplemental intravenous analgesia is required in patients who are receiving or have received epidural or intrathecal opioids within the past 24 hours. (See Chapter 3 for a full discussion of neuraxial opioids.) The respiratory depression that can occur with the combination of intravenous and neuraxial opioids may be less severe if an agonist/antagonist is used rather

Table 8-5. Opioid Classification According to Chemical Structure

1. Naturally Occurring Agents
   Morphine
2. Semi-synthetic Agents
   Codeine, hydromorphone, oxycodone, oxymorphone
3. Synthetic Agents
   Fentanyl, sufentanil, alfentanil, remifentanil, meperidine, methadone

Table 8-6. Potency and Half-life of Opioids

Agent	Potency	Half-life	Active Metabolites
Agonists			
Morphine	1	2-3 h	Yes
Meperidine	0.1	2-3 h	Yes
Hydromorphone	5	2-4 h	No
Oxymorphone	10	2-4 h	No
Methadone	1	12-24 h	No
Fentanyl	100	20-30 min	No
Sufentanil	1000	20-30 min	No
Alfentanil	20	10-15 min	No
Remifentanil	100	5 min	No
Agonist/antagonists			
Butorphanol	5	2 to 4 h	No
Nalbuphine	1	5 h	No
Pentazocine	0.3 to 0.4	2 to 3 h	No

than a pure agonist, such as morphine. In these situations, incremental doses of nalbuphine (0.02-0.03 mg/kg) are administered every 5 to 10 minutes as needed until the desired level of analgesia is achieved.

Agent, Mode, and Route of Administration

There is relatively little information concerning which opioid is best for postoperative analgesia. Several acceptable alternatives are available, all of which provide equivalent analgesia when equipotent doses are administered. Respiratory depression is not more likely with any specific opioid when equipotent doses are administered.

In the patient with compromised cardiovascular status or at risk for pulmonary hypertension, such as an infant with a large preoperative systemic-to-pulmonary (left-to-right) shunt or any neonate following cardiopulmonary bypass, the synthetic opioids (fentanyl, sufentanil, alfentanil, remifentanil) with their cardiovascular stability, beneficial effects on pulmonary vascular resistance, and ability to blunt the sympathetic stress response may be advantageous. Because synthetic opioids have short plasma half-lifes (less than 30 minutes), they generally are administered by a continuous infusion to maintain a plasma concentration adequate to provide analgesia. There seems to be no inherent advantage to using any of the currently available synthetic opioids, except that fentanyl is the least expensive. Remifentanil, metabolized by plasma esterases, has the shortest half-life of any of the synthetic opioids (approximately 5-10 minutes). Unlike the other opioids that are dependent on hepatic metabolism, there is no difference in the clearance of remifentanil across age ranges so that its half-life is consistent, even in neonates. Given these properties, it has become a popular agent for intraoperative use with limited application outside the operating room. The synthetic opioids are used most commonly in critically ill patients in the intensive care unit, usually in conjunction with mechanical ventilation. Alternatively, given its short duration of action, intermittent doses of intravenous fentanyl are sometimes used to provide analgesia during brief, painful invasive procedures.

While the synthetic opioids can be expected to maintain stable hemodynamics in patients with compromised cardiovascular function, other alternatives, such as morphine, are acceptable in patients with normal cardiovascular function. For most patients, morphine generally is the first-line agent. The dosing regimen depends on the mode of administration that is chosen (Table 8-7). Due to decreased hepatic metabolism and increased permeability of the blood-brain barrier with an increased risk of respiratory depression, dosing with any opioid should start at 50% of the listed dose in infants younger than 6 months. Respiratory function monitoring with continuous pulse oximetry is recommended when opioids are used in this age group or in patients with compromised cardiorespiratory status.

Morphine can cause venodilatation, resulting in decreased blood pressure, especially in hypovolemic patients. Morphine is metabolized in the liver to morphine-6-glucuronide (M6G), which is significantly more potent than the parent compound. Because it is water-soluble, M6G penetrates the CNS poorly and, therefore, in most circumstances,

Table 8-7. Morphine Dosing Guidelines*

Initial intravenous titration for acute, moderate-severe pain 0.01-0.02 mg/kg every 5 minutes, titrate to effective analgesia
PRN or fixed interval dosing 0.05 mg/kg every 3 hours
Continuous infusion 0.01-0.03 mg/kg/h
Patient-controlled analgesia bolus: 0.02 mg/kg every 10 minutes basal infusion: 0.004-0.005 mg/kg/h

*The doses listed are guidelines for starting doses in patients that have not previously been receiving opioids. These doses should be adjusted up or down as necessary to achieve the desired level of analgesia while limiting adverse effects. When opioids are used in infants younger than 6 months or patients with severe systemic illnesses (see Table 8-9), the starting dose should be 50% of the above-listed doses and monitoring of cardiorespiratory function is recommended.

is of little consequence. However, because it is cleared by the kidneys, M6G can accumulate in patients with renal failure or insufficiency and lead to respiratory depression. In such patients, alternative opioids such as hydromorphone (see following text), which has no active metabolites, should be considered.

Other opioids that have been used in the treatment of acute pain include hydromorphone (Dilaudid), meperidine (Demerol), and methadone (Dolobid). Hydromorphone may be used when adverse effects related to histamine release, such as pruritus, occur with morphine. Pruritus may be more common in adolescents and young adults. Therefore, the author's practice includes the use of hydromorphone as a first-line agent for control of severe pain in this population. Hydromorphone is 5 to 7 times as potent as morphine (Table 8-6) and, therefore, one fifth to one seventh of the morphine dose is used. Patient-controlled analgesia solutions can be prepared so that an equipotent amount of the opioid is present in each milliliter of the solution. This includes 1 mg/mL for morphine, 1 mg/mL for nalbuphine, 0.15 mg/mL for hydromorphone, and 10 mg/mL for meperidine.

Meperidine, also known as pethidine in Europe and Great Britain, is approximately one tenth as potent as morphine. It is associated with a relatively high incidence of adverse CNS effects, including dysphoria, agitation, and seizures. In older children and adults, the dysphoric response may manifest itself as complaints of "not feeling well" and restlessness, while agitation and uncontrollable crying may be the only manifestation in the younger child or infant. The CNS toxicity (including seizures) results from the accumulation of normeperidine that is produced following hepatic N-methylation of the parent compound. Normeperidine has a long half-life (15-20 hours) and is dependent on renal clearance. High or toxic levels occur more commonly in cases of renal failure or insufficiency, with the coadministration of drugs such as phenobarbital that stimulate hepatic microsomal enzymes, and with large doses (>2 g/d in an adult). Toxicity may be a significant problem in the patient who is receiving opioids long term in whom dose escalations are needed to provide effective analgesia. Because meperidine offers no particular advantage over other opioids and may be less effective than morphine in controlling acute pain,[23] morphine or hydromorphone is preferred.

Methadone has a potency similar to that of morphine with a plasma half-life of 12 to 24 hours. Its long plasma half-life provides a prolonged steady state serum concentration following a single bolus administration, thereby providing prolonged analgesia without the need for a continuous infusion or PCA device. Berde et al[24] found that a single intraoperative dose of intravenous methadone (0.2 mg/kg) in children aged 3 to 7 years resulted in lower pain scores and decreased the need for supplemental opioid analgesic agents during the initial 36 postoperative hours. Although there is still limited experience with methadone in children, its longer duration of action offers certain advantages over the intermittent administration of agents with shorter half-lifes. It may be useful in situations where PCA devices or continuous infusions are not available. However, the intravenous preparation may not be readily available in many institutions. Given its long half-life, methadone should only be administered by physicians who have significant experience with its use.

Mode of administration options include on demand ("as needed" or PRN dosing), fixed interval administration, continuous infusion, or PCA. To provide optimal analgesia, opioids should be administered in a manner that maintains a steady-state serum concentration. For moderate to severe pain, PRN or "on demand" administration generally does not provide adequate analgesia. With PRN dosing, a significant delay can occur from the time it is recognized that the child is in pain until the medication is drawn up, administered, and takes effect. Patient-controlled analgesia remains the optimal mode for the delivery of opioids to provide analgesia. It allows the patient to administer a preset amount of opioid at specific intervals. These devices may be used in children as young as 5 to 6 years.[25]

Prior to instituting PCA, the pain must be controlled. An opioid is titrated in small, intravenous bolus doses (morphine 0.02 mg/kg every 5 minutes) to the desired level of analgesia, then the PCA device is started. Although any opioid can be used with PCA, morphine is most commonly used, at a starting dose of 0.01 to 0.02 mg/kg every 10 minutes as needed. Patient-controlled analgesia needs to be instituted immediately after analgesia has been achieved with a "loading dose" of opioid as previously outlined so that the serum concentration of opioid does not diminish. A frequent problem is that patients are not provided with a PCA pump soon enough after leaving the post-anesthesia care unit and must repeatedly push the PCA button to reestablish an analgesic plasma concentration of the opioid. In the author's institution, the PCA pump is delivered to the recovery room and started prior to discharge to the floor.

Patient-controlled analgesia also may include a low basal infusion rate in addition to the patient-administered bolus doses. This represents one of the most controversial issues concerning PCA. It has been suggested that the use of a basal infusion rate contradicts the safety factor of PCA—"If a patient is too sleepy to push the button, no opioid is infused." With the basal infusion rate, opioid is infused regardless of the patient's demands. Different results have been reported in pediatric patients depending on the dose used for the basal infusion rate. Doyle et al[26] compared PCA (morphine 0.02 mg/kg every 5 minutes as needed) with and without a basal infusion rate of 0.02 mg/kg/h. There was no difference in the pain scores between the 2 groups. However, there were more adverse effects including nausea, sedation, and hypoxemia in the patients who received the basal infusion rate. In a follow-up study, the same investigators compared 3 different regimens of PCA that included morphine 0.02 mg/kg every 5 minutes as needed with no basal infusion rate (group 1), a basal infusion of 0.01 mg/kg/h (group 2), and a basal infusion rate of 0.004 mg/kg/h (group 3).[27] Pain scores were equivalent in all 3 groups.

There was increased time spent sleeping during the first 2 postoperative nights in groups 2 and 3, with no difference in time asleep during the day. There was an increased incidence of nausea and vomiting in the group that received the basal infusion rate of 0.01 mg/kg/h (group 2). The authors concluded that a low basal infusion of 0.004 mg/kg/h (4 μg/kg/h) improved the sleep pattern when compared with no basal infusion rate.

When used in its "classic sense," PCA requires an awake, cooperative patient who is able to comprehend its purpose and is able to push the button when additional analgesia is required. As such, its use may be limited in certain patients due to age, underlying illness, or mental capabilities. However, in these patients, many centers still use PCA, but allow the device to be activated by the bedside nurse. In this setting, the PCA device eliminates the delay in opioid administration that occurs as the nurse signs out the medication and draws it up. Murphy et al[28] demonstrated equivalent levels of analgesia and equivalent opioid consumption when comparing patient-controlled analgesia with nurse-controlled analgesia. Although they noted no difference in the incidence of adverse effects, when used in this fashion, the inherent safety factor of PCA (see previous text) is lost. Although practices vary, the author currently uses nurse-controlled analgesia in patients who are unable to activate the device, but does not ask or allow family members to activate the PCA device.

The Non-intravenous Administration of Opioids

While most moderate to severe acute pain is treated with intravenous opioids, certain situations may arise that limit or preclude intravenous administration. In these situations, non-intravenous routes of administration may become necessary to provide ongoing analgesia. Non-intravenous routes may include subcutaneous, oral, transdermal, and transmucosal (sublingual, buccal, intranasal, rectal, inhaled) administration.[29] Refer to Reference 29 for a full review of alternative, non-intravenous routes of delivery for opioids. Many of the techniques are still considered investigational and have a limited role in the day-to-day management of acute pain in children. The intramuscular route should be avoided because variability in uptake and absorption leads to erratic serum levels and ineffective analgesia. Additionally, children will deny pain to avoid a "shot."

The simplest and cheapest of the non-intravenous routes remains oral administration. Although this route is frequently chosen for outpatients (see previous text), its use remains limited in hospitalized patients. The oral administration of the "weak opioids," including codeine and oxycodone, has been discussed previously in this chapter. This technique is a viable option even in hospitalized patients, provided the pain is considered mild to moderate. Other opioids, including morphine, hydromorphone, and methadone, can be administered orally. Decreased oral bioavailability necessitates the use of larger doses and, when compared with intravenous administration, there is a significant delay in the onset of action. Although the use of these opioids via the oral route is common practice for controlling cancer-related pain in the outpatient setting, there is limited information about this technique for controlling moderate to severe pain in the inpatient setting. Litman and Shapiro[30] described oral PCA (hydromorphone or morphine) to treat acute pain related to medical illnesses in 4 children. Regardless of the opioid, problems that arise with oral administration include a delay in onset of action, the need for larger doses due to decreased bioavailability, and underlying medical/surgical problems that preclude the use of the GI tract.

Subcutaneous administration also generally has been reserved for the terminal cancer patient. However, preliminary studies outside the cancer population suggest its efficacy for controlling acute pain. Doyle and colleagues[31] investigated the efficacy of PCA by the subcutaneous route in children following appendectomy. The patients were randomized to either intravenous or subcutaneous administration. The PCA regimen included morphine with bolus doses of 0.02 mg/kg every 5 minutes as needed with a basal infusion rate of 0.005 mg/kg/h. The subcutaneous PCA was delivered through a 22-gauge intravenous cannula that was placed into the subcutaneous tissue over the deltoid muscle. There was no difference in the pain scores at rest or with activity between the 2 groups. There were significantly more hypoxemic events (oxygen saturation <90%) with intravenous versus subcutaneous administration.

Lamacraft et al[32] evaluated the efficacy of subcutaneous morphine in the control of postoperative pain in a cohort of 220 pediatric patients. Morphine was administered via an indwelling catheter placed into the subcutaneous tissue after the induction of anesthesia. The patients denied pain on administration of subcutaneous morphine. When compared with intermittent intramuscular administration of opioids, 95% of the nurses preferred the subcutaneous route and 74% stated that they would give morphine more readily via the subcutaneous route compared to intramuscular administration. The author's experience has demonstrated similar efficacy with the use of subcutaneous opioids.[33] In a cohort of 24 children, subcutaneous opioids were administered during gradual weaning of opioid administration following prolonged intensive care unit stays, for acute pain problems, and during terminal care. The reason for using subcutaneous administration included lack of venous access and drug incompatibilities that limited venous access.

For subcutaneous administration, a butterfly needle or a standard intravenous catheter is inserted into the subcutaneous tissue of the thigh, abdominal wall, subclavicular area, or deltoid. Dosing regimens including basal infusions, continuous infusions, and boluses are the same as for intravenous administration. Plasma concentrations of the opioid during subcutaneous administration can be expected to be equivalent to those achieved with intravenous administration. However, the peak plasma concentration will not be achieved as rapidly following subcutaneous administration when compared with intravenous bolus dosing. The fluid volume used to deliver the opioid should be restricted to a maximum of 3 mL/h. The site should be changed every 7 days or sooner if erythema or local tissue reaction is noted. Several different opioids can be administered subcutaneously, including morphine, hydromorphone, and fentanyl. Methadone can cause significant tissue reaction with erythema and is not recommended for subcutaneous administration.

Adverse Effects of Opioids

Several adverse effects may occur with opioids, thereby interfering with the delivery of effective analgesia (Table 8-8). Respiratory depression is directly related to potency and occurs with all opioids. Equianalgesic doses of opioids produce equivalent degrees of respiratory depression. Factors that may predispose patients to respiratory depression include extremes of age, severe underlying systemic diseases, preexisting altered

Table 8-8. Adverse Effects of Opioids and Treatment Strategies*

Adverse Effect	Treatment Strategy
Respiratory depression	Stop opioid Airway management as needed Naloxone 2 µg/kg every 3 minutes up to 10 µg/kg
Constipation/ileus	Stool softeners Cathartic agents Motility agent (metoclopramide)
Nausea/vomiting	Phenothiazine (promethazine 0.25 mg/kg up to 25 mg)* or ondansetron (0.1 mg/kg up to 4 mg)
Pruritus	Diphenhydramine (0.5 mg/kg up to 25 mg) Change opioid

*Monitoring of respiratory status is suggested when opioids are used in conjunction with the phenothiazines because there may be a potentiation of opioid-induced respiratory depression.

Table 8-9. Patients at Risk for Opioid-Related Adverse Effects*

1. Extremes of Age (infants <6 months of age)
2. Patients with severe underlying systemic illness
   - Cardiorespiratory dysfunction
   - Hepatic insufficiency
   - Renal insufficiency
   - Altered mental status
   - Airway obstruction
   - Central or obstructive apnea
3. Concomitant Use of Other Medications
   - Barbiturates
   - Phenothiazines
   - Benzodiazepines

*The presence of the above-mentioned problems does not preclude opioid administration. When opioids are used in these patients, 50% of the usual dose is recommended in addition to continuous monitoring of cardiorespiratory function.

mental status, and the addition of other medications that potentiate the central respiratory depressant effects of opioids (Table 8-9). The presence of such problems does not preclude the use of opioids; however, initial doses should start at approximately 50% of the usual regimens and monitoring of cardiorespiratory function is suggested.

Respiratory depression also may occur in the presence of renal failure in patients receiving morphine. While the parent compound (morphine) undergoes primarily hepatic metabolism, one of the metabolites (M6G) possesses respiratory depressant and analgesic activity several times that of the parent compound and is dependent on renal excretion. When renal function is altered, an opioid such as hydromorphone may be a safer alternative because it does not have active metabolites that are dependent on renal function.

Following appropriate airway management with provision of supplemental oxygen or bag-mask ventilation, naloxone is recommended for treating severe respiratory depression related to opioids. Naloxone is available in several different dilutions. Therefore, particular attention must be paid to the individual ampule. Standard pediatric ampules contain either 0.4 or 1.0 mg/mL. Naloxone should be administered in incremental doses of 1 to 2 μg/kg (up to a total dose of 10 μg/kg), repeated every 3 minutes as needed. These small incremental doses are suggested because it is possible to reverse respiratory depression without reversing analgesia. Using the doses recommended in many reference texts (10-15 μg/kg) will result in a precipitous reversal of all analgesia, which may lead to agonizing consequences for the patient. Such large doses are used only for reversing opioid effects in the setting of an acute overdose. Once respiratory depression is reversed, continued monitoring of the patient is important because the half-life of naloxone is only 20 to 30 minutes compared with 2 to 3 hours or longer for many of the opioids such as morphine, meperidine, or hydromorphone. Although there are 2 other, longer-acting opioid antagonists (naltrexone and nalmefene), there is limited information regarding their use in children.

Although life-threatening effects of opioids, such as respiratory depression, are most worrisome, it is more commonly the non–life-threatening problems that interfere with the delivery of effective analgesia. Inadequate analgesia may occur in younger children and infants because of health care providers' unfounded fears of addiction. The incidence of addiction in patients receiving opioids for acute pain management is exceedingly rare. What does occur following the prolonged administration (>5-7 days) of opioids and sedative agents is physical dependence. (See Chapter 7 for a full discussion of tolerance, dependency, and withdrawal.) The possibility of physical dependence should not limit the use of opioids, but rather remind us of the need to slowly taper use following prolonged administration.

Additional adverse effects of opioids include sedation, constipation, pruritus, nausea, and vomiting. Careful attention to the patient's bowel habits and the concurrent use of stool softeners may help to avoid constipation. Although tolerance to some of the other adverse effects of opioids, such as sedation, may develop, tolerance to the effects on

GI motility does not occur. Cathartic or osmotic agents (Milk of Magnesia, 70% sorbitol) may be needed for refractory cases or when constipation already has developed. Preventing constipation with a daily dose of Milk of Magnesia during outpatient opioid therapy is easier than treating the problem once it has occurred. Patients receiving opioids for acute pain frequently are inactive and may have less than normal fluid intake, which only serves to aggravate the problem of constipation.

Nausea and vomiting are probably the most bothersome of the non–life-threatening adverse effects of opioids. Three different mechanisms may be involved, including a direct stimulation of the central chemoreceptor trigger zone of the medulla, decreased GI motility with increased pyloric tone, and sensitization of the vestibular apparatus. Regardless of the mechanism involved, treatment is primarily symptomatic and may include phenothiazines, metoclopramide, and ondansetron. Phenothiazines, such as promethazine, are available in a preparation for rectal administration, while ondansetron recently has been released in a wafer that dissolves in the mouth, thereby offering an alternative to oral administration for outpatient treatment. Although phenothiazines are used most commonly (promethazine 0.25-0.5 mg/kg up to 25 mg), adverse effects may occur, including dystonic reactions, lowering of the seizure threshold, alteration of cardiac repolarization, and potentiation of opioid-induced respiratory depression. When phenothiazines are used to treat nausea in patients receiving PCA, it may be appropriate to stop the PCA for 30 minutes before and after the dose, due to the potential for opioid-induced respiratory depression. Other options to treat nausea and vomiting include metoclopramide (0.1 mg/kg, up to 10 mg) or serotonin antagonists (ondansetron, dolasetron, or granisetron). Ondansetron is administered intravenously in a dose of 0.15 mg/kg (maximum of 4 mg) intravenously every 6 hours as needed. Unlike the phenothiazines, ondansetron, dolasetron, and granisetron do not cause sedation or potentiate the respiratory depressant effects of opioids. If nausea or vomiting persists despite symptomatic treatment, changing opioids may be helpful. There does not seem to be any particular opioid that has a higher incidence of nausea and vomiting.

Pruritus may occur as an isolated symptom or in association with urticaria. The mechanisms of opioid-induced pruritus are multifactorial and include a direct central effect as well as histamine release. Strategies to control pruritus include the administration of an antihistamine such as diphenhydramine (0.5 mg/kg up to 25 mg) or changing to another opioid. The sedative properties of diphenhydramine also may potentiate opioid-induced sedation. When pruritus is not controlled with antihistamines, changing to another opioid with fewer histamine-releasing properties may be helpful. For intravenous use, these include hydromorphone, oxymorphone, and the synthetic agent fentanyl. Given the higher incidence of pruritus in some patient populations (adolescents, patients with sickle cell disease), the author initiates PCA with hydromorphone in these patients. Patients with severe skin diseases, such as cutaneous involvement of graft-versus-host disease, may be particularly likely to develop opioid-induced pruritus. In this group of patients, it may be necessary to use fentanyl to provide analgesia and prevent pruritus.[34] To determine dosing guidelines in such circumstances, consultation with the anesthesiology department or pain service is suggested.

Measurement of Pain

One of the more difficult aspects of acute pain management in children is deciding when to treat pain and how to grade the responses to pain therapy. Older patients can tell you when they feel pain. Preverbal children or those with cognitive impairment, however, cannot communicate effectively, which complicates pain management. Generalized irritability and agitation may be related to pain, but also may be related to other factors, such as absence of parents or hunger. Various pain scales and assessment tools have been introduced into clinical practice.

These tools can be divided into 3 groups: self-report, observational, and physiologic. Self-report techniques rely on the patient's ability to assess and report pain. Variations of the self-report pain scales that make them more user friendly and applicable in younger children (5-7 years old) include the use of poker chips, a ladder, colored crayons, or pictures of children in varying degrees of distress.[35] With the poker chip scale, the child expresses pain as a certain number of red poker chips (1-4). "A little bit of hurt" is 1 poker chip while 4 poker chips indicate "the most hurt" the child could have. The pain ladder is a picture of a ladder with 9 steps or rungs. At the bottom of the ladder is "no hurt" and at the top of the ladder is "hurt as bad as it could be." Pain severity also can be expressed by selecting a colored crayon, with red indicating severe pain and blue indicating little or no pain. The use of colors to express pain has been shown to have some variability because the association of blue with calm or no pain and red with pain is not consistent among all ethnic groups. Another self-report technique uses the Faces Pain Scale described by Bieri et al,[36] which has drawings of a child in various degrees of distress. Although not validated for this purpose, some centers have used the Faces Pain Scale as an observational tool. The health care provider assesses the child and selects the face and, hence, the degree of pain they determine the patient is manifesting. Beyer and Wells[37] used actual photographs placed beside a corresponding 0- to 10-point vertical scale to develop what is known as the Oucher Scale.

A more involved assessment tool frequently used in clinical research is the CHEOPS (Children's Hospital of Eastern Ontario Pain Score) developed by McGrath et al.[38] The scale assigns a score of 0 to 2 for 6 categories, including cry, facial expression, verbal complaints or pain, position of the torso, whether the child is touching the wound, and position of the legs. Although generally observational (assigned by a health care professional) the scale requires verbalization of the child for 1 of the 6 elements.

Assessment of pain is difficult in patients too young or who have some type of cognitive impairment and, therefore, cannot express the severity of their pain. The tools used to assess pain in those types of patients combine observational and physiologic factors. Observational tools may include an assessment of the patient's facial features or body posture, or the presence or absence or crying. Physiologic parameters include heart rate, blood pressure, respiratory rate, and even oxygen saturation in some systems. Although not practical for everyday bedside use, clinical research into pediatric pain also may include physiologic parameters such as neurohumoral changes, including elevations in endogenous production of stress hormones such as adrenocorticosteroids, norepinephrine, and epinephrine.

Various observational tools have been described and validated for neonates,[39,40] preterm infants,[41] and patients with cognitive impairment.[42] These tools have excellent inter-observer reliability and are quick and easy to use, thereby not significantly increasing the time required for patient evaluations. One of the keys to effective pain management is an ongoing assessment of the patient's response to the therapy. Therefore, it is our philosophical belief that the actual tool used is not the crucial factor. It is, rather, to ensure that pain is evaluated in all hospitalized patients, especially those receiving analgesic agents. The author's institution considers pain to be the fifth vital sign and asks the nursing staff to assign a pain score for all hospitalized patients as often as the other vital signs are checked. Ongoing education and auditing of inpatient records has resulted in a remarkably high (>90%) acceptance rate of this practice.

Summary

Ongoing evidence continues to demonstrate the deleterious physiologic effects of pain and the beneficial results of effective postoperative analgesia. As previously outlined, a 3-step approach is recommended, depending on the severity of pain. This approach uses a combination of

NSAIDs and/or acetaminophen, weak opioids (codeine, oxycodone, hydrocodone), and intravenous opioids. In the setting of moderate to severe pain, acetaminophen or an NSAID should be continued on a fixed interval basis as a means of decreasing total opioid consumption and opioid-related adverse effects. Decisions regarding opioid use include the choice of opioid, its route of administration, and its mode of administration. For severe pain in the hospitalized patient, PCA is the preferred mode of administration. Although the intravenous administration of opioids remains the primary route of administration for moderate and severe pain in the hospital setting, future formulations and developments may allow for the increased use of non-parenteral routes. In addition to the appropriate choice of medications, an integral aspect of pain management is the assessment of the patient's pain to judge the response to therapy and the need to adjust the level of analgesia.

References

1. Mather L, Mackie J. The incidence of postoperative pain in children. *Pain.* 1983;15:271-282
2. Schug SA, Zech D, Dorr U. Cancer pain management according to WHO analgesic guidelines. *J Pain Symptom Manage.* 1990;5:27-32
3. Tobias JD. Weak analgesics and nonsteroidal anti-inflammatory agents in the management of children with acute pain. *Pediatr Clin North Am.* 2000;47:527-543
4. Tobias JD, Lowe S, Hersey S, et al. Analgesia after bilateral myringotomy and placement of pressure equalization tubes in children: acetaminophen versus acetaminophen with codeine. *Anesth Analg.* 1995;81:496-500
5. Birmingham PK, Tobin MJ, Henthorn TK, et al. Twenty-four-hour pharmacokinetics of rectal acetaminophen in children. *Anesthesiology.* 1997;87:244-252
6. Rivera-Penera T, Gugig R, Davis J, et al. Outcome of acetaminophen overdose in pediatric patients and factors contributing to hepatotoxicity. *J Pediatr.* 1997;130:300-304
7. Williams DG, Patel A, Howard RF. Pharmacogenetics of codeine metabolism in an urban population of children and its implications for analgesic reliability. *Br J Anaesth.* 2002;89:839-845

8. Tobias JD. Tramadol for postoperative analgesia in adolescents following orthopedic surgery in a third world country. *Am J Pain Manage.* 1996;6:51-53
9. Viitanen H, Annila P. Analgesic efficacy of tramadol 2 mg kg (-1) for paediatric day-case adenoidectomy. *Br J Anaesth.* 2001;86:572-575
10. Rose JB, Finkel JC, Arquedas-Mohs D, et al. Oral tramadol for the treatment of pain of 7-30 days' duration in children. *Anesth Analg.* 2003;96:78-81
11. Tobias JD. Seizure after overdose of tramadol. *South Med J.* 1997;90:826-827
12. Bosenberg AT, Ratcliffe S. The respiratory effects of tramadol in children under halothane anaesthesia. *Anaesthesia.* 1998;53:960-964
13. Maunuksela EL, Ryhanen P, Janhunen L. Efficacy of rectal ibuprofen in controlling postoperative pain in children. *Can J Anaesth.* 1992;39:226-230
14. Sims C, Johnson CM, Bergesio R, et al. Rectal indomethacin for analgesia after appendectomy in children. *Anaesth Intens Care.* 1994;22:272-275
15. Vetter TR, Heiner EJ. Intravenous ketorolac as an adjuvant to pediatric patient-controlled analgesia with morphine. *J Clin Anesth.* 1994;6:110-113
16. Dsida RM, Wheeler M, Birmingham PK, et al. Age-stratified pharmacokinetics of ketorolac tromethamine in pediatric surgical patients. *Anesth Analg.* 2002;94:266-270
17. Burd RS, Tobias JD. Ketorolac for pain management after abdominal surgical procedures in infants. *South Med J.* 2002;95:331-333
18. Reuben SS, Connelly NR, Lurie S, et al. Dose-response of ketorolac as an adjunct to patient-controlled analgesia with morphine in patients after spinal fusion surgery. *Anesth Analg.* 1998;87:98-102
19. Foster PN, Williams JG. Bradycardia following intravenous ketorolac in children. *Eur J Anaesthesiol.* 1997;14:307-309
20. Glassman SD, Rose SM, Dimar JR, et al. The effect of postoperative nonsteroidal anti-inflammatory drug administration on spinal fusion. *Spine.* 1998;23:834-838
21. Bonabello A, Galmozzi MR, Canaparo R, et al. Dexibuprofen [S(+)-isomer ibuprofen] reduces gastric damage and improves analgesic and anti-inflammatory effects in rodents. *Anesth Analg.* 2003;97:402-408
22. Joshi W, Connelly NR, Reuben SS, Levin CR, Sethna NF. An evaluation of the safety and efficacy of administering rofecoxib for postoperative pain management. *Anesth Analg.* 2003;97:35-38
23. Vetter TR. Pediatric patient-controlled analgesia with morphine versus meperidine. *J Pain Symptom Manage.* 1992;7:204-208
24. Berde CB, Beyer JE, Bournaki MC, Levin CR, Sethna NF. Comparison of morphine and methadone for prevention of postoperative pain in children. *J Pediatr.* 1991;119:136-141

25. Berde CB, Lehn BM, Yee JD, et al. Patient-controlled analgesia in children and adolescents: a randomized, prospective comparison with intramuscular administration of morphine for postoperative analgesia. *J Pediatr.* 1991;118:460-466
26. Doyle E, Robinson D, Morton NS. Comparison of patient controlled analgesia with and without a background infusion after lower abdominal surgery in children. *Br J Anaesth.* 1993;71:670-673
27. Doyle E, Harper I, Morton NS. Patient-controlled analgesia with low dose background infusions after lower abdominal surgery in children. *Br J Anaesth.* 1993;71:818-822
28. Murphy DF, Graziotti P, Chaldiadis G, McKenna M. Patient-controlled analgesia: a comparison with nurse-controlled intravenous opioid infusion. *Anaesth Intens Care.* 1994;22:589-592
29. Tobias JD. The non-intravenous administration of opioids in children. *Am J Anesthesiol.* 1997;24:254-263
30. Litman RS, Shapiro BS. Oral patient-controlled analgesia in adolescents. *J Pain Symptom Manage.* 1992;7:78-81
31. Doyle E, Morton NS, McNicol LR. Comparison of patient controlled analgesia in children by i.v. and s.c. routes of administration. *Br J Anaesth.* 1994;72:533-536
32. Lamacraft G, Cooper MG, Cavalletto BP. Subcutaneous cannulae for morphine boluses in children: assessment of a technique. *J Pain Symptom Manage.* 1997;13:43-49
33. Dietrich CC, Tobias JD. Subcutaneous fentanyl infusions in the pediatric population. *Am J Pain Manage.* 2003;13:146-150
34. Tobias JD. Patient-controlled analgesia using fentanyl in pediatric patients with sickle cell vaso-occlusive crisis. *Am J Pain Manage.* 2000;10:149-153
35. Hester NO, Foster R, Kristensen K. Measurement of pain in children: generalizability and validity of the pain ladder and the poker chip tool. *Adv Pain Res Ther.* 1990;15:79-84
36. Bieri D, Reeve RA, Champion GD, et al. The Faces Pain Scale for the self-assessment of the severity of pain experience by children: development, initial validation, and preliminary investigation for ratio scale properties. *Pain.* 1990;41:139-150
37. Beyer JE, Wells N. The assessment of pain in children. *Pediatr Clin North Am.* 1989;36:837-854
38. McGrath PJ, Johnson G, Goodman JT, et al. CHEOPS: a behavioral scale for rating postoperative pain in children. *Adv Pain Res Ther.* 1985;9:395-402

39. Taddio A, Nulman I, Koren BS, et al. A revised measure of acute pain in infants. *J Pain Symptom Manage.* 1995;10:456-463
40. Krechel SW, Bildner J. CRIES: a new neonatal postoperative pain measurement score. Initial testing of validity and reliability. *Paediatr Anaesth.* 1995;5:53-61
41. Stevens B, Johnson C, Petryshen P, Taddio A. Premature Infant Pain Profile: development and initial validation. *Clin J Pain.* 1996;12:13-22
42. Breau LM, Finley GA, McGrath PJ, Camfield CS. Validation of the Non-communicating Children's Pain Checklist—Postoperative Version. *Anesthesiology.* 2002;96:528-535

Chapter 9

Neonatal Pain Management

Constance S. Houck, MD, FAAP

Assessment of Acute Pain in Neonates
- Neonatal Facial Coding System
- Neonatal Infant Pain Scale
- Premature Infant Pain Profile

Analgesia for Painful Medical Procedures
- Eutectic Mixture of Local Anesthetics
- Nonnutritive Sucking and Sucrose Pacifiers

Analgesia for Circumcision
- Dorsal Penile Nerve Block
- Subcutaneous Ring Block
- Eutectic Mixture of Local Anesthetics
- Adjunctive Techniques

Pharmacologic Pain Management for Acute Pain and Surgery
- Opioid Analgesics
- Acetaminophen
- Epidural Analgesia

Introduction

Over the past 15 years there has been increasing evidence that neonates and infants have the neuroanatomical, neurochemical, and functional ability to respond vigorously to painful stimuli, and that early pain experiences may alter responses to pain later in life.[1] Preterm and term neonates in the neonatal intensive care unit (NICU) are exposed to numerous sources of pain and stress, including heel lances, intravenous and arterial line insertions, lumbar punctures, and bladder taps; many times without the administration of analgesia. Because of the immaturity of inhibitory pathways in the central nervous system in preterm and term neonates, tissue-damaging procedures may be particularly painful. Untreated pain can lead to a number of adverse physiologic consequences, including increased physiologic energy expenditure, increased secretion of adrenal stress hormones, altered cerebral blood flow, and disturbed sleep/wake cycles.[2] Strategies for treating and preventing pain in the NICU and newborn nursery, particularly for commonly performed neonatal procedures such as heel lance and circumcision, recently have been developed, and preliminary studies have suggested that early aggressive pain control and stress reduction strategies may minimize long-term effects on pain thresholds and behavior.[3]

Assessment of Acute Pain in Neonates

Despite active research over the last 10 to 15 years, there is still no easily administered, widely accepted system for assessing pain in neonates and infants. Most scales that have been developed rely on behavioral measures, physiologic measures, or a combination of both. Behavioral measures that have been accurately correlated with pain include facial expression, cry, gross motor movements, changes in behavioral state, and changes in behavior patterns such as sleep. Heart rate, blood pressure, and oxygen saturation are the most widely used physiologic measures of pain. Although there are more than a dozen scales that are considered valid for measuring neonatal and infant pain, the 3 most commonly used pain scales for both preterm and term infants are the Neonatal Facial Coding System (NFCS), the Neonatal Infant Pain Scale (NIPS), and the Premature Infant Pain Profile (PIPP). The CRIES (crying, requirement for oxygen supplementation, increases in heart rate and blood pressure, facial expression, and sleeplessness) scale has demonstrated a high reliability for assessing postoperative pain in term infants, for which it was specifically designed.[4]

Neonatal Facial Coding System

Facial expression is the most comprehensively studied pain assessment measure and is the most reliable and consistent indicator of pain across populations and ethnic groups.[5] Facial expressions of neonates and infants experiencing acute pain include the following characteristics: eyes forcibly closed; brows lowered and furrowed; nasal roots broadened and bulged; deepened nasolabial furrow; a square mouth; and a taut, cupped tongue. Though not currently widely used except for research purposes, the complete NFCS has been used reliably at the bedside in the NICU.[6]

Neonatal Infant Pain Scale

The NIPS is another tool that relies on behavioral assessment for measuring pain in both preterm and term neonates.[7] It can be used to monitor pain before, during, and after a painful procedure such as venipuncture. The NIPS scores pain by assessing facial expression, cry, breathing patterns, limb movements, and arousal. It is scored at 1-minute intervals before, during, and after procedures. The complete NIP scale is shown in Table 9-1.

Premature Infant Pain Profile

The PIPP measures 7 items, including behavioral, physiologic, and contextual factors.[8] The gestational age and behavioral state of neonates are taken into consideration in the scoring, which means this scale can be reliably used in preterm infants of all ages as well as term infants.

Analgesia for Painful Medical Procedures

Painful procedures such as heel lance, venipuncture, and circumcision are routinely performed on neonates and infants in the NICU and the newborn nursery. Intravenous boluses of opioid analgesics, such as morphine and fentanyl (see following text), can be used routinely for painful procedures in intubated neonates and infants in the NICU, but may not be appropriate for spontaneously breathing newborns who, due to their immature central respiratory control systems, are at high

Table 9-1. Neonatal/Infant Pain Scale

Pain Assessment	
Facial Expression	
0–Relaxed muscles	Restful face, neutral expression
1–Grimace	Tight facial muscles; furrowed brow, chin, jaw, (negative facial expression–nose, mouth, and brow)
Cry	
0–No cry	Quiet, not crying
1–Whimper	Mild moaning, intermittent
2–Vigorous cry	Loud scream; rising, shrill, continuous (Note: Silent cry may be scored if baby is intubated as evidenced by obvious mouth and facial movement.)
Breathing Patterns	
0–Relaxed	Usual pattern for this infant
1–Change in breathing	Indrawing, irregular, faster than usual; gagging; breath holding
Arms	
0–Relaxed/restrained	No muscular rigidity; occasional random movements of arms
1–Flexed/extended	Tense, straight legs; rigid and/or rapid extension, flexion
Legs	
0–Relaxed/restrained	No muscular rigidity; occasional random leg movement
1–Flexed/extended	Tense, straight legs; rigid and/or rapid extension, flexion
State of Arousal	
0–Sleeping/awake	Quiet, peaceful sleeping or alert random leg movement
1–Fussy	Alert, restless, and thrashing
Total Score*	

*A score of greater than 3 indicates need for pain management
Adapted from *Neonatal Netw.* 1993;12:59-66.

risk for respiratory depression. Recent studies have demonstrated the safety and efficacy of local anesthetics, pacifiers dipped in sucrose, and non-opioid analgesics in providing pain relief for procedures in which opioid analgesics are not indicated.

Eutectic Mixture of Local Anesthetics

Several topical local anesthetic agent preparations are available; although most experience in the neonatal population has been with the use of eutectic mixture of local anesthetics (EMLA) (Astra-Zeneca, Wilmington, DE). This eutectic mixture of lidocaine and prilocaine has been commonly used for various procedures in term neonates without significant side effects. A theoretical concern is the potential of the local anesthetic agent, prilocaine, to induce methemoglobinemia (when the iron molecule in hemoglobin is oxidized from the ferrous to the ferric state, thereby interfering with the oxygen carrying capacity of the hemoglobin). Fetal hemoglobin is more sensitive to the oxidizing effects of various medications, and newborns have lower levels of methemoglobin reductase. Therefore, neonates and infants may be at higher risk for methemoglobinemia with the systemic absorption of prilocaine. Taddio and colleagues[9] measured methemoglobin plasma concentrations in a group of full-term neonates who received EMLA for circumcision and found no increased levels. Additionally, a recent systematic review found EMLA to be safe and effective at reducing the pain associated with circumcision, venipuncture, arterial puncture, and venous catheter placement in neonates.[10] However, EMLA was not effective for heel lance, leading to the recommendation that, whenever possible, newborn screening should be performed via venous puncture rather than the more painful heel lance procedure.[11]

Nonnutritive Sucking and Sucrose Pacifiers

Nonnutritive sucking provides calming and pain-relieving effects in both preterm and term neonates, though its mechanism of action is not known. It is speculated that sucking triggers the release of serotonin, which may modulate transmission and processing of nociception. In neonatal rat studies, nonnutritive sucking has been found to be antinociceptive and to reduce vocalizations by non-opioid mechanisms.[12] In human neonates and infants, pain responses and crying can be significantly reduced by nonnutritive sucking during heel lance procedures.[13-15] Adding a solution of sucrose seems to enhance these antinociceptive effects.[13] This improved analgesia with sucrose is speculated to be mediated through the effects of endogenous opioids released in response to the sweet taste. Human milk, lactose, and substances found in milk do not seem to be nearly as effective as sucrose in reducing pain.[16,17] It is unclear whether the coadministration of sucrose with nonnutritive sucking is additive or synergistic, but pacifiers dipped in sucrose seem to be more effective than sucrose given orally or via a nasogastric tube.[18,19] A recent systematic review of 271 infants demonstrated a statistically and clinically significant reduction in crying with the use of the "sucrose pacifiers" during painful procedures in term and preterm neonates.[20] Two milliliters of 12% to 24% sucrose solution administered approximately 2 minutes before the painful stimulus was the most effective in reducing crying. Although no adverse effects have been reported with intraoral administration of small amounts of sucrose for single events, one report suggests that frequent small amounts of a 20% sucrose solution given by nasogastric tube in very low birth weight infants could have contributed to a higher incidence of necrotizing enterocolitis.[21]

Analgesia for Circumcision

Circumcision is one of the most painful procedures performed routinely in neonates and infants. Despite a number of studies more than 20 years ago demonstrating the physiologic consequences of circumcision performed without analgesia,[22-25] many neonates still undergo circumcision without analgesia. A 1998 survey of pediatricians, family practitioners, and obstetricians who perform circumcision revealed that only

45% routinely used procedural analgesia.[26] The longer-term effects of this procedure on pain response only recently have been determined. Taddio and colleagues[27] demonstrated lower pain thresholds and more crying during immunization at 4 to 6 months in circumcised infants compared with those infants who had not undergone the procedure, and that the use of local anesthesia ameliorated these effects. In response to these and other studies demonstrating the adverse effects of neonatal circumcision without analgesia, the American Academy of Pediatrics (AAP) issued a policy statement in 1999 that declared that, "if a decision for circumcision is made, procedural analgesia should be provided."[28] The AAP recommended that topical anesthetics (ie, EMLA) and/or nerve blocks with lidocaine should be used to reduce the pain associated with this procedure. Pacifiers dipped in a sucrose solution (see previous text) and acetaminophen also can be used to provide adjunctive pain relief. Additionally, different circumcision techniques are associated with less pain (eg, Mogen clamp) and more physiologic positioning can reduce the stress of this procedure.

Dorsal Penile Nerve Block

Kirya and Werthmann[29] first reported the effectiveness of dorsal penile nerve block for infant circumcision in 1978. The technique involves injecting 0.4 mL of 1% lidocaine (it is imperative that epinephrine not be added to the solution) using a 27-gauge needle at the 10- and 2-o'clock positions (0.8 mL total) at the base of the penis. The needle is directed posteriomedially to a depth of 3 to 5 mm, and a slight "pop" is felt when Buck's fascia is entered. Careful aspiration is performed before injection of the local anesthetic to avoid intravascular injection. Using this technique, complications are quite rare. In one study of 491 patients, slight bruising at the injection site was noted in 11% of infants.[30] Bruising had resolved in all infants when they were reevaluated at 2 weeks of age. Hematoma or bleeding at the injection site was noted in 1.2% of infants after circumcision in a retrospective study of more than 1,000 infants.[31]

Subcutaneous Ring Block

Subcutaneous ring block for neonatal circumcision was described by Broadman et al[32] in 1987. This technique is easily performed by injecting 0.8 mL of 1% lidocaine subcutaneously around the midshaft of the penis. A recent study suggested that this block is more effective than the more traditional dorsal penile nerve block.[33] Lander and colleagues[33] demonstrated significantly less crying and a lower heart rate throughout the procedure after subcutaneous ring block compared with either dorsal penile nerve block, EMLA, or a topical placebo. In response to this, and the recommendations in the AAP policy statement on circumcision, a training video was recently produced at the Massachusetts General Hospital to demonstrate this technique. It is available through the AAP Web site at www.aap.org.

Eutectic Mixture of Local Anesthetics

Eutectic mixture of local anesthetics has been shown to significantly reduce facial activity, crying time, and heart rate increases compared with placebo when applied 60 to 80 minutes before circumcision.[9] One milliliter of the cream is drawn into a 3-mL syringe and one third of the dose is applied to the lower abdomen. The penis is then extended upward and gently pressed against the abdomen. The remainder of the drug is applied to a bio-occlusive dressing (Tegaderm) to cover the dorsal side of the penis and then secured to the abdomen. This allows for prolonged circumferential exposure to the topical anesthetic cream. Despite theoretical concerns in this age group, no increases in methemoglobin levels were found in any of these infants.[9]

Adjunctive Techniques

Pacifiers dipped in a sucrose solution also have been shown to significantly reduce crying during circumcision.[34] Acetaminophen can improve postoperative comfort when given orally every 6 hours after the procedure, although it does not reduce pain responses during circumcision.[36] A padded physiologic restraint chair significantly reduced crying time when compared with the traditional hard plastic restraint device.[35] In infants given EMLA cream for analgesia, the use of a Mogen clamp, compared with a Gomco clamp, reduced crying and grimacing, perhaps, in part, due to the decreased time needed to perform the procedure.[37] As with postoperative analgesia, using a multimodal analgesic approach seems to provide the best analgesia for circumcision. A recent study found significantly reduced crying time when a Mogen clamp technique was used in conjunction with EMLA, dorsal penile nerve block, and a sucrose pacifier compared with the Gomco clamp procedure and analgesia with EMLA cream.[38]

Pharmacologic Pain Management for Acute Pain and Surgery

Although a number of recent studies have helped to better define the pharmacokinetics and pharmacodynamics of opioids, acetaminophen, and local anesthetics in neonates and infants, because most analgesic agents are conjugated in the liver and excreted through the kidneys, there remains a great deal of variability in clearance of the drugs in preterm and term neonates. With the maturation of hepatic enzyme systems and improved glomerular filtration rate in the weeks after birth, dosing intervals for intermittent boluses often require frequent adjustment. The therapeutic window for pain relief without respiratory compromise also can be quite narrow, necessitating careful titration to effect and the use of continuous infusions whenever possible. Recent pharmacokinetic studies in newborns have made it easier to know where to start with bolus drugs and analgesic infusions, but titration based on clinical response remains the cornerstone of pain treatment in newborns.

Opioid Analgesics

The response to opioid analgesics can be quite variable in neonates and infants, making the treatment of severe postoperative pain problematic. The pharmacodynamic issues surrounding opioid administration in the neonatal period remain controversial despite a number of animal and human investigations. Early studies in newborn rats suggested that newborns were less sensitive to the analgesic effects of morphine, but more sensitive to the respiratory depressant effects of this drug than older rats.[39] However, more recently, McLaughlin and Dewey[40] have shown that infant rats are more sensitive to the analgesic effects of morphine, meperidine, buprenorphine, and fentanyl when evaluating the suppression of responses to mechanical or thermal pain. In dogs, respiratory depression from morphine decreases markedly in the first month of life, but the ventilatory effects of fentanyl did not show age-related changes.[41] Ventilatory response curves in infants who received continuous infusions of morphine did not show age-related changes when the infusion rate was adjusted to maintain equivalent plasma morphine concentrations, suggesting that delayed clearance of the drug is age-related and responsible for differences in age-related respiratory effects of opioids.[42] However, in less well-controlled studies, significantly more episodes of apnea and respiratory depression were noted when infants received opioid analgesia postoperatively.[43,44] The additional effect of the anesthetic agents or the type of surgery on respiratory depression is unknown.

In the first week of life, the elimination half-life of morphine is more than twice as long in newborns when compared with older children or adults, and even longer in preterm infants.[45,46] The prolongation of the elimination half-life seems to be due to several factors, the most important of which is the immaturity of the newborn infant's hepatic enzyme systems. Clearance of morphine is dependent on conjugation of the drug to the inactive metabolite morphine-3-glucuronide and the active metabolite morphine-6-glucuronide. The rate of conjugation also is dependent on hepatic blood flow, which can be markedly reduced in neonates and infants undergoing abdominal procedures such as gastroschisis, omphalocele, duodenal atresia, or malrotation repair.[47] Even in children who do not undergo surgery, the reduced glomerular filtration rate in the first week of life leads to slow elimination of both of the metabolites as well as the unchanged drug.

Because the therapeutic window for pain relief without respiratory depression can be narrow in neonates and infants and the clearance quite variable, adequate treatment of severe postoperative pain with intermittent boluses of morphine or fentanyl may lead to wide swings in plasma concentrations. Therefore, continuous intravenous infusions generally are preferred to provide a more constant level of pain relief. Neonates and infants require an initial loading dose of morphine that is similar to older children (0.05-0.1 mg/kg) followed by an infusion at a lower rate to avoid accumulation. Recent pharmacokinetic studies in newborns by Lynn and colleagues[48] suggest that this rate should be approximately 0.01 mg/kg/h, about one third that used for older children. Neonates and infants undergoing cardiac surgery require even smaller infusion rates—approximately 0.005 mg/ kg/h. Infusion rates can then be adjusted based on clinical signs of either inadequate pain relief or increased somnolence. Both an infant pain score and a sedation score generally are needed to determine the most appropriate infusion rate. Starting infusion rates for the most commonly used opioid analgesics in infants are outlined in Table 9-2.

With the safe and effective use of nurse-controlled analgesia in infants and young children outside of the NICU, this technique is

Table 9-2. Suggested Starting Infusion Rates for Morphine and Fentanyl*

	Morphine	Fentanyl
Preterm infants	5-10 μg/kg/h	0.5-1 μg/kg/h
Term neonates <30 d	10 μg/kg/h	1 μg/kg/h
Term neonates <30 d (cardiac)†	5 μg/kg/h	0.5-1 μg/kg/h
Term infants >30 d	20 μg/kg/h	1-2 μg/kg/h
Term infants >30 d (cardiac)†	15 μg/kg/h	0.5-2 μg/kg/h

*Adapted from *Anesth Analg.* 1998;86:958-963.

†Infants undergoing cardiac surgery require lower infusion rates to maintain acceptable plasma levels of morphine. Rates should be adjusted downward for infants with sepsis, decreased hepatic blood flow, abdominal surgery, or evidence of cardiac dysfunction. (see text).

beginning to be used in the NICU. Morphine concentrations of 0.1 mg/mL are used to minimize the effect of catheter flushes and potential overdose of the medication.

Acetaminophen

Acetaminophen can provide significant adjunctive pain relief and reduce opioid requirements after major surgery. In the United States, it is administered as a rectal suppository or as an oral elixir, because the intravenous formulation is not currently available. Hepatic toxicity results from increased levels of a metabolite of acetaminophen, and infants and young children seem to be less susceptible.[49] It is unclear whether this is due to lower production of this metabolite or increased binding by glutathione peroxidase (GSH). Animal studies suggest that neonates and infants have elevated GSH levels as a part of hepatic growth; therefore, more efficiently shunting the toxic metabolite of acetaminophen metabolism into the GSH pathway.[50] Weanling rats in one study demonstrated a 24-fold increase in GSH conjugate production and less histopathologic damage than adult rats when a toxic dose of acetaminophen was administered. Fasting, however, can lower GSH production and should be considered when long-term dosing of acetaminophen is anticipated.

Acetaminophen is well absorbed orally in neonates and infants, but the elimination half-life is approximately 50% longer than in older children.[51] Therefore, the appropriate dosing interval for oral administration in the first 2 weeks of life should be no more frequent than every 6 to 8 hours. Appropriate dosing by the rectal route is somewhat controversial, but can be extrapolated from studies with older children and several recent studies in neonates. Studies in the late 1980s and early 1990s showed that doses of 20 to 25 mg/kg of acetaminophen administered rectally to children led to subtherapeutic plasma levels.[52,53] Subsequent pharmacokinetic studies revealed that single doses of 35 to 45 mg/kg resulted in plasma levels in the therapeutic range.[54,55] However, these doses were associated with a longer elimination half-life, mandating less frequent dosing. Several recent studies have examined the pharmacokinetics of rectal acetaminophen in neonates and preterm infants. Lin and colleagues[56] first demonstrated that rectal acetaminophen doses of 20 mg/kg administered to 5 preterm neonates led to serum blood levels below the generally accepted therapeutic range of 10 to 20 μg/mL. A subsequent and more comprehensive study evaluating several different age groups revealed that 20 mg/kg administered rectally led to therapeutic concentrations in 16 of 21 of neonates between 28 and 32 weeks gestational age, but only 1 of 7 in the 32- to 36-week gestational age group.[57] These and 4 other studies were included in a recent pooled population analysis of 124 preterm and term neonates to assess the developmental pharmacokinetics of this drug.[58] This study suggested that absorption via the rectal route is somewhat more efficient in preterm neonates than older infants and that dosing should be less frequent in younger infants. Guidelines based on this study for both oral and rectal acetaminophen dosing for preterm and term neonates are outlined in Table 9-3. These dosing guidelines include recommendations for maximum daily dosing at various gestational ages.

Epidural Analgesia

Epidural analgesia can provide excellent postoperative analgesia for neonates and infants undergoing thoracic, abdominal, and lower extremity surgery. It can be particularly useful for surgeries where early resumption of spontaneous ventilation is desired to avoid barotrauma (eg, diaphragmatic hernia repair). The use of epidural analgesia in neonates and infants has been facilitated by the discovery that a catheter can be reliably threaded to the thoracic region from the simpler caudal approach.[59] This technique tends to be quite reliable in neonates and infants weighing less than 5 kg.[60] Because proper alignment of the tip of the epidural catheter can be crucial to the success of this technique, placement should be verified by injecting 0.5 mL of radioopaque dye (Omnipaque 180 or Isovue 200) through the catheter, followed by radiography (Figure 9-1).[61] Radioopaque catheters (Theracath™, Arrow International, Redding, PA) also are available that allow the level of the catheter tip to be detected with a plain radiograph. The advantage of these catheters is that placement can be easily verified throughout the duration of the infusion.

Continuous infusions of bupivacaine can provide excellent pain relief, but clearance of local anesthetics can vary in neonates and infants. Bupivacaine is an amide local anesthetic requiring conjugation to inactive metabolites in the liver and excretion in the kidneys. Clearance may, therefore, be delayed in neonates and infants, especially after abdominal surgery. Early pharmacokinetic studies demonstrated that infants younger than 4 months receiving infusions of 0.1%

Table 9-3. Acetaminophen Dosing in Preterm and Term Neonates*

Preterm Neonates (28-32 wk)†	
Oral	12 mg/kg every 12 h
Rectal	15 mg/kg every 12 h
Maximum daily dose	30 mg/kg/d
Preterm Neonates (32-36 wk)	
Oral	10-15 mg/kg every 8 h
Rectal	30 mg/kg loading dose‡ then 20 mg/kg every 8 h
Maximum daily dose	60 mg/kg/d
Full-term Neonates <30 Days of Age	
Oral	10-15 mg/kg every 6–8 h
Rectal	30 mg/kg loading dose‡ then 20 mg/kg every 8 h
Maximum daily dose	60 mg/kg/d
Full-term Infants >30 Days of Age	
Oral	10-15 mg/kg every 4-6 h
Rectal	30 mg/kg loading dose‡ then 20 mg/kg every 6-8 h
Maximum daily dose	80-90 mg/kg/d

*Caution should always be observed in administering acetaminophen to neonates who have evidence of severe systemic illness (eg, sepsis, bowel obstruction, dehydration) or who have other evidence of liver dysfunction.
†There are currently no pharmacokinetic data for preterm neonates <28 weeks, so no recommendation was made for these neonates.
‡Loading doses are not included in maximum daily dose calculations.

bupivacaine can have steadily rising bupivacaine plasma levels, in contrast to the steady-state levels seen in older infants.[62] Subsequent studies focusing specifically on neonates demonstrated that at 48 hours of an infusion at 0.2 mg/kg/h, rising bupivacaine levels are seen in 60% of patients.[63] For this reason, it is recommended that infusion rates in infants younger than 2 months should not exceed 0.2 mg/kg/h for the initial infusion and should be lowered as tolerated during the first several days of infusion. To provide adequate spread of the local anesthetic and still maintain bupivacaine levels below this range, an infusion of 0.05% bupivacaine mixed with 1 μg/mL of fentanyl has been used at rates of 0.2 to 0.4 mL/kg/h (0.1–0.2 mg/kg/h of bupivacaine) with

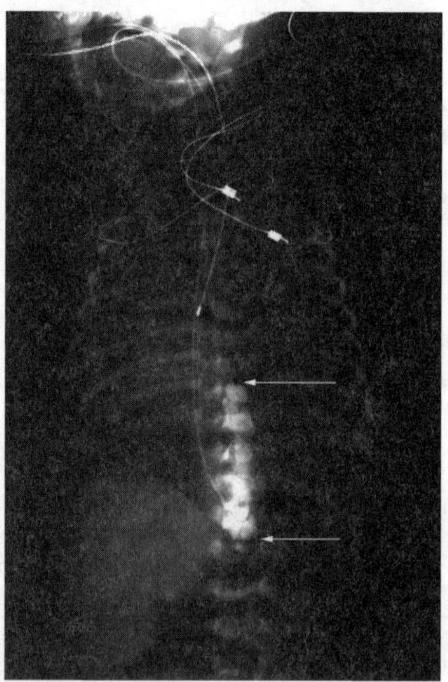

Figure 9-1
Radiograph of infant showing radiocontrast dye within the epidural space. The tip of the catheter is presumed to be at the midpoint of the dye at approximately the level of the tenth thoracic vertebrae.

success. When the tip of the epidural catheter is properly placed, infusion rates often can be further reduced to 0.1 mg/kg/h (0.2 mL/kg/h) on the second or third postoperative day without significantly affecting pain relief. Lidocaine also has been used for continuous epidural infusions in neonates and infants with the possible advantage of allowing plasma blood levels to be easily obtained during the infusion. Concern about the rapid development of tolerance to lidocaine in laboratory animals has limited its widespread use.

More recently, some practitioners have recommended using 2-chloroprocaine for epidural infusions in neonates.[64,65] Because 2-chloroprocaine is an ester local anesthetic, it is metabolized by plasma cholinesterases and rapidly cleared from the circulation. Theoretically, higher infusion rates can be administered with less likelihood of accumulation. A study by Henderson and colleagues[64] supported this and showed rapid clearance in infants even at high infusion rates (1.0 mL/kg/h of 3% chloroprocaine). However, the activity of plasma cholinesterase enzymes is diminished in the first 6 months of life, suggesting that clearance of the ester local anesthetics may be prolonged under certain circumstances. Further studies are needed to assess the efficacy and safety of long-term infusions of 2-chloroprocaine in neonates and infants because the limited data that are available in the adult and pediatric populations[64,65] have included intraoperative infusions with a maximum duration of 3 to 4 hours.

Summary

The recent understanding that painful experiences in neonates and infants can have long-term physiologic and potentially adverse neurologic effects makes it imperative to find strategies to reduce pain. Recent pharmacologic and behavioral studies have made it easier to provide analgesia for many of the routine procedures that newborns undergo. Neonates are just now beginning to receive the same attention to their pain and distress that older children and adults have had for years. These neonates deserve our continued focus on providing developmentally appropriate analgesia for the many painful procedures that are a part of modern medical care.

Effective techniques for relief of procedural pain include topical anesthetic creams, infiltration with local anesthetic agents, regional anesthetic techniques, and nonnutritive sucking. For mild to moderate postsurgical and acute pain, acetaminophen can provide effective pain relief, but higher initial doses may be required when it is administered via the rectal route. For more severe pain, intravenous opioids or regional anesthetic techniques should be considered.

References

1. Porter FL, Grunau RE, Anand KJ. Long-term effects of pain in infants. *J Dev Behav Pediatr.* 1999;20:253-261
2. Grunau R. Early pain in preterm infants. A model of long-term effects. *Clin Perinatol.* 2002;29:373-394
3. Stevens B, Gibbins S, Franck LS. Treatment of pain in the neonatal intensive care unit. *Pediatr Clin North Am.* 2000;47:633-650
4. Krechel SW, Bildner J. CRIES: a new neonatal postoperative pain measurement score. Initial testing of validity and reliability. *Paediatr Anaesth.* 1995;5:53-61
5. Craig KD. The facial display of pain in infants and children. *Pain Res Manag.* 1998;10:103-121
6. Grunau RE, Oberlander T, Holsti L, Whitfield MF. Bedside application of the Neonatal Facial Coding System in pain assessment of premature neonates. *Pain.* 1998;76:277-286
7. Lawrence J, Alcock D, McGrath P, Kay J, MacMurray SB, Dulberg C. The development of a tool to assess neonatal pain. *Neonatal Netw.* 1993;12:59-66
8. Stevens B, Johnston C, Petryshen P, Taddio A. Premature Infant Pain Profile: development and initial validation. *Clin J Pain.* 1996;12:13-22
9. Taddio A, Stevens B, Craig K, et al. The efficacy and safety of lidocaine-prilocaine cream for pain during circumcision. *N Engl J Med.* 1997;336:1197-1201
10. Taddio A, Ohlsson A, Emerson T, et al. A systematic review of lidocaine-prilocaine cream (EMLA) in the treatment of acute pain in neonates. *Pediatrics.* 1998;101:1-14

11. Larsson BA, Tannfeldt G, Lagercrantz H, Olssen GL. Venipuncture is more effective and less painful than heel lancing for blood tests in neonates. *Pediatrics.* 1998;101:882-886
12. Blass EM, Schide DJ, Zaw-Mon C, et al. Mother as shield: differential effects of contact and nursing on pain responsivity in infant rats—evidence for nonopioid mediation. *Behav Neurosci.* 1995;109:342-353
13. Stevens B, Johnson C, Franck L, Petryshen P, Jack A, Foster G. The efficacy of developmentally sensitive behavioral interventions and sucrose for relieving procedural pain in very low birth weight neonates. *Nurs Res.* 1999;48:35-43
14. Field T, Goldson E. Pacifying effects of nonnutritive sucking on term and preterm neonates during heelsticks. *Pediatrics.* 1984;74:1012-1015
15. Shiao SY, Chang YJ, Lannon H, Yarandi H. Meta-analysis of the effects of non-nutritive sucking on heart rate and peripheral oxygenation: research from the past 30 years. *Issues Compr Pediatr Nurs.* 1997;20:11-24
16. Ors R, Ozek E, Baysoy G, et al. Comparison of sucrose and human milk on pain response in newborns. *Eur J Pediatr.* 1999;158:63-66
17. Blass EM. Milk-induced hypoalgesia in human newborns. *Pediatrics.* 1997;99:825-829
18. Ramenghi LA, Evans DJ, Levene MI. Sucrose analgesia: absorptive mechanism or taste perception? *Arch Dis Child Fetal Neonatal Ed.* 1999;80:F146-F147
19. Skogsdal Y, Eriksson M, Schollin J. Analgesia in newborns given oral glucose. *Acta Paediatr.* 1997;86:217-220
20. Stevens B, Taddio A, Ohlsson A, et al. The efficacy of sucrose for relieving pain in neonates: a systematic review and meta-analysis. *Acta Paediatr.* 1997;86:837-842
21. Willis D, Chabot J, Radde IL, Chance GW. Unsuspected hyperosmolarity of oral solutions contributing to necrotizing enterocolitis in very-low birth weight infants. *Pediatrics.* 1977;60:535-538
22. Holve RL, Bronberger Pj, Groveman HD, Klauber MR, Dixon SD, Snyder JM. Regional anesthesia during newborn circumcision: effect on infant pain response. *Clin Pediatr.* 1983;22:813-818
23. Maxwell LG, Yaster M, Wetzel RC, Niebyl JR. Penile nerve block for newborn circumcision. *Obstet Gynecol.* 1987;70:415-419
24. Stang HJ, Gunnar MR, Snellman L, Condon LM, Kestenbaum R. Local anesthesia for neonatal circumcision. Effects on distress and cortisol response. *JAMA.* 1988;259:1507-1511

25. Dixon S, Snyder J, Holve R, Bromberger P. Behavioral effects of circumcision with and without anesthesia. *J Dev Behav Pediatr.* 1984;5:246-250
26. Stang HJ, Snellman LW. Circumcision practice patterns in the United States. *Pediatrics.* 1998;101:e5
27. Taddio A, Katz J, Ilersich AL, Koren G. Effect of neonatal circumcision on pain responses during subsequent routine vaccination. *Lancet.* 1997;349:599-603
28. American Academy of Pediatrics Task Force on Circumcision. Circumcision policy statement. *Pediatrics.* 1999;103:686-693
29. Kirya C, Werthmann MW. Neonatal circumcision and penile dorsal nerve block—a painless procedure. *J Pediatr.* 1978;92:998-1000
30. Snellman LW, Stang HJ. Prospective evaluation of complications of dorsal penile nerve block for neonatal circumcision. *Pediatrics.* 1995;95:705-708
31. Fontaine P, Dittberner D, Scheltema KE. The safety of dorsal penile nerve block for neonatal circumcision. *J Fam Pract.* 1994;39:243-248
32. Broadman LM, Hannallah RS, Belman AB, Elder PT, Ruttiman U. Post-circumcision analgesia—a prospective evaluation of subcutaneous ring block of the penis. *Anesthesiology.* 1987;67:399-402
33. Lander J, Brady-Fryer B, Metcalfe JB, et al. Comparison of ring block, dorsal penile nerve block, and topical anesthesia for neonatal circumcision: a randomized clinical trial. *JAMA.* 1997;278:2157-2162
34. Blass EM, Hoffmeyer LB. Sucrose as an analgesic in newborn infants. *Pediatrics.* 1991;87:215-218
35. Stang HJ, Snellman LW, Condon LM, et al. Beyond dorsal penile nerve block: a more humane circumcision. *Pediatrics.* 1997;100:e3
36. Howard CR, Howard FM, Weitzman ML. Acetaminophen analgesia in neonatal circumcision: the effect on pain. *Pediatrics.* 1994;93:641-646
37. Kaufman GE, Cimo S, Miller LW, Blass EM. An evaluation of the effects of sucrose on neonatal pain with 2 commonly used circumcision methods. *Am J Obstet Gynecol.* 2002;186:564-568
38. Taddio A, Pollock N, Gilbert-MacLeod C, Ohlsson K, Koren G. Combined analgesia and local anesthesia minimize pain during circumcision. *Arch Pediatr Adolesc Med.* 2000;154:620-623
39. Pasternak GW, Zhang AZ, Tecott L. Developmental differences between high and low affinity opiate binding sites: their relationship to analgesia and respiratory depression. *Life Sci.* 1980;27:1185-1190
40. McLaughlin CR, Dewey WL. A comparison of the antinociceptive effects of opioid agonists in neonatal and adult rats in phasic and tonic nociceptive tests. *Pharmacol Biochem Behav.* 1994;49:1017-1023

41. Bragg P, Zwass MS, Lau M, Fisher DM. Opioid pharmacodynamics in neonatal dogs: differences between morphine and fentanyl. *J Appl Physiol.* 1995;79:1519-1524
42. Lynn AM, Nespeca MK, Opheim KE, Slattery JT. Respiratory effects of intravenous morphine infusions in neonates, infants, and children after cardiac surgery. *Anesth Analg.* 1993;77:695-701
43. Purcell-Jones G, Dormon F, Sumner E. The use of opioids in neonates. A retrospective study of 933 cases. *Anaesthesia.* 1987;42:1316-1320
44. Vaughn PR, Townsend SF, Thilo EH, McKenzie S, Moreland S, Denver KK. Comparison of continuous infusion of fentanyl to bolus dosing in neonates after surgery. *J Pediatr Surg.* 1996;31:1616-1623
45. Lynn AM, Slattery JT. Morphine pharmacokinetics in early infancy. *Anesthesiology.* 1987;66:136-139
46. Bhat R, Chari G, Gulati A, Aldana O, Velamati R, Bhargava H. Pharmacokinetics of a single dose of morphine in preterm infants during the first week of life. *J Pediatr.* 1990;117:477-481
47. Gauntlett IS, Fisher DM, Hertzka RE, Kuhls E, Spellman MJ. Pharmacokinetics of fentanyl in neonatal humans and lambs: effects of age. *Anesthesiology.* 1988;69:683-687
48. Lynn A, Nespeca MK, Bratton SL, Strauss SG, Shen DD. Clearance of morphine in postoperative infants during intravenous infusion: the influence of age and surgery. *Anesth Analg.* 1998;86:958-963
49. Rumack BH, Peterson RG. Acetaminophen overdose: incidence, diagnosis, and management in 416 patients. *Pediatrics.* 1978;62:898-903
50. Allameh A, Vansoun EY, Zarghi A. Role of glutathione conjugation in protection of weanling rat liver against acetaminophen-induced hepatotoxicity. *Mech Ageing Develop.* 1997;95:71-79
51. Levy G, Khanna NN, Soda DM, Tsuzuki O, Stern L. Pharmacokinetics of acetaminophen in the human neonate: formation of acetaminophen glucuronide and sulfate in relation to plasma bilirubin concentration and D-glutaric acid excretion. *Pediatrics.* 1975;55:818-825
52. Gaudreault P, Guay J, Nicol O, Dupuis C. Pharmacokinetics and clinical efficacy of intrarectal solution of acetaminophen. *Can J Anaesth.* 1988;35:149-152
53. Hopkins CS, Underhill S, Booker PD. Pharmacokinetics of paracetamol after cardiac surgery. *Arch Dis Child.* 1990;65:971-976
54. Montgomery CJ, McCormack JP, Reichert CC, Marsland CP. Plasma concentrations after high-dose (45 mg/kg) rectal acetaminophen in children. *Can J Anaesth.* 1995;42:982-986

55. Birmingham PK, Tobin MJ, Henthorn TK, et al. Twenty four hour pharmacokinetics of rectal acetaminophen in children: an old drug with new recommendations. *Anesthesiology.* 1997;87:244-252
56. Lin YC, Sussman HH, Bentz WE. Plasma concentrations after rectal administration of acetaminophen in preterm neonates. *Paediatr Anaesth.* 1997;7:457-459
57. Van Lingen RA, Deinum JT, Quak JME, et al. Pharmacokinetics and metabolism of rectally administered paracetamol in preterm neonates. *Arch Dis Child Fetal Neonatal Ed.* 1999;80:F59-F63
58. Anderson BJ, van Lingen RA, Hansen TG, Lin YC, Holford NH. Acetaminophen developmental pharmacokinetics in premature neonates and infants: a pooled population analysis. *Anesthesiology.* 2002;96:1336-1345
59. Bosenberg AT, Bland BA, Schulte-Steinberg O, Downing JW. Thoracic epidural anesthesia via the caudal route in infants. *Anesthesiology.* 1988;69:265-269
60. Blank JW, Houck CS, McClain BC, Berde CB. Cephalad advancement of epidural catheters: radiographic correlation. *Anesthesiology.* 1994;81:A1345
61. Valairucha S, Seefelder C, Houck CS. Thoracic epidural catheters placed by the caudal route in infants: the importance of radiographic confirmation. *Paediatr Anaesth.* 2002;12:424-428
62. Luz G, Innerhofer P, Bachmann B, et al. Bupivacaine plasma concentrations during continuous epidural anesthesia in infants and children. *Anesth Analg.* 1996;82:231-234
63. Larsson BA, Lonnqvist PA, Olsson GL. Plasma concentrations of bupivacaine in neonates after continuous epidural infusion. *Anesth Analg.* 1997;84:501-505
64. Henderson K, Sethna NF, Berde CB. Continuous caudal anesthesia for inguinal hernia repair in former preterm infants. *J Clin Anesthesia.* 1993;5:129-133
65. Tobias JD, Rasmussen GE, Holcomb GW III, et al. Continuous caudal anaesthesia with chloroprocaine as an adjunct to general anaesthesia in neonates. *Can J Anaesth.* 1996;43:69-72

Chapter 10

Treatment of Acute Pain Associated With Medical Illnesses

Stephen R. Hays, MD, FAAP
Jayant K. Deshpande, MD, MPH, FAAP
Joseph D. Tobias, MD, FAAP

Headache Pain
Pain Associated With Otitis Media
Chest Pain
Pain Related to Acute Traumatic Injury
Pain Related to Burns
Pain Related to Hemoglobinopathies, Including Sickle Cell Disease

Introduction

Pain is a common presenting complaint during pediatric health care encounters. At times, the pain may be the reason for seeking medical attention while, in other instances, pain is associated with the primary malady (eg, ear pain associated with fever and otitis media) that necessitates evaluation by a physician. Regardless of the presentation, it often is helpful to follow a general algorithm when evaluating the child who has acute pain associated with a medical illness. The initial step is to determine if the child's pain represents an emergent underlying condition that mandates immediate evaluation and intervention, such as headache pain from a brain tumor and increased intracranial pressure, or abdominal pain heralding visceral catastrophe. In the emergent situation, although initial pain control measures should be undertaken,[1,2] immediate evaluation and referral to appropriate subspecialty care should not be delayed. In other scenarios, elective subspecialty evaluation may be helpful in managing less emergent, but potentially significant, or complex processes leading to pain. For example, the child with headaches consistent with migraines may benefit from referral to a pediatric neurologist, while the teenager with chronic abdominal pain, weight loss, and bloody diarrhea suggestive of inflammatory bowel disease merits evaluation by a pediatric gastroenterologist.

At times, there may be recurrent, acute pain (eg, sickle cell vaso-occlusive crisis), the progression of acute pain to chronic pain (eg, reflex sympathetic dystrophy or chronic regional pain syndrome type I), or chronic pain such as that associated with oncologic diseases. In such cases, effective pain control may require more aggressive or elaborate interventions, which can only be provided by long-term, multidisciplinary pain management teams. (See Chapter 12 for a discussion of the treatment of chronic pain in children.) Most commonly, pain in children represents an acute, non–life-threatening process that can be managed by the primary health care provider. Despite the myriad conditions that cause acute pain, the treatment strategies are relatively similar with a progression from nonsteroidal anti-inflammatory agents (NSAIDs) for mild pain to weak opioids, such as oxycodone for moderate pain, and the use of potent opioids for severe pain. This chapter outlines the approach to some of the more commonly seen types of acute pain in the pediatric population. See Chapter 8 for suggested dosing regimens of the various agents discussed in the chapter.

Headache Pain

Headaches have existed since the dawn of civilization, with reports of the disorder dating back 25 to 30 centuries to the time of the ancient Egyptians. However, little information was available on the potential impact of headache disorders in children until 1873, when British pediatrician William Henry Day, MD, included an entire chapter on headache disorders in his book, *Essays on Diseases in Children.* Although much has been learned about headaches since then, many of Dr Day's impressions are applicable today, including the basic premises that nonvascular headaches are most common and that many headache disorders in children are related to psychosocial stresses. The potential effect of headaches on the activities of daily living of a child should not be underestimated. Headache disorders can be chronic, recurrent problems that interfere with usual childhood activities, including school attendance. More than 30% of children report having headaches by age 6, and up to 75% by age 15. In fact, children miss more than a million days of school each year because of headaches. Foremost in the minds of many parents and health care providers is the fear that some underlying problem is responsible for the headache (eg, brain tumor). In most cases, no life-threatening problem is found, but a thorough history and physical examination is necessary to rule out potentially life-threatening problems. In many cases, especially when evaluating recurrent headache problems, neurologic imaging (computed tomography [CT] or magnetic resonance imaging) is obtained.

Various nocioceptive pathways may be involved in the pathogenesis of headache pain. The brain and the meninges have no pain fibers. Headache pain comes from the innervation of the vasculature inside the brain and outside the skull or from the muscles of the head and neck. Migraine pain typically is related to innervation of the vasculature, while tension-type headache pain is related to the muscles in the head and neck. Although the exact cause has not been determined, pain and other symptoms (eg, nausea, tingling, sensitivity to light and sound) that occur during migraine headaches are related to changes in blood flow to structures within the brain. The changes in blood flow, in turn, affect neurons within the central nervous system (CNS). Blood flow changes and alterations in the function of the affected neurons can change the concentration of neurotransmitters (eg, nitric oxide, serotonin, substance P) in the CNS. Serotonin concentrations are low between migraine attacks and increase significantly during migraine headaches, although the exact chemicals (neurotransmitters) responsible for migraine pain have not been delineated. Medications that alter serotonin levels play a crucial role in the treatment of migraine (see following text).

The potential differential diagnosis of headache can be vast (Table 10-1); however, the history and physical examination, most importantly the specific characteristics regarding the headache, can significantly limit the differential diagnosis and frequently provide a specific diagnosis without the need for additional testing. Specific characteristics may be indicative of potentially emergent underlying conditions that require prompt evaluation, merit imaging of the CNS, and suggest the need for subspecialty referral (Table 10-2). Headache associated with major traumatic injury, any alteration in the level of consciousness, focal neurologic deficits, headaches that awaken the child from sleep, headaches occurring only in the morning, loss of developmental milestones, inappropriate increase in head circumference, worsening of headache when the child is supine, and physiologic changes suggestive of increased intracranial pressure (any component or combination of Cushing's triad: bradycardia, hypertension, altered respiratory pattern) mandate a careful evaluation for significant underlying disease. Additionally, the

Table 10-1. Differential Diagnosis of Headache Pain in Children

Increased Intracranial Pressure
- Hydrocephalus
- Intracranial mass
- Pseudotumor cerebri
- Hypertension
- Cerebrovascular accident
- Sinus thrombosis

Infection
- Meningitis
- Sinusitis
- Otitis (media or externa)
- Mastoiditis
- Pharyngitis
- Dental caries/abscess

Traumatic Injury
- Laceration, abrasion
- Skull fracture
- Concussion, contusion
- Intracranial hemorrhage

Primary Headache Syndromes
- Migraine headache (classic, common, variant)
- Tension headache
- Cluster headache

Functional Headache
- Somatization, conversion reaction
- Avoidance behavior, secondary gain
- Anxiety, stress
- Depression, affective disorder

Miscellaneous
- Postdural puncture headache
- Poisonings or intoxication (eg, carbon monoxide)
- Metabolic disorders
- Ophthalmologic problems (glaucoma, strabismus, refractive error)
- Bony disorders (temporomandibular joint dysfunction, cervical spine disease)
- Cranial nerve neuralgias

failure of headaches to respond to simple analgesics (acetaminophen or ibuprofen) may suggest the need for additional investigation. Such symptomatology may be associated with significant pathology responsible for headache pain and/or increased intracranial pressure such as hydrocephalus, intracranial mass, pseudotumor, hypertension, stroke, sinus thrombosis, or CNS infection. Although these symptoms may be suggestive of life-threatening pathology, they also may be found in the benign causes of headache pain, including migraine and tension headaches.

Table 10-2. Signs and Symptoms Suggestive of Pathology in Headache Pain

Increased frequency of pain
Increased intensity of pain
Constant or daily pain
Morning headaches
Patient awakens from sleep with pain
Nausea and vomiting
Change in pain with change in body position
No family history of migraine disorders
Altered mental status
Seizures
Focal neurologic deficit
Mood swings, irritability
Appetite changes
Change in school performance
Visual disturbances
Gait problems
Failure to respond to simple analgesics
Increased head circumference
Alteration in vital signs (decreased heart rate, increased blood pressure)

One way of classifying headache disorders is to separate them into primary and secondary headaches. Primary headaches are classified as such because the pain or headache is the primary symptom related to a disturbance of the brain or the blood vessels within the brain. Primary headaches include migraine, cluster, and ordinary headaches (a mild form of either migraine or tension headache). Ordinary headaches are the most common form of headache and usually are treated easily with simple analgesics (acetaminophen or NSAIDs such as ibuprofen). In general, ordinary headaches do not significantly interfere with daily activities, have no associated signs and symptoms, produce mild pain, last a few hours, and do not recur at regular intervals. Secondary headaches are related to an underlying problem such as a sinus infection or brain tumor. There are literally hundreds of causes for secondary headaches (Table 10-1), originating in several different organ systems, including head trauma, dental problems, hypertension, carbon monoxide poisoning, and viral illnesses.

Headaches also may be classified as acute; acute, recurrent; chronic, progressive; or chronic, nonprogressive. An acute headache is a one-time event that occurs suddenly and without warning. Possible causes of an acute headache include ordinary headache; the first occurrence of a migraine headache, in which case the headache will recur and become an acute, recurrent headache; tension headache; or a wide range of systemic illnesses, some of which may be life-threatening and require immediate medical attention (eg, infections of the CNS, toxins such as carbon monoxide, hypertension, or a brain tumor).

Acute, recurrent headaches are characterized by moderate to severe pain that occurs suddenly, lasts several hours, and occurs at regular intervals with pain-free periods in between. This type of headache does not increase in intensity or frequency over time. Migraines and tension-type headaches are included in this group. A patient diagnosed with migraine headaches who presents with increasing severity or frequency of pain or a change in the location of the pain warrants additional investigation for a secondary cause of the headache, such as an intracranial mass. In such cases, the patient may move into another category of headache—chronic, progressive headaches, which become more painful and more frequent over time. When accompanied by other signs and symptoms such as nausea, vomiting, or findings on physical examination, a problem, such as a brain tumor, may be present. Chronic, nonprogressive headaches occur at frequent intervals (daily) or are constant, but do not increase in severity. There are no associated clinical signs or symptoms. These headaches frequently are associated with some type of psychosocial stress.

Acute, recurrent headache pain may be related to either a migraine headache disorder or tension headaches. The classic symptom associated with migraine headache is an aura. An aura, which generally precedes a migraine, is a sensation of light or warmth that is caused by vascular alterations within the CNS. Visual changes are the most common type of an aura and may include flashing lights, double vision, partial vision loss, zigzag lines, or size distortions. The aura also may cause sensory changes in an extremity, a peculiar smell, motor weakness, aphasia, or even abdominal pain. Migraine headaches occur equally in boys and in girls. Approximately 30% of migraines in children are associated with an aura. Boys typically experience migraine headaches at a younger age than girls do. Age of onset of migraines with aura is 5 to 7 years in boys and 12 to 13 years in girls. Migraine without aura first occurs at age 10 to 11 years in boys and age 14 to 17 years in girls. Motion sickness is observed in almost half of children with migraines. Other associated conditions include asthma or eczema. Although there may still be some social stigmata associated with migraine headaches, there is no evidence to link the occurrence of migraine with anxiety, depression, or psychiatric problems.

Migraines may be further classified as either migraine without aura (formerly known as "common migraine") or migraine with aura (formerly known as "classic migraine"). Migraine without aura is diagnosed in the child who has at least 5 attacks of headache pain that last from 4 to 72 hours (the duration of pain is decreased to 2 hours in children <15 years old), plus 2 of the following characteristics: 1) unilateral pain; 2) pulsating type of pain; 3) moderate to severe intensity of the pain; 4) pain aggravated by physical activity; and 5) associated symptoms, including nausea, vomiting, photophobia, or phonophobia. Migraine with aura is diagnosed by 2 attacks with the same pain criteria as listed for migraine without aura, plus 1) one or more reversible auras, 2) gradual development of the aura over a 5- to 10-minute period, and 3) onset of the headache within 60 minutes of the aura.

In distinction, tension-type headaches of the acute, recurrent type are diagnosed by headache lasting 30 minutes to days, with 2 of the following characteristics: 1) bilateral location; 2) non-pulsatile, pressing, or tightening quality; 3) mild to moderate intensity; 4) no aggravation by physical activity; and 5) no associated nausea, vomiting, photophobia, or phonophobia. Although these definitions may aid a diagnosis, it also is inevitable that there may be significant overlap between the different categories because many of the signs and symptoms are subjective. Additionally, because worrisome signs and symptoms (Table 10-2) may occur with primary headache disorders, neurologic imaging frequently is obtained in patients with recurrent, acute headaches, even in the absence of positive physical findings.

The effective treatment for childhood headache begins with an accurate diagnosis of the condition. In many cases, this can be made through a history and physical examination. Most importantly, a negative physical examination, including a fundoscopic examination and a blood-pressure check to rule out hypertension, can help eliminate many of the secondary, life-threatening causes of headache. Treatment, or at least elimination of provocative factors, may be achieved by asking the patient to keep a headache diary, documenting the frequency of the headaches; duration; intensity; factors that might lead to the headache, such as certain foods and environmental factors, such as stress and lack of sleep; and the child's response or lack of response to the treatments tried at home. Treatment options include the use of simple analgesics (acetaminophen or ibuprofen) and, in the case of migraine headaches, abortive or prophylactic medications (see following text). Alternative routes of administering analgesics, including suppository forms of acetaminophen or indomethacin, should be considered when headaches are accompanied by nausea and vomiting that prevent a child from taking oral medications. Although these simple analgesics are effective even in most children diagnosed with migraine headaches, there will be a percentage of patients in whom simple analgesics fail, thereby necessitating the use of other medications. Additional medications include abortive medications taken during the aura of migraines with aura or at the onset of pain in migraine without aura. These agents work specifically to reverse blood flow changes that are thought to cause migraine headaches. Although effective, significant acute and chronic problems may result from the use of such medications and, therefore, a physician with significant experience in this area should direct the prescribing of such medications. These agents include direct vasoconstrictors such as the ergotamine derivatives (dihydroergotamine) that cause constriction of the dilated intracranial vessels. Dihydroergotamine can be administered via nasal spray, injection, or the sublingual routes. The $serotonin_1$ receptor agonist sumatriptan (Imitrex, GlaxoSmithKline, Reasearch Triangle Park, NC) is available and may relieve pain related to migraine. This medication is available as a nasal spray, injection, or tablet. These types of medications may lead to adverse side effects, including hypertension and, rarely, coronary or distal vascular ischemia. Children who experience recurrent migraine headaches also may be treated with prophylactic medications such as β-adrenergic antagonists, calcium channel blockers, or antidepressants. In addition to pharmacologic therapy, children with recurrent headaches may achieve success with nonpharmacologic techniques used in other chronic pain conditions, including acupuncture, transcutaneous electrical nerve stimulation (TENS), biofeedback, hypnosis, and other so-called "nontraditional" methods. These options are discussed in greater detail in Chapters 11 and 12.

Pain Associated With Otitis Media

The innervation of the ear is complex. The auriculotemporal nerve, a branch of the third or mandibular division of the trigeminal nerve (V cranial nerve), supplies the anterior portion of the external ear, as well as the interior of the auditory canal. The great auricular nerve, which arises from branches of the cervical plexus, supplies the inferior and posterior aspects of the external ear. The nerve of Arnold, or auricular branch of the vagus nerve (X cranial nerve), innervates the external auditory meatus behind the tragus, as well as a small portion of the posteromedial surface of the pinna. The inferior portion of the tympanic membrane also is innervated by the vagus, while the medial aspect of the tympanic membrane and the mucosa of the Eustachian tube are supplied by a branch of the glossopharyngeal nerve (IX cranial nerve).[3]

Acute otitis media and acute otitis externa both cause moderate to severe otalgia or ear pain.[4] In acute otitis media, eustachian tube dysfunction causes loss of normal pressure regulation in the middle ear, allowing accumulation of middle-ear fluid that may then become secondarily infected, causing moderate to severe pain. Acute otitis externa also causes moderate to severe pain, including exquisite tenderness on manipulation of the pinna. In both conditions, toxins elaborated by infectious agents likely contribute to otalgia. Acetaminophen or ibuprofen often is sufficient for adequate analgesia. Combined use of these agents can be synergistic. As with any type of acute pain, around-the-clock administration (not "as needed" dosing) may further increase efficacy. Oral administration of one of the "weak" opioids may occasionally be needed for effective analgesia until the underlying inflammation has abated. Codeine, hydrocodone, or oxycodone are reasonable options. Combination products with acetaminophen are available, but can result in dose limitations because of the acetaminophen dose.

In addition to parenteral therapy, topical therapy with otic drops may have a role in the management of pain associated with acute otitis media or otitis externa. These topical solutions contain a combination of an anti-inflammatory and local anesthetic agent in a glycerin base. One of the more commonly used agents (Auralgan, Wyeth Pharmaceuticals, Philadelphia, PA) contains a combination of antipyrine, benzocaine, and glycerin. These agents may provide additional analgesia when combined with the oral administration of simple analgesics (ibuprofen or acetaminophen). Alternatively, otic solutions containing various herbal extracts, such as allium sativum, vervascum thapsus, calendula flores, and hypericum perforatum, are frequently available as "over-the-counter" medications.

In addition to acute otitis media or externa, a frequent cause of acute ear pain in children is operative myringotomy with placement of pressure equalization tubes for recurrent otitis media or serous otitis. Although generally considered a minor surgical procedure, patients frequently experience significant postoperative pain that may require oral opioids. Although it is a brief operative procedure of less than 5 minutes in most patients, the procedure usually requires general anesthesia. Intravenous access is not obtained in most institutions, thereby mandating the use of the non-intravenous route for analgesic delivery. Oral acetaminophen and/or ibuprofen in standard doses may be administered preoperatively, along with the premedication (midazolam in most institutions). Administration of preoperative opioid (codeine in a dose of 1 mg/kg), along with acetaminophen, may improve postoperative analgesia when compared with acetaminophen alone.[5] Alternatively, rectal acetaminophen 40 mg/kg and/or intramuscular ketorolac 0.5 to 1 mg/kg may be administered after the induction of general anesthesia.[6] More recently intraoperative nasal fentanyl (1-2 μg/kg) has emerged as an effective means of improving analgesia following this procedure.[7]

Chest Pain

Chest pain is a common complaint in pediatric patients, particularly among school-aged children and adolescents. As with many of the other acute pain complaints in children, chest pain can be related to one of several conditions (Table 10-3). In distinction to adults in whom chest pain can be worrisome, given the potential for its relationship with myocardial ischemia, chest pain in children only rarely represents a life-threatening disease.[8] However, the pain may be significant and its management may be challenging.

The innervation of the chest arises from the thoracic spinal cord. Each intercostal nerve courses within a neurovascular bundle along a groove on the inferior aspect of each rib, supplying sensation to the overlying chest wall. The thoracic viscera and the pleurae are innervated by sympathetic fibers originating from upper thoracic spinal segments, as well as by parasympathetic nerves originating in the brainstem. The peritoneal surface of the diaphragm and abdominal viscera also receive considerable thoracic sympathetic innervation, thereby explaining the frequent referral of abdominal gastrointestinal (GI) pain to the chest.[9]

Most causes of chest pain in children are musculoskeletal in origin, particularly in athletes,[10] and tend to present with relatively localized pain. Muscle spasm or strain and traumatic injury generally cause little diagnostic difficulty. The possibility of non-accidental trauma must be considered in appropriate settings. Acetaminophen or NSAIDs often provide adequate analgesia. Occasionally, treatment with oral opioids and/or medications to relieve muscle spasm may be necessary.

Costochondritis causes characteristic pain that can be elicited with pressure applied to the costochondral junctions. The pain is reproducible with direct palpation or with compression of the rib cage. Slipping rib syndrome (Cyriax syndrome),[11] first described by Cyriax in 1919, involves disruption of the anterior fibrous attachments of the lower ribs with resulting instability of the anterior costochondral junction. The intermittent subluxation of the affected costal cartilage causes

Table 10-3. Partial Differential Diagnosis of Chest Pain in Children

Musculoskeletal
Muscle spasm or strain
Traumatic injury
Costochondritis
Precordial catch syndrome
Slipping rib syndrome
Fibromyalgia, amplified musculoskeletal pain syndromes
Gastrointestinal
Gastroesophageal reflux
Erosive esophagitis
Esophageal spasm
Gastric distention
Gastritis
Peptic ulcer disease
Constipation
Pulmonary
Pneumonia
Pleural effusion
Pleuritis
Empyema
Pneumothorax
Asthma
Cardiac
Dysrhythmias
Pericarditis
Pericardial effusion or tamponade
Myocardial contusion
Myocardial ischemia
Aortic injury/dissection
Functional Chest Pain
Somatization, conversion reaction
Avoidance behavior, secondary gain
Anxiety, stress
Depression, affective disorders
Miscellaneous Causes
Sickle cell disease and other hemoglobinopathies
Cystic fibrosis
Herpes zoster
Familial Mediterranean fever
Intercostal neuralgia

severe pain. Slipping rib syndrome is suggested by history and may be confirmed by demonstrating costochondral instability on examination (the "hooking maneuver"). Intercostal nerve block with local anesthetic agents may provide transient relief and has been used diagnostically for slipping rib syndrome. Surgery may be considered in refractory cases.

Precordial catch syndrome (Texidor's twinge),[12] first described by Miller and Texidor in 1955, involves intermittent episodes of well-localized, sharp, stabbing, needle-like chest pain unrelated to activity and without additional symptomatology. The pain invariably resolves spontaneously within several minutes. No specific treatment is necessary other than reassurance about the benign nature of the condition. Fibromyalgia and other amplified musculoskeletal pain syndromes[13] are diagnosed increasingly in children, particularly adolescents. These poorly understood conditions seem to involve heightened sensitivity to pain and, generally, are best treated in a center with expertise in chronic pain syndromes involving a multidisciplinary approach with psychosocial interventions, aggressive physical therapy and rehabilitation, adjuvant medications, non-pharmacologic techniques, and avoidance of opioids.

Gastrointestinal etiologies of chest pain are common in children. Pain may originate in the esophagus,[14] particularly from gastroesophageal reflux, esophagitis, or esophageal spasm. Gastrointestinal pain from gastric distension, gastritis, ulcer disease, and even constipation[15] also may be referred to the chest. A careful history and thorough physical examination usually will suggest a possible GI cause for chest pain in children.[16] Therapy is directed at the underlying process with analgesic agents as required.

Pulmonary processes also represent a common cause of chest pain in children. As with GI pain referred to the chest, a pulmonary cause of chest pain usually is apparent from the patient's history and examination. Pleuritic pain, or chest pain aggravated by inspiration, suggests a process involving diaphragmatic or pleural irritation, such as pneumonia, pleural effusion, pleuritis, empyema, or pneumothorax. Although much less common than in adults, pulmonary embolism may occur in pediatric patients,[17] particularly in patients with a history of tobacco and/or oral contraceptive use. The possibility of pulmonary embolism should be considered in the setting of acute chest pain, shortness of breath, and hypoxemia without other obvious cause. Reactive airway disease also can cause chest pain.[18] Treatment is aimed at the underlying process, and analgesic agents are titrated as required.

True cardiac chest pain is rare in children, but concerns about it can be frightening for patients, families, and care providers. The possibility that the chest pain is related somehow to the heart is a frequent reason that patients and parents seek medical attention and why primary care health providers refer such patients to a cardiologist. Ischemic coronary artery disease is often well known to children and their families from the experience of older relatives, and reports of sudden cardiac death in previously healthy athletes and adolescents often are given significant media exposure. Therefore, chest pain in children often is assumed to represent cardiac disease, generating frequent referrals for subspecialty evaluation despite the rarity of such disease in the general pediatric population.[19]

Cardiac causes of chest pain include dysrhythmia, pericarditis, pericardial effusion, pericardial tamponade, myocarditis, and myocardial ischemia. Numerous medications (eg, theophylline, caffeine, inhaled bronchodilators); structural heart disease, including mitral valve prolapse; and primary cardiac dysrhythmia may generate dysrhythmias with subjective discomfort from palpitations. Various inflammatory conditions, including the collagen vascular diseases, are associated with pericarditis and pericardial effusion. The progression of such effusions or trauma may lead to cardiac tamponade. Myocarditis in children is most often idiopathic, but may be secondary to certain viral infections and metabolic disorders. Atherosclerotic coronary artery disease in children is seen almost exclusively in the setting of disorders of lipid metabolism or in patients who are status post-cardiac transplantation. Myocardial ischemia in children is, more commonly, due to congenital heart disease (particularly anomalous origin of the left coronary artery), cocaine exposure, or conditions such as Kawasaki disease.[20] The evaluation to rule out cardiac pathology should include a careful patient history and thorough physical examination. Chest radiography and a 12-lead electrocardiogram are reasonable initial investigations,[21] with subspecialty referral for evaluation if significant abnormalities are noted. In most cases, no underlying cardiac etiology is found, and reassurance and expectant management are appropriate.

In many cases, pediatric chest pain has no obvious etiology in any organ system, leading to the probable diagnosis of functional chest pain. Functional chest pain is quite common in children and can be associated with a wide range of psychological disorders.[22] The management of functional chest pain can be quite challenging. Recognition of the condition, a trusting relationship between the patient (and family) and health care provider, avoidance of inappropriate investigations and therapies, and early involvement of mental health services for persistent cases can be of significant benefit. Finally, a number of specific disease states, including sickle cell disease and other hemoglobinopathies, cystic fibrosis,[23] herpes zoster, familial Mediterranean fever,[24] and intercostal neuralgia, can potentially cause significant chest pain. Specific therapy for many of these underlying conditions is symptomatic, with an aggressive attempt to manage the primary disease.

A significant problem in the management of chest pain associated with chronic conditions, resulting in the progressive deterioration of pulmonary function, is the need to balance prevention of respiratory compromise secondary to the pain itself with prevention of respiratory depression from opioid analgesia. Significant chest pain is more likely to cause respiratory compromise secondary to splinting and poor respiratory effort, and more likely to require opioid therapy for satisfactory analgesia. Using lower-potency analgesics, such as acetaminophen and NSAIDs, can help minimize the use of opioids and, therefore, decrease the risk of opioid-mediated respiratory depression. Oral or even intravenous opioid therapy may be required, and should be titrated to clinical effect. Patient-controlled analgesia (PCA) should be considered for patients requiring multiple doses of intravenous opioid, because PCA modalities have been shown to improve analgesia while reducing total opioid requirement. In patients too young to activate a demand device appropriately, nurse-controlled analgesia can be safe and effective, provided the lockout interval is increased appropriately. Opioid pharmacology is discussed in greater detail in Chapter 2, and the specifics of acute pain management, including suggested dosing regimens for PCA, are discussed in Chapter 8.

Children with severe acute chest pain unresponsive to intravenous opioids, or with inadequate analgesia secondary to opioid side effects, may benefit from peripheral regional or neuraxial blockade. For patients with a chest tube, a local anesthetic agent may be administered through the tube. The tube should be clamped for 1 to 2 hours after local anesthetic delivery to ensure effective analgesia. Analgesia may be further potentiated by repositioning the patient with the chest tube clamped to encourage spread of local anesthetic within the pleural space and into the paravertebral area. The chest tube is then returned to suction and the procedure repeated at intervals as needed. When using this technique, the physician must be aware that the plasma concentrations of local anesthetics are highest following this technique when compared with any other regional anesthetic technique. Therefore, careful calculation of the dose on a mg/kg basis is necessary to prevent local anesthetic toxicity. See Chapter 3 for a discussion of dosing regimens of local anesthetic agents during regional anesthetic techniques. Any technique requiring repeated injections is labor intensive and may be impractical, depending on the resources available. Chest tube removal also can cause considerable pain, which can be lessened by administering local anesthetic through the chest tube as described, by peripheral regional or neuraxial blockade, by supplemental systemic opioids, or by the application of a topical anesthetic cream such as eutectic mixture of local anesthetics (EMLA, AstraZeneca Pharmaceuticals, Wilmington, DE) around the chest tube insertion site.[25]

Intercostal nerve blockade can provide excellent relief of rib and chest wall pain, but entails the risk of pneumothorax. See Chapter 4 for a full description of the technique of intercostal nerve blockade. Additionally, in young children, blocks generally must be performed under general anesthesia. The duration of analgesia is limited by the properties of the local anesthetic used, requiring that the procedure be repeated every 6 to 12 hours for ongoing pain problems or that an intercostal catheter be placed to allow for the repeated administration of the local anesthetic agent. As with local anesthetic administration through a chest tube, repeated injections require significant time and resources. Additionally, given the high vascularity of the intercostal spaces, repeated injections and continuous infusions increase the risk for local anesthetic toxicity secondary to vascular absorption. Techniques of intrapleural[26] and retropleural or paravertebral[27] catheters for continuous infusion analgesia in children also have been described. Peripheral regional blockade in children is discussed in greater detail in Chapter 4. Neuraxial blockade (epidural and spinal analgesia) also may be used for the management of chest pain in children and is discussed in greater detail in Chapter 3.

Pain Related to Acute Traumatic Injury

Traumatic injury is a leading cause of morbidity and mortality among children, and a significant cause of pain related both to the initial injury and to the subsequent surgical procedures. Although awareness and understanding of pain in pediatric trauma have grown, children with painful injuries are still less likely than their adult counterparts to receive appropriate analgesia,[28] particularly if very young[29] or a member of a minority or economically disadvantaged population.[30]

Acute pain caused by trauma is a physiologic response to tissue damage, and may provide important information about the location and nature of the injury. Traditionally, there has been some reluctance to provide potent analgesia to trauma patients, particularly children, until a complete examination is performed to detect possible injuries. It is now increasingly recognized that such an approach causes dramatic undertreatment of pain, particularly in children.[31] Furthermore, judiciously titrated analgesia not only improves pain scores and reduces patient distress, but also actually may allow a more thorough and accurate evaluation, particularly in frightened and uncooperative pediatric patients.

Pain localized to different parts of the body may be reported and treated quite differently. As listed in Table 10-1, various types of traumatic injury may cause headache. Lacerations and abrasions to the scalp usually are very painful, and have potential for causing extensive blood loss that is often underestimated. Skull fractures may be present with or without scalp injuries, but generally are not as painful as more superficial trauma. Contusions characteristically are not painful because the brain parenchyma has no pain sensation. An epidural or subdural hematoma may be reported simply as a headache, but not necessarily as severe pain.

Closed head injury in the pediatric patient may lead to an altered mental status, often with agitation or combativeness, rendering both assessment and treatment of pain challenging. Administration of potent sedative or analgesic agents to the patient with closed head injury not only carries risk for respiratory depression with increasing partial pressure of carbon dioxide and exacerbation of increased intracranial pressure, but may cloud the serial physical assessments that may be necessary for the patient's ongoing evaluation and treatment. If such a patient requires significant sedation or analgesia, as for an imaging procedure, definitive airway control with endotracheal intubation and mechanical ventilation may be the safest alternative.

Ongoing control of pain related to acute musculoskeletal trauma in such patients frequently requires avoiding agents that may alter the patient's level of consciousness. The use of NSAIDs (provided that there are no contraindications given their effects on platelet function) or acetaminophen is acceptable; however, these agents may not provide effective analgesia for moderate to severe pain. In this setting, peripheral nerve blockade (eg, femoral nerve block for a femoral shaft fracture) can be an effective means of providing analgesia, while avoiding the systemic effects of opioids.

Neck pain also can have multiple etiologies in the trauma patient, the most ominous of which is injury to the cervical spine. Neck pain in a trauma patient is assumed to represent cervical spinal injury until proven otherwise. Standard of care for any victim of multisystem or high-energy trauma mandates cervical spine immobilization, pending evaluation for cervical spine injury. In patients with neck pain or altered mental status, which precludes a clear physical examination, anterior-posterior, lateral, and odontoid radiographs of the neck with or without cervical spine computed tomography should be obtained to assess for bony injury. Spinal cord injury without radiologic abnormality is far more common in children 8 years old or younger compared with adults, owing to the greater relative size and weight of the pediatric head, and to the greater flexibility of the ligaments of the vertebral column in children. Neck pain secondary to trauma also may indicate musculoskeletal strain, or may represent referred pain from the shoulder or chest.

The differential diagnosis of chest pain in children after traumatic injury includes many entities (Table 10-3). Traumatic musculoskeletal injuries to the thorax are common and may cause significant pain. Pulmonary processes, including pleural effusion, pneumothorax, and pulmonary embolism, may produce chest pain following trauma, as may esophageal injury or referred pain from the upper abdominal viscerae. Various cardiac processes, including dysrhythmias, pericardial effusion, tamponade, myocardial contusion, and myocardial ischemia, also may cause chest pain following trauma. Of particular concern in high-energy trauma is the possibility of aortic injury, including dissection, suggested on radiologic studies by a widened mediastinum.

Abdominal pain following trauma usually is related to superficial laceration or abrasion of the abdominal wall, and/or to GI or genitourinary injury Traumatic abdominal pain often is vague, diffuse, and poorly localized, rendering clinical diagnosis difficult, particularly in children. Judicious analgesia, including opioids if necessary, should be administered during the evaluation process. Recent advances in pediatric trauma radiology, particularly CT and ultrasonography, have reduced the incidence and necessity of surgical exploration following abdominal trauma in children.[32] Surgical intervention following trauma, however, is always a possibility. Children wearing lap seat belts without a shoulder belt are at risk for lap belt injury, which characteristically includes transverse abdominal contusion, abdominal visceral injury, and lumbar spinal injury. Extremity pain following trauma is usually due to bone or soft tissue injury, although direct nerve injury and resultant neuropathic pain may occur. As with scalp injury, blood loss secondary to extremity laceration or fracture may be significant, but is often underestimated or occult. In the setting of spinal cord injury or other traumatic denervation, extremity pain may not be reported, despite significant limb damage.

Treatment of the underlying injury is the most important step in the management of traumatic pain. As appropriate evaluations and interventions are pursued, appropriate analgesia should be provided. In patients able to tolerate oral medication, acetaminophen and NSAIDs may provide adequate analgesia for mild pain and also will serve to minimize the dose of opioid required. Most NSAIDs adversely affect platelet function and should be avoided in patients at risk for hemorrhagic complications. Choline magnesium trisalicylate, however, does not affect platelet function and is an alternative in such patients. Rectal administration may be used in patients unable to take oral medications, while ketorolac is available for intravenous administration. Future studies with the newer cyclooxygenase-2 inhibitors, particularly with the anticipation of the introduction of a parenteral preparation for intravenous administration, may provide information about the potential role of these agents in the pediatric population. Nonpharmacologic techniques, such as distraction, also are effective in managing traumatic pain in children.[33]

Opioids often are required to control severe traumatic pain. These potent analgesic agents should be titrated appropriately (morphine 0.02 mg/kg every 10 minutes or fentanyl 0.5 µg/kg every 5 minutes) and should be used cautiously in head injury or other injuries requiring careful serial evaluation. Oral opioids may be sufficient in patients able to tolerate oral medication. When intravenous opioid therapy is required, intermittent bolus dosing or PCA regimens may be employed. Patient-controlled analgesia modalities have been shown to improve analgesia while reducing overall opioid requirement, and usually are preferable in any patient requiring multiple doses of intravenous opioid. Patients with bilateral hand injuries may be physically unable to activate the PCA machine, and very young patients may not be able to activate a demand dose appropriately. As in other acute pain settings, nurse-controlled analgesia is a safe and effective alternative.

Certain types of traumatic pain in children may be managed with peripheral regional or neuraxial blockade. Advantages of these techniques include superior pain control,[34] improved pulmonary function,[35] and avoidance of the adverse effects associated with parenteral opioid therapy. Peripheral regional blockade may be helpful in managing extremity[36] and chest pain,[37] and is discussed in greater detail in Chapter 4. Neuraxial blockade (epidural and spinal analgesia) may be helpful in the management of lower extremity pain, abdominal pain, and chest pain, and is discussed in greater detail in Chapter 3. Central types of neuraxial blockade are contraindicated in patients with coagulation disturbances or alterations in intracranial pressure. There often is reluctance to pursue peripheral regional or neuraxial blockade in the context of extremity injury or surgery for fear that the dense analgesia may mask a developing compartment syndrome.[38] Although pain is not the only sign of a compartment syndrome and the severe pain of a compartment syndrome cannot be expected to be totally relieved by the dilute concentrations of local anesthetic agents (0.01%-0.2% bupivacaine, ropivacaine, or levobupivacaine) used in peripheral blockade to provide analgesia, such concerns serve as a reminder that the risks and benefits of any treatment must be weighed carefully in each patient.

Pain Related to Burns

Burn patients who do not succumb to asphyxia or acute thermal injury often face a long and painful hospitalization, followed by months or even years of physical therapy, rehabilitation, and repeated surgical procedures. Physical pain frequently is accompanied by emotional anguish over disfigurement. Appropriate analgesia is essential.

Acute pain from burn injury results from the stimulation of nociceptors at the burn site, causing pain transmission via A-δ and various subtypes of C fibers to the dorsal horn of the spinal cord and then to the thalamus and cerebral cortex. The traditional belief that third-degree burns are not painful because of destruction of nociceptors is now considered false.[39] Even third-degree burns may be excruciatingly painful from the transmission of nocioceptive impulses via damaged yet viable nerve endings at the margins of the burn.[40] Burn victims also are at risk for chronic pain syndromes from the continuous acute pain secondary to the burn injury and its treatment, in addition to neuropathic and even phantom pain.[41]

The treatment of an acute burn injury is multifaceted. Pain management should be integrated into the total care plan.[42] In general, burn patients have 2 components to their pain: a static baseline level of pain related to the underlying thermal injury and a dynamic component related to procedures such as debridements and dressing changes. Appropriate analgesia for burns should include a baseline regimen, titrated to achieve acceptable patient comfort with supplemental analgesic measures as needed for breakthrough pain, including procedure-related pain.

Acetaminophen and NSAIDs are appropriate analgesics in the management of burn pain, particularly when administered on a regular basis. These agents improve analgesia, reduce opioid requirements, and assist in temperature control. The role of NSAIDs may be limited by their adverse effects on platelet function and by their potential to cause nephrotoxicity. Therefore, opioids remain the mainstay of analgesia in the burn patient. The opioid dose should be adjusted as needed for each patient, rather than based on any specific guidelines. An appropriate dose is one that provides adequate analgesia without intolerable side effects. Burn pain is, in general, responsive to opioid therapy, but remarkably large doses may be required secondary to altered metabolism and an increased volume of distribution that occurs in patients with large body surface area burns. Burn patients also frequently develop rapid tolerance to opioids, requiring escalating doses to achieve adequate analgesia. In such patients, there should be an ongoing assessment using pain scales that are age-appropriate and titration of the opioid dose as needed.

In some patients, particularly those with lower extremity or abdominal burns, epidural analgesia may be appropriate. Neuraxial blockade is discussed in greater detail in Chapter 3. Contraindications to regional anesthetic techniques include burn at the proposed insertion site, coagulopathy, and bacteremia, all of which may occur in the burn patient. Some components of burn pain may be neuropathic secondary to nerve injury. Neuropathic pain is characteristically unresponsive to conventional analgesics such as opioids. Control of neuropathic pain may require alternative agents, including anticonvulsants (gabapentin, carbamazepine), tricyclic antidepressants (nortritptyline, amitriptyline), and agents with local anesthetic effects (lidocaine, mexiletine).

Pain associated with procedures such as dressing changes may be difficult to manage, especially because adding other agents to the baseline analgesic regimen may potentiate respiratory depression. Prevention of procedure-related pain is discussed in Chapter 5. Intubated patients may receive supplemental opioid as required, with little concern for respiratory depression, whereas spontaneously breathing patients present a greater challenge. Opioids, even when carefully titrated, may cause respiratory depression at the doses required. Ketamine is an extremely useful agent because it confers sedation and analgesia with minimal respiratory depression. However, ketamine is a general anesthetic agent and, as with the use of any sedative agent, the personnel and equipment for emergent airway management must be immediately available. Ketamine causes increased secretions. Therefore, its administration should be preceded by the administration of an antisialogogue such as glycopyrrolate. Ketamine also may cause dysphoria and hallucinations, which usually are preventable with simultaneous administration of a benzodiazepine such as midazolam or lorazepam. Tolerance to ketamine necessitating dose escalation may develop after repeated administration. Propofol recently has gained popularity as an anesthetic for painful procedures in burn patients. Because of its brief duration of action, it generally is administered by continuous infusion, except for the briefest procedures. Although spontaneous respiration may be preserved at lower doses, propofol also is a general anesthetic, and induces loss of airway reflexes and apnea at higher doses. Hypotension related to negative inotropic and vasodilatory properties may occur, particularly in the hypovolemic patient. Although a potent sedative-hypnotic, propofol does not provide analgesia and, therefore, is not suitable as a sole agent for the management of burn pain.

Coping with the physical pain and emotional turmoil of burn injury may be difficult for the patient, especially school-aged children and adolescents, given the profound loss of control inherent to such injuries. Patient-controlled analgesia modalities may be helpful in restoring a degree of control to the patient. Self-participation in dressing changes is another method to increase patient involvement.[43] Ongoing mental health services should be available, and it always should be remembered that successful management of burn pain in children is a multidisciplinary effort.[44]

Pain Related to Hemoglobinopathies, Including Sickle Cell Disease

Sickle cell disease affects approximately 8% of Americans of African, Hispanic, and Mediterranean descent. Two common clinical manifestations of sickle cell disease are chronic hemolytic anemia and recurring painful crises. The severity and frequency of pain is unpredictable and shows components of acute and chronic pain syndromes. In some African languages, sickle cell disease has various descriptive names, such as "body biting" and "body chewing." The chronicity is onomatopoetically described in the Ga language as "Chwe-chwe-chwe" to connote the repetitive nature of the painful crisis. About 20% of patients with sickle cell disease have frequent and severe painful crises. Most hospitalizations for sickle cell pain involve this group. About 30% rarely have crisis pain, while the remaining 50% have intermediate disease with rare severe crises and/or multiple mild crises that generally do not require repeated hospitalization.

Because there are often no outward signs of pathology or accurate subjective indicators of pain magnitude, caregivers must rely on patient reports, as well as nonspecific clinical signs to guide analgesic therapy. Management of patients with sickle cell disease is complicated by many factors. Patients and families may experience frustration and helplessness because of the incurable nature of the disease and its highly unpredictable clinical course. Potentially chronic opioid therapy causes concern over side effects and fear of addiction. Particularly in adolescents, there may be suspicion for drug-seeking behavior. Racial and ethnic differences among patients and caregivers may exacerbate misunderstandings and miscommunications, contributing to adversarial interactions.

There are many causes of pain in sickle cell disease. Bone pain related to vaso-occlusive crisis and bony infarctions are the most frequent. Splenic infarction and cholecystitis can cause visceral pain. Patients with chronic pain complicating sickle cell disease frequently have intermittent acute pain superimposed on their chronic pain, and express both acute and chronic pain behaviors. Although the pain experience of patients with sickle cell disease is well described,[45] specific management guidelines for the pain of sickle cell disease remain elusive.[46] The care of patients with sickle cell disease should involve a multidisciplinary approach.

Sickle cell disease results from the substitution of a single amino acid at position 6 on the β chain of the hemoglobin molecule. This locus is normally glutamic acid, which has a charged side chain. In sickle hemoglobin, this glutamic acid is replaced by an uncharged valine, resulting in a net attractive force between sickle hemoglobin molecules. Deoxygenated sickle hemoglobin polymerizes, causing deformation and eventually sickling of erythrocytes, at a rate dependent on the concentration of sickle hemoglobin. Other hemoglobinopathies resulting from other amino acid substitutions also can result in sickling and painful crises, although the severity of these other hemoglobinopathies is generally less than that of sickle cell disease.[47] The incidence and severity of painful crises is greatest in patients who are homozygous for sickle cell disease (SS) followed by hemoglobin SC disease, hemoglobin S-β thalassemia, and least in patients with sickle cell trait (AS).

Fetal hemoglobin (hemoglobin F) inhibits polymerization of deoxygenated sickle hemoglobin. Fetal hemoglobin has α and γ chains but no β chain. It can, functionally, substitute for defective sickle hemoglobin. Agents that induce fetal hemoglobin production, such as butyrate[48] and hydroxyurea,[49] have the potential to ameliorate the clinical severity of sickle cell disease. Fetal hemoglobin levels of 20% or greater seem to be required for this protective effect. Although initial trials were promising, results have been inconsistent and such therapy is by no means the standard of care. Several chemotherapeutic agents have been shown to increase hemoglobin F production, but the cytotoxicity of such drugs may preclude their long-term administration. Erythropoietin, alone or in combination with hydroxyurea, has not had a significant effect on the percentage of hemoglobin F. Larger trials to determine long-term tolerance, efficacy, and adverse effects of these agents are ongoing.

Vaso-occlusive crises result from the sludging in the microcirculation secondary to erythrocyte sickling with resultant tissue hypoxia and, eventually, ischemia. The cascade of events may be triggered by many factors, including dehydration, acidosis, marked temperature changes, or hypoxemia. Frequently, no specific inciting event can be identified. Little is known about the epidemiologic features of vaso-occlusive episodes or risk factors for their occurrence, although dactylitis, severe anemia, and leukocytosis before age 2 years seem to correlate with more severe disease later in life.[50] Conversely, increased frequency of painful crises correlates with increased mortality later in life, but not before age 20 years.[51] Chronic transfusion protocols suppress endogenous production of sickle hemoglobin and have been shown to reduce the incidence and severity of most clinical manifestations of sickle cell disease,[52] but entail the metabolic (iron overload) and infectious disease risks of chronic transfusion. Bone marrow transplantation for sickle cell disease is currently under investigation.[53]

The management of pain in sickle cell disease must address the clinical and pathophysiologic manifestations of the disease. Rehydration, correction of acidosis, treatment of hypoxia or infection, and adequate analgesia are the foundations of therapy for painful crises. Transfusions are indicated for the management of severe anemia or for conditions unresponsive to other therapies (eg, acute chest syndrome, priapism). Mild or moderate pain often can be managed on an outpatient basis with acetaminophen and NSAIDs. Low-potency oral opioids, such as codeine, hydrocodone, or oxycodone, may be added if required. As in other conditions, scheduled acetaminophen and NSAIDs improve analgesia and minimize opioid doses. More severe pain is better managed with hospitalization and intravenous opioids such as fentanyl, hydromorphone, methadone, or morphine. Historically, intramuscular meperidine was a common choice for analgesia in patients with sickle cell disease. Intravenous therapy is now recognized to be more reliable and humane. Given its potential for toxicity, including seizures from the metabolite normeperidine, the use of meperidine is no longer recommended. Its use may have originated, at least in part, from the perception that it caused fewer side effects, in particular less respiratory depression and less hepatobiliary spasm, than other opioids. It is now understood, however, that in equianalgesic doses, meperidine has no significant advantage over any other opioid and its use as a first-line analgesic is no longer recommended.

As in other conditions associated with acute pain, the use of PCA modalities in sickle cell disease will optimize analgesia and reduce overall opioid requirement. Initial dosing guidelines are similar to those for postsurgical analgesia, although frequent adjustments in regimen may be necessary because of the highly variable nature of painful crises. As pain subsides, patients are eventually converted back to oral opioid therapy. Opioid-mediated CNS depression and hypoventilation, with resultant hypoxia and hypercarbia, can further exacerbate the vaso-occlusive crisis. Careful monitoring with frequent dose adjustments may be necessary to ensure patient safety. Treating sickle cell pain with appropriate potent analgesia has been shown to reduce the length of hospitalization of patients,[54] and intravenous opioid therapy is now recognized as the mainstay of therapy for severe sickle cell crisis pain.[55] Fear of addiction in patients with sickle cell disease often is expressed by health care providers, as well as by patients and their families. The fear is exacerbated by perceptions of increased tendency toward addiction in the minority populations. Studies, however, have not demonstrated a higher risk of addiction among adolescents with sickle cell disease.

As with any complex disease, pain management in children with sickle cell disease is best undertaken with a multidisciplinary team approach.[56] To preserve continuity of care, the patient should remain on the primary care provider's service, with consultation as appropriate from various members of the multidisciplinary care team. As suggested by the World Health Organization's Analgesic Ladder, adjuvant techniques should be used whenever possible. Self-hypnosis and biofeedback have been reported to improve analgesia in sickle cell disease.[57] High-dose methylprednisolone has been shown to decrease the duration of severe pain in children and adolescents with sickle cell disease, but with increased frequency of rebound pain after the steroid was discontinued.[58] Given the preliminary nature of these reports, the beneficial effects of corticosteroids on the course of pain must be weighed against the potential adverse effects.

Techniques for peripheral regional and neuraxial blockade offer several theoretic advantages in the management of sickle cell crises. In addition to pain control with minimal respiratory depression, the sympathectomy induced by such blockade should cause vasodilatation, thereby reducing sludging and enhancing blood flow in the microcirculation of the anesthetized area. Epidural analgesia for the management of sickle cell pain was first described in a parturient in 1988,[59] and has since been reported for the management of both severe crisis pain[60] and priapism.[61] As with other diseases, regional anesthetic techniques should be considered in patients with sickle cell crisis when conventional intravenous opioids fail to provide adequate analgesia or cause unacceptable complications. Despite the numerous theoretic advantages, the use of regional anesthetic techniques in the management of sickle cell crisis pain remains primarily anecdotal.

Summary

Headache in children may arise from numerous medical conditions, but is most commonly caused by non–life-threatening processes, including tension or migraine. Chest pain in children has many possible causes but, again, is not usually indicative of serious cardiopulmonary disease. Traumatic injuries, including burns, often cause significant pain requiring more aggressive evaluation and management. Hemoglobinopathies, including sickle cell disease, are complex conditions often requiring repetitive analgesic interventions. The challenge in all of these settings is to differentiate between the rare instances of pain heralding emergent potentially life-threatening processes, the less critical painful conditions that may require subspecialty referral, and the more common straightforward medical illnesses causing pain in children. Appropriate analgesia must be individualized to each child and illness, ideally using an incremental, titrated approach with the ultimate goal being freedom from pain.

References

1. Kim MK, Strait MT, Sato TT, Hennes HM. A randomized trial of analgesia in children with acute abdominal pain. *Acad Emerg Med.* 2002;9:281-287
2. Thomas SH, Silen W, Cheema F, et al. Effects of morphine analgesia on diagnostic accuracy in emergency department patients with abdominal pain: a prospective, randomized trial. *J Am Coll Surg.* 2003;196:18-31
3. Rareshide E, Amedee RG. Referred otalgia. *J La State Med Soc.* 1990;142:7-10
4. Leung AK, Fong JH, Leong AG. Otalgia in children. *J Natl Med Assoc.* 2000;92:254-260
5. Tobias JD, Lowe S, Hersey S, Rasmussen GE, Werkhaven J. Analgesia after bilateral myringotomy and placement of pressure equalization tubes in children: acetaminophen versus acetaminophen with codeine. *Anesth Analg.* 1995;81:496-500

6. Korpela R, Korvenoja P, Meretoja OA. Morphine-sparing effect of acetaminophen in pediatric day-case surgery. *Anesthesiology.* 1999;91:442-447
7. Galinkin JL, Fazi LM, Cuy RM, et al. Use of intranasal fentanyl in children undergoing myringotomy and tube placement during halothane and sevoflurane anesthesia. *Anesthesiology.* 2000;93:1378-1383
8. Leung AK, Robson WL, Cho H. Chest pain in children. *Can Fam Physician.* 1996;42:1156-1164
9. Berezin S, Medow MS, Glassman MS, New LJ. Chest pain of gastrointestinal origin. *Arch Dis Child.* 1988;63:1457-1460
10. Gregory PL, Biswas AC, Batt ME. Musculoskeletal problems of the chest wall in athletes. *Sports Med.* 2002;32:235-250
11. Saltzman DA, Schmitz ML, Smith SD, Wagner CW, Jackson RJ, Harp S. The slipping rib syndrome in children. *Paediatr Anaesth.* 2001;11:740-743
12. Gumbiner CH. Precordial catch syndrome. *South Med J.* 2003;96:38-41
13. Sherry DD. Diagnosis and treatment of amplified musculoskeletal pain in children. *Clin Exp Rheumatol.* 2001;19:617-620
14. Glassman MS, Medow MS, Berezin S, Newman LJ. Spectrum of esophageal disorders in children with chest pain. *Dig Dis Sci.* 1992;37:663-666
15. Luder AS, Segal D, Saba N. Hypoxia and chest pain due to acute constipation: an underdiagnosed condition? *Pediatr Pulmonol.* 1998;26:222-223
16. Sabri MR, Ghavanini AA, Haghighat M, Imanich MH. Chest pain in children and adolescents: epigastric tenderness as a guide to reduce unnecessary work-up. *Pediatr Cardiol.* 2003;24:3-5
17. Goldsby RE, Saulys AJ, Helton JG. Pediatric pulmonary artery thromboembolism: an illustrative case. *Pediatr Emerg Care.* 1996;12:105-107
18. Wiens L, Sabath R, Ewing L, Gowdamarajan R, Portnoy J, Scagliotti D. Chest pain in otherwise healthy children and adolescents is frequently caused by exercise-induced asthma. *Pediatrics.* 1992;90:350-353
19. Tunaoglu FS, Olgunturk R, Akcabay S, Oguz D, Gucuyener K, Demirsoy S. Chest pain in children referred to a cardiology clinic. *Pediatr Cardiol.* 1995;16:69-72
20. Burns JC, Shike H, Gordon JB, Malhotra A, Schoenwetter M, Kawasaki T. Sequelae of Kawasaki disease in adolescents and young adults. *J Am Coll Cardiol.* 1996;28:253-257
21. Swenson JM, Fischer DR, Miller SA. Are chest radiographs and electrocardiograms still valuable in evaluating new pediatric patients with heart murmurs or chest pain? *Pediatrics.* 1997;99:1-3
22. Hotopf M, Mayou R, Wadsworth M, Wessely S. Psychosocial and developmental antecedents of chest pain in young adults. *Psychsom Med.* 1999;61:861-867

23. Ravilly S, Robinson W, Suresh S, Wohl ME, Berde CB. Chronic pain in cystic fibrosis. *Pediatrics.* 1996;98:741-747
24. Bakkaloglu A. Familial Mediterranean fever. *Pediatr Nephrol.* 2003;18:853-859
25. Rosen DA, Morris JL, Rosen KR, et al. Analgesia for pediatric thoracostomy tube removal. *Anesth Analg.* 2000;90:1025-1028
26. Semsroth M, Plattner O, Horcher E. Effective pain relief with continuous intrapleural bupivacaine after thoracotomy in infants and children. *Paediatr Anaesth.* 1996;6:303-310
27. Gibson MP, Vetter T, Crow JP. Use of continuous retropleural bupivacaine in postoperative pain management for pediatric thoracotomy. *J Pediatr Surg.* 1999;34:199-201
28. Brown JC, Klein EJ, Lewis CW, Johnston BD, Cummings P. Emergency department analgesia for fracture pain. *Ann Emerg Med.* 2003;42:197-205
29. Alexander J, Manno M. Underuse of analgesia in very young pediatric patients with isolated painful injuries. *Ann Emerg Med.* 2003;41:617-622
30. Hostetler MA, Auinger P, Szilagyi PG. Parenteral analgesic and sedative use among ED patients in the United States: combined results from the National Hospital Ambulatory Medical Care Survey (NHAMCS) 1992-1997. *Am J Emerg Med.* 2002;20:83-87
31. O'Donnell J, Ferguson LP, Beattie TF. Use of analgesia in a paediatric accident and emergency department following limb trauma. *Eur J Emerg Med.* 2002;9:5-8
32. Vane DW. Imaging of the injured child: important questions answered quickly and correctly. *Surg Clin North Am.* 2002;82:315-323
33. Tanabe P, Ferket K, Thomas R, Paice J, Marcantonio R. The effect of standard care, ibuprofen, and distraction on pain relief and patient satisfaction in children with musculoskeletal trauma. *J Emerg Nurs.* 2002;28:118-125
34. Luchette FA, Radafshar SM, Kaiser R, Flynn W, Hassett JM. Prospective evaluation of epidural versus intrapleural catheters for analgesia in chest wall trauma. *J Trauma.* 1994;36:865-870
35. Cicala RS, Voeller GR, Fox T, Fabian TC, Kudsk K, Mangiante EC. Epidural analgesia in thoracic trauma: effects of lumbar morphine and thoracic bupivacaine on pulmonary function. *Crit Care Med.* 1990;18:229-231
36. Davidson AJ, Eyres RL, Cole WG. A comparison of prilocaine and lidocaine for intravenous regional anesthesia for forearm fracture reduction in children. *Paediatr Anaesth.* 2002;12:146-150

37. Matsota P, Livanios S, Marinopoulou E. Intercostal nerve block with Bupivacaine for post-thoracotomy pain relief in children. *Eur J Pediatr Surg.* 2001;11:219-222
38. Dunwoody JM, Reichert CC, Brown KL. Compartment syndrome associated with bupivacaine and fentanyl epidural analgesia in pediatric orthopaedics. *J Pediatr Orthop.* 1997;17:285-288
39. Atchison NE, Osgood PF, Carr DB, Szyfelbein SK. Pain during burn dressing change in children: relationship to burn depth, area and analgesic regimen. *Pain.* 1991;47:41-45
40. Choiniere M, Melzack R, Papillon J. Pain and paresthesia in patients with healed burns: an exploratory study. *J Pain Symptom Manage.* 1991;6:437-444
41. Thomas CR, Brazeal BA, Rosenberg L, Robert RS, Blakeney PE, Meyer WJ. Phantom limb pain in pediatric burn survivors. *Burns.* 2003;29:139-142
42. Stoddard FJ, Sheridan RI, Saxe GN, et al. Treatment of pain in acutely burned children. *J Burn Care Rehabil.* 2002;23:135-156
43. Kavanagh CK, Lasoff E, Eide Y, et al. Learned helplessness and the pediatric burn patient: dressing change behavior and serum cortisol and beta-endorphin. *Adv Pediatr.* 1991;38:335-363
44. Martin-Herz SP, Paterson DR, Honari S, Gibbons J, Gibran N, Heimbach DM. Pediatric pain control practices of North American burn centers. *J Burn Care Rehabil.* 2003;24:26-36
45. Jacob E. The pain experience of patients with sickle cell anemia. *Pain Manag Nurs.* 2001;2:74-83
46. Ballas SK. Sickle cell anemia: progress in pathogenesis and treatment. *Drugs.* 2002;62:1143-1172
47. Williams S, Maude GH, Serjeant GR. Clinical presentation of sickle cell-hemoglobin C disease. *J Pediatr.* 1986;109:586-589
48. Perrine SP, Olivieri NF, Faller DV, Vichinsky EP, Dover GJ, Ginder GD. Butyrate derivatives. New agents for stimulating fetal globin production in the beta-globin disorders. *Am J Pediatr Hematol Oncol.* 1994;16:67-71
49. Ferster A, Tahriri P, Vermylen C, et al. Five years of experience with hydroxyurea in children and young adults with sickle cell disease. *Blood.* 2001;97:3628-3632
50. Miller ST, Sleeper LA, Pegelow CH, et al. Prediction of adverse outcomes in children with sickle cell disease. *N Engl J Med.* 2000;342:83-89
51. Platt OS, Thorington BD, Brambilla DJ, et al. Pain in sickle cell disease. Rates and risk factors. *N Engl J Med.* 1991;325:11-16

52. Miller ST, Wright E, Abboud M, et al. Impact of chronic transfusion on incidence of pain and acute chest syndrome during the Stroke Prevention Trial (STOP) in sickle-cell anemia. *J Pediatr.* 2001;139:785-789
53. Walters MC, Storb R, Patience M, et al. Impact of bone marrow transplantation for symptomatic sickle cell disease: an interim report. Multicenter investigation of bone marrow transplantation for sickle cell disease. *Blood.* 2000;95:1918-1924
54. Brookhoff D, Polomano R. Treating sickle cell pain like cancer pain. *Ann Intern Med.* 1992;116:364-368
55. Cole TB, Sprinkle RH, Smith SJ, Buchanan GR. Intravenous narcotic therapy for children with severe sickle pain crisis. *Am J Dis Child.* 1986;140:1255-1259
56. Shapiro BS, Cohen DE, Covelman KW, Howe CJ, Scott SM. Experience of an interdisciplinary pediatric pain service. *Pediatrics.* 1991;88:1226-1232
57. Cozzi L, Tyron WW, Sedlacek K. The effectiveness of biofeedback-assisted relaxation in modifying sickle cell crises. *Biofeedback Self Regul.* 1987;12:51-61
58. Griffin TC, McIntire D, Buchanan GR. High-dose intravenous methylprednisolone therapy for pain in children and adolescents with sickle cell disease. *N Engl J Med.* 1994;330:733-737
59. Finer P, Blair J, Rowe P. Epidural analgesia in the management of labor pain and sickle cell crisis—a case report. *Anesthesiology.* 1988;68:799-800
60. Yaster M, Tobin JR, Billett C, Casella JF, Dover G. Epidural analgesia in the management of severe vaso-occlusive sickle cell crisis. *Pediatrics.* 1994;93:310-315
61. Labat F, Dubousset AM, Baujard C, Wasier AP, Benhamou D, Cucchiaro G. Epidural analgesia in a child with sickle cell disease complicated by acute abdominal pain and priapism. *Br J Anaesth.* 2001;87:935-936

Chapter 11

Non-pharmacologic Techniques for the Management of Pediatric Pain

John T. Algren, MD, FAAP
Chris L. Algren, RN, MSN, EdD

Cognitive-Behavioral Techniques
- Preparation
- Distraction
- Music Therapy
- Relaxation and Imagery

Biophysical Techniques
- Nonnutritive Sucking
- Cutaneous Stimulation
- Cold and Heat Therapy
- Massage
- Therapeutic Exercise
- Transcutaneous Electrical Nerve Stimulation
- Acupuncture

Introduction

Non-pharmacologic techniques are essential components of effective pain management regimens. Pain perception is a dynamic phenomenon, influenced by cognitive, emotional, social, and behavioral factors. Children seem to be especially sensitive to the influence of these factors. Analgesics and anesthetics offer the most direct and immediate interventions for relieving pain, but do not address associated anxiety and emotional distress. Furthermore, relying on drug therapy alone, especially in managing chronic and recurrent pain disorders, increases the likelihood that patients will develop drug-related adverse effects, including tolerance. Comprehensive pain management programs integrate the expertise of many practitioners and therapists, including physicians, nurses, psychologists, physical therapists, massage therapists, and child-life specialists, who use cognitive and behavioral, biophysical, and alternative treatment techniques.

Cognitive and behavioral techniques reduce fear, anxiety, and emotional distress; enhance the effectiveness of analgesics; and decrease pain perception.[1] Cognitive and behavioral techniques also help patients develop coping skills and gain a sense of control, thereby promoting psychological and emotional well-being. Biophysical techniques, such as cold or heat therapy and exercise, are useful adjuncts to managing acute, recurrent, and chronic pain. Comprehensive physical therapy regimens designed to restore and maintain musculoskeletal function are essential to managing chronic pain disorders that compromise physical activity. So-called complementary and alternative medicine therapies, such as chiropractic manipulation, massage, yoga, and acupuncture, are popular among adult patients, and many of these techniques are gaining acceptance among traditional medical practitioners.[1] The potential benefit of alternative pain management techniques is of increasing interest to patients and families as well as pediatric pain management practitioners.

Cognitive-Behavioral Techniques

Pain is more than a sensory event and includes cognitive, affective, and behavioral components. Each person experiences pain differently. Physical, cognitive, emotional, cultural, and social factors influence how children and adults experience pain and how they respond to various methods of pain control. Helping children cope with pain gives them a sense of mastery and self-control they can apply to other situations and to future health-related pain. While many first consider pharmacologic interventions to control pain, children often are highly responsive to pain control strategies that involve their natural imagination, high degree of suggestibility, and sense of play. Although cognitive and behavioral interventions share common outcomes in pain management, cognitive strategies center on changing the way the patient perceives pain, whereas behavioral interventions focus on changing the patient's response to pain. These strategies are simple to learn, safe, effective, inexpensive, and may be employed for acute, recurrent, and chronic pain problems (Table 11-1). Cognitive approaches are most effective in children 8 years and older; younger children require a coach, usually a parent. Basic principles apply to all cognitive strategies. For the technique to be effective, the child must be a willing participant. Second, learning the strategies requires concentration and energy. Seriously ill children may not have sufficient energy to learn new skills. Children who have previously mastered the skills, however, often will use them regardless of their energy level.

Preparation

Because stress and anxiety intensify the sensation of pain, any strategy that reduces fear and anxiety can alter the child's perception of pain. Age-appropriate preparation is one of the most widely used interventions for reducing anxiety in children undergoing painful or operative procedures. Using preparatory information is based on the belief that fear of the unknown is worse than the fear of the known and causes tension and a lowered pain threshold. Providing the child with information can change his or her perception of pain.

Four types of information seem to be most helpful: 1) why the procedure is being performed; 2) what is going to be done; 3) sensations or feelings that might be experienced; and 4) suggestions for how the child may cope with the procedure, which enable the child to practice strategies and allow parents to rehearse supportive roles. Preparatory information should be age-appropriate; however, it is most effective for the preschool, school-aged, and adolescent population. Various methods, such as hospital tours, coloring books, dolls, puppets, and play therapy, can be used to prepare the child. Active participation promotes the effectiveness of medications and becomes part of the therapy itself, so the child should be encouraged to express fears and concerns and to ask questions.

Distraction

The simplest technique, and probably the one most often used instinctively by parents, is distraction. Pain intensity actually increases when

Table 11-1. Cognitive-Behavioral Techniques for Children

Preparation	Age-appropriate explanation about reason for procedure, description of procedure, expected sensations or feelings, coping strategies.
Distraction	Various age-appropriate and patient-oriented techniques to refocus attention: view videos, read, color pictures, sing, count, tell stories, play video games, listen to music with headphones.
Music	Provides distraction and relaxation, reducing pain perception. Select music according to age, culture, patient's preference.
Relaxation	Promotes muscle relaxation and reduces anxiety. Technique appropriate for age and developmental level: holding and rocking, rhythmic deep breathing, muscle contraction-relaxation exercise, images associated with relaxed state.
Guided Imagery	Patients imagine being secure and comfortable in a favorite place (eg, in bed at home, relaxing on a beach, floating on a cloud).
Hypnosis	Altered state of consciousness produced by focused attention and relaxation; state of high suggestibility. Guided imagery is an effective method to induce hypnotic state in children. Focus on relief of pain (eg, with a switch to turn off pain or with ice to relieve a burning sensation).

the individual concentrates on pain.[2] Therefore, pain perception can be modified by other stimulation. Distraction engages the child in an activity that helps the child to refocus attention on something other than the painful stimulus. Although it does not reduce the intensity of the noxious stimulus, it reduces pain perception and improves pain tolerance.

Parents and staff can play an important role in distraction techniques. After assessing the child's chronological age, developmental level, and interests, finding strategies involving hearing, vision, movement, and touch are most effective. Infants and young children require concrete objects on which to focus their attention, while older children can be distracted by mental games and tasks. "Active" distraction techniques include playing games, telling or listening to jokes, blowing bubbles, viewing kaleidoscopes, singing or counting, listening to stories or music with headphones, or reading books. Interactive computer and video games also provide excellent distraction for older children and adolescents. The perception of pain is only altered, however, during the distracting activity. When the child is no longer distracted, pain awareness, fatigue, and irritability may increase. A recent study implemented distraction strategies for children with chronic illnesses of different ages undergoing repeated needle sticks.[2] Reductions in behavioral distress were observed and improvements in parental reports of child distress and nurse reports of child cooperation were sustained over 16 weeks of therapy.[2]

Music Therapy

Music, as a means of providing distraction and relaxation and decreasing anxiety and discomfort, has been used in health care settings, including operating rooms, post-anesthesia care units, and neonatal intensive care units.[3,4] Music therapy involves singing, playing, listening, or moving to music for therapeutic results. Positive effects of music include anxiolysis, relaxation, and pain reduction. Like other cognitive-behavioral techniques, music decreases pain perception in several ways.

Music provides a distraction from the focus of pain, produces relaxation, reduces anxiety, and creates a feeling of well-being. Music should be meaningful to the patient, so music selections should be based on the patient's age, cultural and religious background, and personal preference.

Relaxation and Imagery

For children who are capable of abstract thinking, relaxation and imagery are effective adjunctive therapies for pain management. Anxiety and fear produce a heightened state of tension and an increase in sympathetic nervous system activity. As anxiety intensifies, tolerance to pain decreases, and children become trapped in the cycle of anxiety and pain. As relaxation occurs, pain becomes more tolerable. These techniques do not need to be complex to be effective. Muscle tension, which intensifies pain, can be alleviated by simple relaxation methods such as holding or rocking a young child. Older children benefit from rhythmic deep breathing, progressive muscle contraction-relaxation exercise, and imagery. Relaxation techniques may be ineffective in patients from cultures that accept and expect dramatic displays of pain behaviors.

Controlled breathing may be used alone or with other techniques to promote relaxation. The child is taught to take slow, deep breaths through the nose and to exhale slowly through pursed lips. "Blowing away the pain" is a form of controlled breathing. The child is taught to blow as hard as he or she can at the first sensation of pain. Young children are especially receptive to this technique.

Imagery is a popular cognitive strategy used to minimize pain in children. It dulls the awareness of reality by encouraging the child to use his or her imagination to focus on something familiar or pleasurable and unrelated to pain. It may be most effective when preceded by relaxation exercises. Some experts consider imagery a form of self-hypnosis. Although the child is fully awake, attention is deflected from the pain. Children 3 years or older actively use their imaginations and usually are able to participate in imagery.

Guided imagery is the intentional use of imagery for a therapeutic effect. Children can be coached to visualize themselves in a favorite place, playing on a beach, or floating on a cloud or magic carpet. Imagery seems to be more effective when several senses are incorporated. For example, the child can be asked to imagine how the water feels, what kind of smell is in the air, how the waves sound, and how the child feels. Children may use their fantasies to imagine medication traveling through the body to the pain site, their favorite super heroes attacking the pain, or a "pain switch" that is used to gradually turn off the pain.

Hypnosis has been suggested as a valuable tool for managing procedural and cancer pain in children. Relaxation or guided imagery can induce a hypnotic state, during which the patient's attention is intensely focused and he or she becomes highly receptive to suggestions. The hypnotherapist may suggest that the patient is becoming more relaxed and less anxious. Children respond to suggestions that their pain is less and that the site of the pain is getting numb so that they can no longer feel the pain. Like other cognitive strategies, hypnosis modifies factors that have been shown to alter nociceptive responses and pain perception.[5-8] Hypnotic techniques have been used in children with cancer during bone marrow aspirations and lumbar punctures, and have been shown to be consistently more effective than distraction and supportive counseling.[5] Hypnosis also has been successfully used for pain associated with the reduction of fractures, burns, laceration repair, and vaso-occlusive crisis.[6-8]

Mindfulness meditation, a complementary therapy, is a skill that can be learned to reduce anxiety and pain. It is a process of purposefully paying attention to the present moment without thinking about what has happened or will happen in the future. Although studies document its usefulness for stress reduction in adults, there is no research with its use in children. Anecdotal reports, however, demonstrate that children can learn mindfulness meditation to reduce stress and lessen pain.[9]

Biophysical Techniques

Biophysical techniques useful in pain management range from relatively simple techniques, such as cutaneous stimulation and cold or heat therapy, to comprehensive physical therapy regimens (Table 11-2). Nurses and physicians routinely employ cutaneous stimulation and cold or heat therapy to relieve mild pain. Massage and hydrotherapy may be used by many practitioners, including physical therapists, massage therapists, nurses, chiropractors, and physicians, as well as patients

Table 11-2. Biophysical Techniques for Children

Technique	Description
Cutaneous Stimulation	Non-painful stimulation (eg, stroking or rubbing skin and tissue near painful area) interferes with transmission of pain impulse through spinal cord interneurons.
Cold and Heat Therapy	Cold packs reduce nerve activation and conduction, retard inflammation, and reduce swelling. Avoid extreme cooling, which is painful and may cause tissue injury.
	Hot packs or whirlpool treatments promote circulation and muscle relaxation, and reduce swelling and joint stiffness. Avoid high temperature.
	"Fluidotherapy" is useful in sickle cell pain crises and chronic regional pain syndrome.
Massage Therapy	Reduces muscle tension, improves flexibility, produces relaxation, and improves sleep. Can be focused on muscle "trigger points" to relieve spasm and pain.
Transcutaneous Electrical Nerve Stimulation (TENS)	Non-painful electrical stimulus interferes with transmission of pain by altering spinal cord "gating" mechanism; may cause endorphin release. Use as adjunct for moderate to severe chronic pain disorders. Usually tolerated well by school-aged children.
Acupuncture	Technique of traditional Chinese medicine; seems to alter spinal cord gating mechanism and causes release of endorphins. Insertion of fine needles is relatively painless.
Therapeutic Exercise	Guided exercise program to restore and maintain joint flexibility, muscle strength, coordination, and function. Essential aspect of management of chronic regional pain syndromes.

and family members. These techniques must be coordinated with other facets of the patient's pain management program to best benefit the patient and avoid adverse effects.

Physical therapists are important members of the pain management team. They rely on a sound foundation in anatomy and physiology, and training in therapeutic exercise and other treatment modalities to provide individualized treatment regimens. Goals of these regimens include pain relief as well as restoration and maintenance of musculoskeletal function. Physical therapy is useful in treating acute and recurrent pain problems and is essential to managing chronic pain disorders that compromise musculoskeletal function and interfere with the activities of daily living.

Nonnutritive Sucking

The concept of developmental care for preterm and term infants is consistent with enhancing comfort and reducing stress during therapeutic procedures (Table 11-3). Some interventions used during developmental care have been studied to determine their efficacy for the management of pain. During painful procedures, nonnutritive sucking, such as sucking a pacifier, can help attenuate behavioral responses such as cry duration and heart rate changes. The calming effect terminates almost immediately when sucking ceases.[10]

Table 11-3. Non-pharmacologic Techniques for Infants

Nonnutritive Sucking	Sucking a pacifier or nipple attenuates behavioral responses to pain.
Sucrose	2 mL of 12%-24% sucrose by syringe, dropper, or pacifier.
Cutaneous Stimulation	Stroking or massage of head and back comforts and relaxes.
Swaddling or Holding	Comforts, limits movement and activity, quiets, and relaxes.
Rocking	Quiets and promotes sleep.

The administration of sucrose, with or without nonnutritive sucking, has been the most frequently studied non-pharmacologic intervention for the relief of procedural pain in neonates.[11] In a variety of doses and concentrations ranging from 24% to 50%, oral sucrose has been shown to significantly decrease heart rate, behavioral pain indicators, and composite pain scores in neonates undergoing various invasive procedures, including heel stick and venipunctures.[11] The administration method does not seem to affect the analgesic effect and sucrose (2 mL of 12%-24% solution) has been shown to be effective when given by syringe, dropper, or a pacifier dipped into the sucrose solution.[12] There also seems to be a significant synergistic effect when sucrose administration is combined with swaddling or hands-on containment throughout the procedure. Adverse effects have not been reported. Sucrose and nonnutritive sucking can be used before mild to moderate procedural pain in infants. Despite its effectiveness, sucrose should be used as an adjunct to, and not a substitute for, analgesic agents.

Cutaneous Stimulation

Light stroking and gentle massage of the head or back is comforting to infants and young children. Swaddling also is a very effective method for calming babies during and after minor procedures such as venipuncture. Cutaneous stimulation, produced by rubbing the skin adjacent to a painful area, diminishes mild pain. According to the "gate theory," proposed by Melzack and Wall,[13] pain perception can be diminished or prevented by inhibiting dorsal horn interneurons, which relay nociceptive transmission from peripheral neurons through the spinal cord to the brain. Concurrent non-painful sensory stimulation activates large-diameter, sensory neurons (A-β fibers) and ascending sensory pathways, interfering with activation of dorsal horn interneurons by pain fibers (A-δ and C fibers). Cutaneous stimulation also may mediate the analgesic effects of transcutaneous electrical nerve stimulation (TENS) and acupuncture.

Cold and Heat Therapy

Cold therapy to the skin reduces local pain perception by retarding chemical reactions associated with inflammation and by reducing nerve activity and conduction velocity.[14] For example, ethyl chloride spray applied to the skin effectively reduces pain during venipuncture. Rubbing an ice cube on the skin following a bee sting has a similar effect. Cold therapy is a key component of the RICE (rest, ice, compression, and elevation) regimen for acute management of soft tissue injuries. Intermittent application of cold packs during the first 24 to 48 hours following sprains, strains, and other soft tissue injuries produces vasoconstriction, prevents edema, decreases inflammation, and reduces associated pain. Ice packs should not be applied directly to the skin because excessive cooling of tissue may cause cellular injury. Furthermore, extremely cold stimuli are painful and are not well tolerated by children.

Heat therapy (hot packs or moist heat) promotes circulation, relaxes muscles, reduces edema, and relieves joint stiffness. It is very useful during the remobilization period following acute injuries and also is effective in chronic inflammatory conditions such as arthritis. Careful attention to temperature and duration of therapy is essential to avoid thermal injury.

Hydrotherapy combines the benefit of heat with swirling or pulsating water. Whirlpool and "hot tub" treatments provide heat, cutaneous stimulation, and superficial massage, which promote circulation and muscle relaxation, reduce pain, and facilitate joint movement. Fluidotherapy transfers heat through air-filtered solids and permits range of motion exercises during treatments. Physical therapists use fluidotherapy to provide heat, cutaneous stimulation, desensitization, and range of motion exercises. Fluidotherapy is useful in managing patients with chronic regional pain syndromes and patients with sickle cell disease complicated by acute vaso-occlusive pain crisis.[15]

Massage

Many adults routinely enjoy the benefits of massage, which reduces muscle tension and associated pain, improves flexibility, and produces relaxation. Popular techniques include Swedish and deep-tissue massage, pressure-point techniques (shiatsu and acupressure), and movement integration. Therapeutic massage reduces muscle tension, improves circulation and flexibility, reduces stress hormones, and promotes relaxation. In addition, it improves sleep and enhances the sense of well-being. Massage techniques also can be focused to relax trigger points, alleviating muscle spasm and associated pain. Massage is underused in managing chronic pediatric pain disorders, even though its benefits have been documented in numerous studies.[16] Specific massage techniques may be employed by physical therapists and massage therapists.

Therapeutic Exercise

Pain provides important feedback that effectively limits activity of an injured area, preventing additional injury. However, ongoing pain may prolong the recovery phase and lead to disuse atrophy and limited joint mobility. Under the guidance of physical therapists, patients can follow individualized exercise programs designed to accelerate mobilization and provide rehabilitation of injured tissue.

Neuropathic pain associated with chronic regional pain syndromes limits activity and, if untreated, leads to muscle atrophy, reduced joint mobility, and progressive disability. Comprehensive physical therapy programs, including modalities such as fluidotherapy and TENS, are integrated with pharmacologic regimens and cognitive-behavioral techniques to maximize therapeutic benefit.[17,18] Physical activity also seems to have a positive emotional effect, counteracting depression that commonly accompanies chronic pain disorders.[18]

Transcutaneous Electrical Nerve Stimulation

Transcutaneous electrical nerve stimulation modulates pain perception by stimulating sensory nerves with a low-intensity electrical current delivered by a portable, battery-powered, programmable generator. This electrical stimulus seems to inhibit nociceptive transmission through the interneurons of the dorsal horn, in accordance with the "gate control theory."[13] The release of endorphins in the brain may mediate inhibition of nociceptive transmission.[19] Transcutaneous electrical nerve stimulation has been shown to have an opioid-sparing effect and may be associated with the development of opioid tolerance.[20]

Physical therapists typically oversee the use of TENS and instruct patients and families regarding its use. Electrodes generally are applied adjacent to the area of pain, but can be applied along the corresponding peripheral nerve or dermatome. Conventional stimulation mode delivers electrical pulses of high frequency (50-100 Hz), short duration (0.05-0.5 ms) and low amperage (10-60 mA). This regimen causes a non-painful tingling sensation. Transcutaneous electrical nerve stimulation can be used during periods of physical therapy and for more extended periods, according to patient tolerance.

Transcutaneous electrical nerve stimulation has been used to treat acute and chronic pain problems in children and adults.[21,22] Analgesia provided by TENS is incomplete, so it should generally be used as an adjunct rather than primary mode of pain relief. Transcutaneous electrical nerve stimulation is usually tolerated well by children old enough to understand a simple explanation of its use.

Acupuncture

Acupuncture, one of the treatment modalities of traditional Asian medicine, has gained acceptance in western medicine and is now practiced by both physician acupuncturists and licensed acupuncturists in the United States.[1] The mechanism by which acupuncture treatments relieve pain is not fully understood, but scientific evidence suggests that it causes an increase in serotonin, endorphins, and enkephalins, which inhibit nociceptive pathways, thereby reducing pain perception.[23]

Acupuncturists insert fine needles (26-36 gauge) into the skin at classic acupuncture points along body meridians. Insertion of acupuncture needles by an experienced acupuncturist is relatively painless. Stimulation is produced by manual movement of the needles or by electroacupuncture, which delivers low-voltage electrical current, similar to TENS. Acupuncture has been used to treat acute and chronic pain in adults. It also has seen potential application in the treatment of postoperative nausea and vomiting. Its application in the management of chronic pain in children is growing, but experience with its use and, therefore, data demonstrating its efficacy are limited.

Summary

Non-pharmacologic techniques are important adjuncts in managing acute, recurrent, and chronic pain in children. Cognitive-behavioral techniques, such as preparation, distraction, relaxation, and guided imagery, seek to enhance a patient's ability to cope with pain, while also modifying pain perception. Intermediate goals include improved understanding of health problems and their management, reduced anxiety and emotional distress, and cooperative behavior. Cognitive-behavioral methods are especially beneficial in managing pain perception and pain behavior during minor procedures. In addition, these methods also improve the patient's ability to cope with chronic pain disorders.

Biophysical techniques, such as cutaneous stimulation, TENS, and acupuncture, modify pain perception by altering nociceptive transmission. These techniques are effective for mild to moderate pain, but should be used as adjunctive modalities in managing more severe pain problems. In addition, many biophysical techniques, including massage therapy, cold and heat therapy, and therapeutic exercise, are highly effective methods for facilitating rehabilitation, maintaining function, and reducing pain during the recovery period. Multimodal management of acute, recurrent, and chronic pain disorders integrates both pharmacologic and non-pharmacologic modalities to optimize pain relief, minimize side effects of treatment, and facilitate recovery of normal activity.

References

1. Rusy LM, Weisman SJ. Complementary therapies for acute pediatric pain management. *Pediatr Clin North Am.* 2000;47:589-599
2. Dahlquist LM, Busby SM, Slifer E, et al. Distraction for children of different ages who undergo repeated needle sticks. *J Pediatr Oncol Nurs.* 2002;19:22-24
3. Moss A. Music and the surgical patient: the effect of music on anxiety. *AORN J.* 1988;48:64-69
4. Collins SK, Kuck K. Music therapy in the neonatal intensive care unit. *Neonatal Netw.* 1991;9:23-26
5. Zeltzer L, LeBaron S. Hypnosis and nonhypnotic techniques for reduction of pain and anxiety during painful procedures in children and adolescents with cancer. *J Pediatr.* 1982;101:1032-1035
6. Serson KV. Hypnosis for pediatric fracture reduction. *J Emerg Med.* 1999;17:53-56
7. Bierman SF. Hypnosis in the emergency department. *Am J Emerg Med.* 1989;7:238-242
8. Ewin DM. Emergency room hypnosis for the burned patient. *Am J Clin Hypn.* 1986;29:1012
9. Ott MJ, Lonobucco-Hynes S, Hynes V. Mindfullness meditation in pediatric clinical practice. *Pediatr Nurs.* 2002;28:487-492
10. Campos R. Rocking and pacifiers: two comforting interventions for heel - stick pain. *Res Nurs Health.* 1994;17:321-331
11. Benis MM. Efficacy of sucrose as analgesia for procedural pain in neonates. *Adv Neonatal Care.* 2002;2:93-100
12. Gibbons S, Stevens B, Hodnett E. Efficacy and safety of sucrose for procedural pain relief in preterm and term neonates. *Nurs Res.* 2002;51:375-382
13. Melzack R, Wall PD. Pain mechanisms: a new theory. *Science.* 1965;50:971-979
14. Ernst E, Fialka V. Ice freezes pain? A review of the clinical effectiveness of analgesic cold therapy. *J Pain Symptom Management.* 1994;9:56-59

15. Alcorn R, Bowser B, Henley EJ, Holloway V. Fluidotherapy and exercise in the management of sickle cell anemia. *Phys Ther.* 1984;64:1520-1522
16. Kemper KJ, Gardiner P. Complementary and alternative medical therapies in pediatric pain management. In: Schechter NK, Berde CB, Yaster M, eds. *Pain in Infants, Children, and Adolescents.* 2nd ed. Philadelphia, PA: Lippincott Williams and Wilkins; 2003:449-461
17. Wilder RT, Berde CB, Wolohan M, Vieyra MA, Masek BJ, Micheli LJ. Reflex sympathetic dystrophy in children. Clinical characteristics and follow-up of seventy patients. *J Bone Joint Surg Am.* 1992;74:910-919
18. Lee BH, Scharff L, Sethna NF, et al. Physical therapy and cognitive-behavioral treatment of complex regional pain syndromes. *J Pediatr.* 2002;141:135-140
19. Sjolund BH, Erickson MBE. The influence of naloxone on analgesia produced by peripheral conditioning stimulation. *Brain Res.* 1979;173:295-301
20. Chandran P, Sluka KA. Development of opioid tolerance with repeated transcutaneous electrical nerve stimulation administration. *Pain.* 2003;102:195-201
21. McCarthy CF, Shea AM, Sullivan P. Physical therapy management of pain in children. In: Schechter NK, Berde CB, Yaster M, eds. *Pain in Infants, Children, and Adolescents.* 2nd ed. Philadelphia, PA: Lippincott Williams and Wilkins; 2003:434-448
22. Bjordal JM, Johnson MI, Ljunggreen AE. Transcutaneous electrical nerve stimulation (TENS) can reduce postoperative analgesic consumption. A meta-analysis with assessment of optimal treatment parameters for postoperative pain. *Eur J Pain.* 2003;7:181-188
23. He LF. Involvement of endogenous opioid peptides in acupuncture analgesia. *Pain.* 1987;31:99-121

Chapter 12

Chronic and Cancer Pain Management

Santhanam Suresh, MD, FAAP
Sally E. Tarbell, PhD

Assessment and Evaluation of Chronic Pain
Psychological Methods in the Management of Chronic Pain in Children
Chronic Pain Syndromes in Children
- Complex Regional Pain Syndrome-1
- Headaches
- Headaches in the Child With a Ventriculoperitoneal Shunt
- Cancer Pain
  - Acute Cancer-Related Pain
  - Pain During the Terminal Stages of Illness

Introduction

Clinical research regarding treatment strategies for and outcomes of children with chronic pain syndromes is limited, especially when compared with the significant research available regarding acute pain management in infants and children and chronic pain in adults. Although some of the techniques used in acute pain management can be applied to chronic pain management, in most cases, the treatment of chronic pain requires a multidisciplinary approach. This is especially important when treating children with chronic pain to evaluate the family dynamics and other psychosocial issues, which may play a significant role in the etiology of the pain.

Assessment and Evaluation of Chronic Pain

As with acute pain, chronic pain cannot be effectively managed unless there is a way to evaluate the severity of pain and gauge a patient's response to therapeutic interventions. Assessing chronic pain in pediatric patients requires a biopsychosocial perspective that takes into account all the factors that may influence pain, including biological, developmental, cognitive, behavioral, affective, social, and situational. The Children's Comprehensive Pain Questionnaire and the Varni-Thompson Pediatric Pain Questionnaire[1] assess the patient's and parents' experience with pain with open-ended questions, checklists, and quantitative pain-rating scales. They also gather information about factors shown to influence the patient's pain, including developmental level and understanding of pain,[2,3] pain treatment history, medical history, and interactions with others in relation to pain complaints.[4-6] There also is an assessment of the impact of the pain on the patient's functional abilities, peer relationships, school performance/attendance, and extracurricular activities. The family environment, stresses, and coping abilities, including prior history of psychiatric and medical problems, also are assessed.

Questionnaires that evaluate how the patient copes with chronic pain, the Waldron/Varni Pediatric Pain Coping Inventory, and the Pain Coping Questionnaire, may provide valuable information for planning specific therapies for the treatment of chronic pain.[7] For example, a patient who exhibits a catastrophizing coping style is at risk for poor adaptation to chronic pain,[8] which can be treated in conjunction with the specific pain problem. If a particular aspect of the pain experience requires assessment in greater depth, such as the exhibition of psychiatric symptoms as well as pain, more specific inventories can be added. Sleep may be a factor in the onset and maintenance of pain. Some studies have found a relationship between sleep quality and migraine activity in children.[9] PedMIDAS is a 6-question tool that assesses headache-related disability,[10] including school absences and participation in social and recreational activities. This type of assessment is relevant to all chronic pain conditions in children. Assessing quality of life also is important and is a potential index of treatment progress in children with chronic pain.[11,12] One study found that the quality of life of children with recurrent headaches is similar to that of children with chronic pain related to rheumatoid arthritis or cancer.[13]

Psychological Methods in the Management of Chronic Pain in Children

Psychological pain management methods are directed toward increasing the patient's and family's understanding of the pain and its treatment, including factors that may reduce or exacerbate the pain symptoms and attempt to enhance the child's cognitive and behavioral coping skills so that pain-related discomfort and disability are reduced. Three principles guide the use of psychological techniques in the management of chronic pain.

1. Patients and their parents should be educated about the multidimensional nature of pain and its treatment. This step is crucial to the success of behavioral approaches.[14-16] The categorization

of pain as organic or functional especially should be avoided. Psychological rehabilitative strategies need to be understood as essential treatment components and not as treatments for pain when no organic basis can be identified or when pain is seen as psychological in origin.[17] Explaining how psychological interventions take advantage of the plasticity of the sensory system involved in the perception of pain and inclusion of psychological and physical strategies to decrease discomfort and disability can help parents better appreciate the value of psychological interventions. Without understanding psychological methods and how they treat pain, patients and parents may refuse such treatments due to concern that health care providers do not see their pain as "real."

2. A rehabilitative approach that emphasizes improving the patient's and family's ability to cope with the chronic condition is essential. The focus shifts from the narrow goal of pain reduction and broadens to include decreasing pain-related emotional and behavioral disability, thereby enhancing functional status.[18]
3. Interventions should be tailored to the patient's individual characteristics, not just to his or her specific pain condition. The child's developmental level will determine what types of assessment tools can be used, how the patient understands his or her pain, the factors that may shape his or her pain experience, options for managing pain, and the most suitable treatment regimen.

An initial comprehensive assessment of the patient's pain guides the treatment chosen. Psychological interventions include a diverse array of techniques that treat chronic pain by modifying the cognitive, affective, and sensory experience of pain; behavior in response to pain; and environmental or social factors that influence the pain (see following text). Some techniques primarily deal with altering situational factors that influence pain expression, such as when a family member is encouraged to acknowledge coping behaviors rather than reinforcing a pain complaint with attention. Others work more specifically to alter the sensory aspects of the pain experience. Techniques aimed at modifying situational factors that exacerbate chronic pain and disabilities include contingency or behavioral management methods, and modification of activity and rest cycles. Problem solving for managing and preventing pain exacerbations or relapses is central to the patient and family assuming an active role in managing chronic pain. Cognitive techniques are targeted at modifying the thoughts about pain, in particular to increase a sense of predictability and control over pain and to alter memories about painful experiences[19]; negative cognitions, especially catastrophizing somatic preoccupation; and pain-related rumination.[20] The teaching of active coping strategies, whereby pain and pain-related behaviors and cognitions are identified and targeted for self-regulation, encourages patients to recognize they are competent at coping.

Methods for managing sensory as well as psychological aspects of pain include relaxation; breathing and imagery exercises; hypnosis; and distraction techniques such as music, videos, bubble blowing, and pop-up books. It seems that at least one way these methods work is by engaging the patient's attention. It has been further hypothesized that the extent to which patients can direct their attention away from pain and pain-related concerns will determine the effectiveness of the psychological pain management techniques, although this latter hypothesis requires further empirical validation.

An essential component of any intervention is ongoing assessment of the patient's pain and pain-related functional disability. This assessment will ultimately determine the effectiveness of the strategies chosen, indicate what different interventions may need to be added, and provide concrete evidence of how treatment is progressing. Recording treatment progress allows the patient and family to see positive change when the increments are small, such as when a patient with a complex regional pain syndrome (CRPS)-1 is able to tolerate 10 minutes of activity on an affected limb after having been able to tolerate only 1 to 2 minutes before treatment was initiated. In contrast to the management of acute pain, the focus in the management of chronic pain is less on pain ratings than functional improvements. The family's help in monitoring progress can encourage taking an active role in treatment, which can increase the family's sense of achievement in dealing with the patient's chronic pain. Family involvement in treatment has been shown to produce superior results to routine pediatric care for children with recurrent abdominal pain.[20,21] It also is helpful to screen parents for psychiatric symptoms and disability, and to assess the family environment with standardized questionnaires and psychological assessment tools to identify parental or family issues that could impede the patient's progress. At times the parents may need to be referred for either rehabilitation or psychiatric treatment to assist them in their efforts to help their child's rehabilitation. The child's school and other caretakers also need to be included in the treatment team to ensure a consistent approach to the child's pain and disability.

The complex nature of chronic pain in children creates many challenges in assessment and treatment, but this same complexity can be exploited to provide optimal methods of pain control and functional rehabilitation. Multidimensional assessment provides the foundation for optimal management of chronic pain in children. Psychological interventions include a diverse array of techniques that treat chronic pain by modifying the cognitive, affective, and sensory experience of pain; behavior in response to pain; and environmental and interactional factors that influence pain. Medical treatment of chronic pain without addressing the situational, psychological, and interactional factors that may contribute to pain and pain-related disability may result in poorer outcomes.

Chronic Pain Syndromes in Children

Complex Regional Pain Syndrome-1

Neuropathic conditions are associated with injury, dysfunction, or altered excitability of portions of the peripheral or central nervous system (CNS). Complex regional pain syndrome-1 or reflex sympathetic dystrophy (RSD) is defined as "a continuous pain in a portion of an extremity after trauma, which may include fracture, but does not involve major nerve lesions and is associated with sympathetic hyperactivity." Complex regional pain syndrome-1 can be caused by any traumatic injury and presents as pain and discoloration in a swollen extremity. The incidence of neuropathic pain is greater in teenaged girls than in boys.[22] Although the general incidence of CRPS-1 in the pediatric population is less than that reported in adults, it is likely that the disorder often is missed or misdiagnosed, thereby significantly affecting its actual incidence. Although CRPS-1 has been reported in a patient as young as 3.5 years, it is generally seen in children older than 9 years and is more frequently seen in 11- to 13-year-old girls. Complex regional pain syndrome-1 is commonly seen in girls of middle-class families; usually overachievers who participate in competitive athletic programs. The onset of the disease may be a way for a competitive athlete to gracefully exit from a sport, which underscores the psychological aspect of the disease. Pain often persists despite the absence of ongoing tissue injury or inflammation, which is a hallmark of the disease. The mechanisms that generate neuropathic pain are varied and complex. Injuries to peripheral nerves may involve crush, transection, compression, demyelination, axonal degeneration, inflammation, ischemia, or other processes. The primary loci of increased irritability following peripheral nerve injury may be at several levels in the nervous system, including axonal sprouts or neuroma, the dorsal root ganglia, the dorsal horn of the spinal cord, or sites more rostral in the CNS.[23,24] Several features may help distinguish neuropathic from nociceptive pain (Table 12-1).

A detailed history of the nature of injury, the type and duration of pain, relieving and aggravating factors, and the dependence on medications is mandatory before evaluation. A thorough and systematic neurologic examination should be obtained. A complete evaluation of motor, sensory, cerebellar, cranial nerve, reflex, cognitive, and emotional functioning is important. A concerted effort must be made to rule out a rare, but possible, malignant or degenerative disorder. The strength of the extremity should be evaluated. The presence of allodynia (innocuous stimulus that elicits excruciating pain) is evaluated. Allodynia is very characteristic of neuropathic pain. Tactile allodynia in the absence of local skin pathology signifies the presence of neuropathic pain. Hyperalgesia or a decreased threshold to pain may be present. Hyperalgesia to cold is seen more frequently than to warmth. The distribution generally is not restricted to particular dermatomes as in an adult but, rather, has a "glove and stocking" distribution. Skin and other local changes, including alopecia or localized edema, may be present. Nerve conduction studies may give some insight into the location and type of nerve injury.[25] However, the use of invasive and painful electromyogram may not be acceptable to children. The diagnosis usually is made on the basis of the history, signs, and symptoms, which may vary according to the stage of the disease. A diagnostic test

Table 12-1. Differences Between Neuropathic and Nociceptive Pain

Characteristic	Neuropathic Pain	Nociceptive Pain
Description of Pain	Burning, lancinating, pins and needles	Varied
Tactile Allodynia*	Present	Absent
Duration and Intensity of Pain	Increases with duration	Decreases
Response to Opioids	Absent	Present
Use of TCAs†	Useful	Not useful

*Allodynia is the sensation of a normally non-painful stimulus (touch) as painful.
†TCAs = tricyclic antidepressants.

with phentolamine (an α-adrenergic blocking agent) has been used to confirm the diagnosis and to predict the response to a sympathetic blockade.[26]

Regardless of its etiology, the management of neuropathic pain such as CRPS-1 can be frustrating for the caregiver, patient, and family. There is no single therapy that uniformly provides relief. The titration of medications may be limited by side effects and complications. One of the main goals is to get the patient back to a functional state and back in school. Complete resolution of pain is not always possible. Most of the management techniques for CRPS-1 are extrapolated from work done in adult patients[27] (Table 12-2). It is important to gain the trust of the patient and their parents. Family dynamics are important, because the added burden of familial disharmony or parental abuse can increase the symptoms. A treatment algorithm is outlined in Figure 12-1.[28]

Table 12-2. Management of Neuropathic Pain

Non-pharmacologic Treatment*
Hypnosis, biofeedback, visual guided imagery (psychologist)
Relaxation and cognitive coping methods
Education about multidimensional pain management techniques
Transcutaneous electrical nerve stimulation and physical therapy
Individual and family therapy

Pharmacologic Therapy
Acetaminophen, nonsteroidal anti-inflammatory agents
Tricyclic antidepressants (amitriptyline, nortriptyline, trazodone, desimipramine)
Anticonvulsants (carbamazepine, phenytoin, clonazepam)
Systemic local anesthetics (mexiletine, lidocaine)
Opioids (oral preferred to parenteral)

Regional Blockade and Associated Techniques
Intravenous regional anesthesia (Bier block)
Continuous epidural analgesia
Neurolytic blockade for cancer
Acupuncture
Sympathetic blockade
- Stellate ganglion block (upper extremity)
- Lumbar sympathetic block (lower extremity)

*Offered to all patients.

Behavioral measures are a key component in managing neuropathic pain. Family therapy helps the family cope with the situation. Consultation with a medical psychologist during the first visit to the pain clinic is encouraged for all patients. A number of techniques can be used, including biofeedback,[29] visual guided imagery, relaxation strategies, and structured counseling on coping skills. Physical therapy is an integral part of the treatment to improve mobility of the affected limb and restore function. Transcutaneous electrical nerve stimulation (TENS) is widely used and has been shown, in many cases, to be efficacious

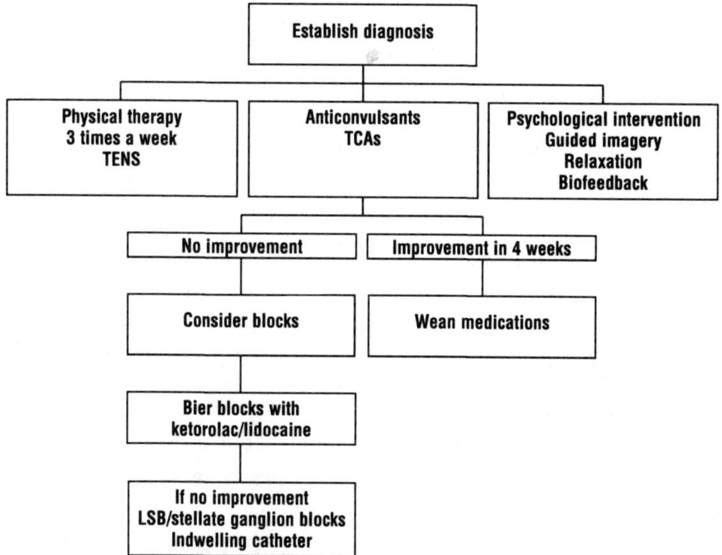

Figure 12-1
Algorithm used in the treatment of CRPS-1 at Children's Memorial Hospital (Chicago, IL). Following the establishment of the diagnosis, multidisciplinary therapy is started that includes 1) physical therapy to maintain and reestablish function; this also may include transcutaneous electrical nerve stimulation (TENS), 2) pharmacologic intervention with either tricyclic antidepressants or anticonvulsants, and 3) psychological intervention with guided imagery, relaxation techniques, and biofeedback. If this therapy is effective, the pharmacologic agent is weaned. If there is no improvement over a 4-week period, regional anesthetic techniques are used (Bier block, lumbar sympathetic block [LSB], or epidural anesthesia).

in adults as well as children.[30] In specific cases, acupuncture also has been helpful.[31]

Although generally of limited efficacy, drug therapy starts with nonsteroidal anti-inflammatory agents (NSAIDs). Specific cyclooxygenase-2 inhibitors, such as celecoxib, rofecoxib, and parecoxib, may be used, given their lower potential for adverse effects with prolonged administration. Opioids can be helpful in the management of neuropathic pain, especially for cancer-related neuropathic pain. Arner and colleagues[32] have shown that there are several types of neuropathic pain that are resistant to the effects of opioids. It is optimal to titrate the opioid in a graded fashion to optimize the effect and limit adverse effects. Sedation is a side effect that may be desirable and, in other cases, may need to be antagonized with the addition of amphetamines.[33] For patients with nonmalignant, neuropathic pain, it is desirable to try non-opioid techniques, including behavior modification, before prescribing large doses of opioids.

The mainstay of pharmacologic management of neuropathic pain remains the tricyclic antidepressants (TCAs) and anticonvulsant drugs. Adults with neuropathic pain frequently are treated with tricyclic antidepressants.[34] Despite the lack of adequate pediatric-controlled studies, TCAs are widely prescribed for several forms of neuropathic pain. The choice of agents depends on its adverse effect profile. If the patient is unable to sleep at night, amitriptyline may be a good choice. However, if the patient experiences anticholinergic side effects, such as dry mouth and morning sleepiness, an agent such as nortriptyline or desimipramine can be used. Amitriptyline and nortriptyline are started at low doses (0.1 mg/kg/dose, once a day) and increased gradually to minimize their adverse effects. A thorough examination of the patient's cardiovascular system is necessary prior to instituting TCA therapy because of associated tachydysrhythmias and other conduction abnormalities such as prolonged QT syndrome. Some patients with neuropathic pain may benefit from drugs in the anticonvulsant class.

Gabapentin, carbamazepine, clonazepam, and phenytoin are the most commonly used medications. Regular monitoring of drug levels, blood counts, and liver function are recommended. Carbamazepine may be quite useful in treating neuropathic pain. More recently, the use of gabapentin has been shown to be very effective in the management of neuropathic pain with a limited adverse effect profile that is favorable compared with other agents.[35,36] Because of the involvement of the sympathetic nervous system with increased sympathetic function leading to vasoconstriction of the affected limb, patients with CRPS-1 also may benefit from vasodilators such as prazosin, nifedipine, and phenoxybenzamine.[37] Significant adverse effects, including orthostatic hypotension, may offset the efficacy of this therapy.

The most common treatment for CRPS-1 is to provide interruption of the apparent pathologic pathways using sympathetic blocks. With serial blocks, the patient typically will notice pain relief that increases with each block and prevents the pain from returning to its original level. If no symptomatic relief is obtained after 2 or 3 blocks, an alternative approach should be instituted. Concurrent physical therapy is indicated to improve range of motion and improve function once the pain has been successfully controlled. In most pediatric patients, these sympathetic regional blocks are performed with sedation or general anesthesia (especially if the patients are younger than 10 years).

Alternatively, intravenous regional (Bier) blocks can be used to manage pain in CRPS-1.[28,38] The technique is easier than direct sympathetic blockade and eliminates the need for precise needle placement near the sympathetic chain or the use of neuraxial (epidural or spinal) blockade. These blocks can be performed with minimal sedation. After venous drainage of the extremity, a tourniquet is placed on the proximal end of the extremity, and intravenous local anesthetic with ketorolac is injected into a distal vein. If the extremity is very painful, elevation may be adequate to provide venous drainage before applying a tourniquet. The tourniquet is kept inflated for 30 minutes and then slowly released. In the authors' experience, a single block has provided total pain relief in some patients. An alternative approach to the management of the peripheral manifestations of neuropathic pain is to use an α-adrenergic antagonist (phentolamine) or medications that deplete norepinephrine from the peripheral sympathetic nervous system (guanethidine or bretylium), using the intravenous regional anesthetic technique. Direct sympathetic blockade (stellate ganglion block for upper extremity or lumbar sympathetic/epidural block for lower extremity CRPS-1) is used when intravenous regional anesthesia fails. Several sympathetic blocks at intervals of 1 to 2 weeks may be necessary to see improvement in symptoms.

Given the limited number of pediatric patients studied, a definitive conclusion regarding the most effective treatment regimen for CRPS-1 and the prognosis of afflicted patients is difficult. Varni[39] reported uniform improvement among their patients using a prolonged program of physical therapy and inpatient rehabilitation programs. Ashwal et al,[40] in a review of CRPS-1 in children, concluded that the prognosis of the disease is more favorable in children than in adults. Wilder et al,[22] from the Boston Children's Hospital, reviewed 70 patients with RSD. There was an average age of 12.5 years and a predominance of females (59 of 70 patients, or 84%). The average time from the initial injury until the diagnosis was 1 year, indicating, in their opinion, that the syndrome remains underrecognized in children. Conservative therapy with physical therapy, TENS, psychological therapies, including cognitive-behavioral management and relaxation training, and TCAs were effective in decreasing pain and improving function in 40 of the 70 patients (57%). Sympathetic blockade was effective in 28 of 37 patients (76%). Despite these therapies, 38 of the 70 patients (54%) continued to have pain and decreased function.

Regardless of its etiology, neuropathic pain can be puzzling and frustrating. Therefore, treatment strategies require a strong alliance with the family and the patient. A multidisciplinary approach with an algorithmic management, using available techniques can be helpful (Figure 12-1). Following the diagnosis, multidisciplinary therapy is initiated and includes 1) physical therapy to maintain and reestablish function; 2) pharmacologic intervention with either TCAs or anticonvulsants; and 3) psychological intervention with guided imagery, relaxation techniques, and biofeedback. If the therapy is effective, the pharmacologic agent is weaned. If there is no improvement in a 4-week period, regional anesthetic techniques are used. Given their ease of placement, this initially includes an intravenous regional anesthetic technique (Bier block) using ketorolac and lidocaine. If this fails, more invasive regional anesthetic techniques (lumbar sympathetic block, stellate ganglion block, or epidural anesthesia) are used.

Headaches

Few physicians discussed headaches in children until 1873, when British pediatrician William Henry Day devoted a chapter to the subject in his book *Essays on Diseases in Children.* In 1967 Freidman and Harms wrote *Headaches in Children.* These early works laid the groundwork for many of the subsequent papers dealing with headaches in children. Each year it is estimated that at least 80% of the population experiences headaches. The difficulty for the practitioner arises because the headache may be functional or due to a minor, non–life-threatening condition, yet missing the rare organic cause, such as a brain tumor, can have devastating consequences. A history and physical examination can help determine the nature of a headache (Table 12-3). Specific questions are asked about signs and symptoms, such as ataxia, lethargy, seizures, poor school performance, and changes in visual acuity, which may signal the presence of associated organic pathology. A history of a severe headache without a previous history of headache, pain that awakens a child from sleep, headaches associated with straining, change in chronic headache patterns, or the presence of a headache with nausea or vomiting also may suggest a pathological origin to the headache.

The classification of headaches is based on the presumed location of the abnormality, its origin, its pathophysiology, or the symptom complex with which the patient presents. The International Headache Society recently has updated its classification. By plotting the severity of a headache over time, headaches can be classified into 5 major categories (Table 12-4). The reader is referred to Chapter 10 for additional information about headache disorders in children, including evaluation and treatment options.

Headaches in the Child With a Ventriculoperitoneal Shunt

As with headaches related to other causes, the management of pain in patients with a ventriculoperitoneal shunt involves a multidisciplinary

Table 12-3. Examination and Investigation of Headache in Children

General Physical Examination
Blood pressure
Skin examination for café-au-lait spots, adenoma sebaceum, hypopigmented lesions, petechiae
Neurologic Examination
Head circumference measurement (comparison of growth charts from birth)
Auscultation of the cranium for bruit (especially in younger children)
Tenderness over the sinuses (maxillary and frontal sinuses)
Presence of occult trauma, indicating a battered child
Funduscopic examination: optic atrophy, papilledema
Cranial nerve examination
Mental status evaluation
Alteration in speech or language skills
Alteration in the gait
Laboratory Tests (not all will be indicated in every patient)
Electroencephalogram: nonspecific
Computed tomography imaging with and without contrast: rapid test to evaluate for intracranial pathology
Magnetic resonance imaging: more sensitive for evaluation of intracranial pathology, especially vascular abnormalities and mass lesions in the sella turcica, posterior fossa, and temporal lobes
Lumbar puncture: rarely indicated except in determining acute infectious causes or to measure intracranial pressure in suspected pseudotumor cerebri, generally performed only after intracranial lesion is ruled out
Psychological Tests to Determine if There Is a Psychological Basis for the Headache

approach, including anesthesiology, neurosurgery, neurology, psychiatry, and physical therapy. In the authors' experience, an aggressive management approach has led to a decrease in operative procedures, school absenteeism, fewer visits to the hospital, and increased self-esteem. Before treatment begins at the author's institution, the patient's clinical status and computed tomography scans are reviewed with a neurosurgeon. Once it has been established by the neurosurgical service that the headaches are not related to increased intracranial pressure, the patient is scheduled for a visit to the Chronic Pain Clinic. A complete history and physical examination are performed. In addition to a complete neurological examination, the physical status of the patient is assessed.

Is the patient actively mobile?

Does the headache prevent the child from performing his or her normal activities?

Table 12-4. Classification of Headaches: Differential Diagnosis

Classification of Headaches
Acute Headaches
Systemic illness
Subarachnoid hemorrhage
Trauma
Toxins (lead or carbon monoxide)
Electrolyte imbalances
Hypertension
Acute Recurrent Headaches
Migraine
Tension-type headache
Chronic Progressive Headaches
Organic brain disease
Ventriculoperitoneal shunt malfunction
Chronic Nonprogressive Headaches
Functional
Mixed Headaches
Combination of any of the above pathologies

Is there school absenteeism?
What is the patient's interaction with the parents and siblings at home?
Are there any relieving factors for the headache?
Has the patient been placed on any medications for pain?
Has there been any improvement at all in the clinical characteristic of pain?
When was the last shunt revision and was the pain any better after the last shunt revision?

Having answered some or all of the questions, various modalities are offered in a stepladder fashion based on the pain status of the patient (Figure 12-2). The authors have treated several pediatric patients who had been debilitated due to headaches and were able to resume normal activity. Most of the patients had associated musculoskeletal problems. Hence, the addition of physical therapy was used to increase muscle strength, thereby helping in the patients' recovery. The intervention of a medical psychologist proficient in pain management was vital to recovery.

Cancer Pain

Managing pain in the pediatric cancer patient combines the understanding of normal childhood development and a knowledge of the natural history and treatment of childhood malignancies.[41-44] Pain in a cancer patient can result from tumor invasion, invasive procedures, and therapy (both surgical and medical), as well as other causes unrelated to cancer. Pain directly related to a malignancy is, most commonly, bone pain, either from a metastasis of the tumor on the bone or from a primary malignancy. Other less common but important causes of cancer-related pain include spinal cord compression, tumor involvement of the central or the peripheral nervous system, and viscus or ureteral obstruction. Procedure-related pain may arise from commonly performed procedures, including bone marrow aspiration, lumbar puncture, and venipuncture. Given the aggressive nature of many chemotherapeutic protocols, these procedures are commonplace during the initial chemotherapy of many childhood malignancies. The type of tumor and its therapy may predict the magnitude of the adverse effects and their resultant pain. Commonly seen problems include mucositis, neuropathy, surgical incisions, corticosteroid-induced bone changes, and gastritis from mucosal damage.

Acute Cancer-Related Pain

As with pain related to other etiologies, effective management of cancer-related pain requires a multidisciplinary approach that includes therapy

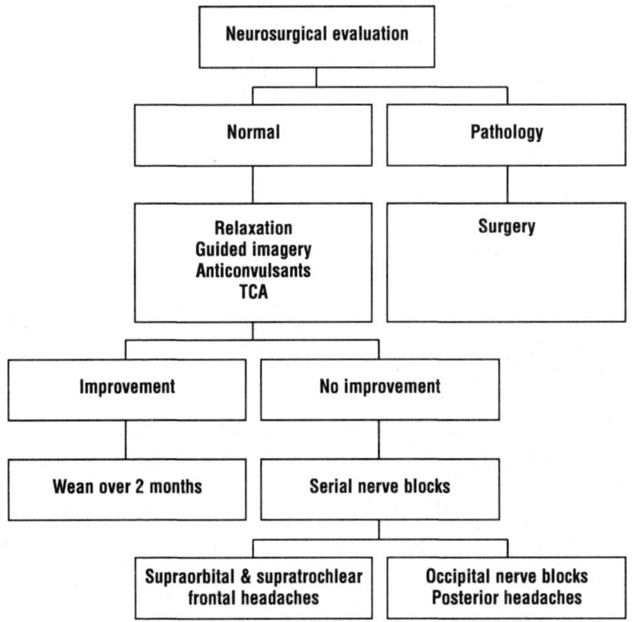

Figure 12-2
Algorithm for the management of headache pain in the child with a ventriculoperitoneal shunt. If the patient experiences nausea, vomiting, or other signs of increased intracranial pressure, the possibility of a shunt malfunction also should be entertained.

directed against the tumor, psychological techniques (see previous text), and pharmacologic management (Table 12-5). The World Health Organization has suggested an analgesic stepladder protocol for the pharmacologic management of pain in cancer patients.[45] Step 1 is the use of non-opioids (acetaminophen and NSAIDs with adjuvants such as TCAs) for mild pain; in step 2, weak opioids such as codeine or oxycodone are added; and, in step 3, potent opioids, such as morphine, are added for severe pain. As treatment progresses from step 1 to 2 to 3, the adjuvants and acetaminophen or NSAIDs are not discontinued. They are used with the weak opioids in step 2 or the potent opioids in step 3 to provide a synergistic effect, thereby decreasing the total opioid requirement and decreasing opioid-related adverse effects. Despite its specific etiology, the medications and techniques are similar to those used for acute pain management in other clinical situations. See Chapter 8 for additional information regarding the pharmacologic approach to the treatment of acute cancer-related pain.

Pain During the Terminal Stages of Illness

Despite improvements in surgical and medical therapies, a cure for cancer in all children is not possible. With the involvement of organizations such as hospices, care of terminally ill children has been developed based on the same philosophy as adults.[46] During the terminal stages of many pediatric malignancies, pain can be a significant problem. Several approaches to pain management are taken based on the state of the patient and the involvement of the disease process (Table 12-5). Patient-controlled analgesia (PCA) has been widely used for hospitalized and homebound patients with terminal cancer.[47] Smaller, more user-friendly pumps have been devised for easy programming and less frequent changing. In patients who do not have venous access, the use of subcutaneous PCA is recommended.

Nonsteroidal anti-inflammatory drugs and steroids are particularly useful in the management of bone pain from metastasis.[48,49] Carbamazepine, gabapentin, and TCAs are useful for managing neuropathic pain.[50] Hypnosis, biofeedback, and distraction techniques can be used very effectively in patients who are not heavily medicated and too sedated.[51-53]

Table 12-5. Approaches to Pain Management in Terminally Ill Patients

Pharmacologic
Nonsteroidal anti-inflammatory agents, including cyclooxygenase-2 inhibitors
Opioid analgesics (oral, transdermal, nebulized, parenteral)
Anticonvulsants (gabapentin, carbamazepine)
Tricyclic antidepressants (trazodone, amitriptyline, nortriptyline)
Corticosteroids
Amphetamines (to combat somnolence associated with opioids)
Chemotherapy
Psychological
Emotional support
Distraction (guided imagery)
Hypnosis
Relaxation techniques
Biofeedback
Regional Anesthetic Techniques
Neuraxial blockade with indwelling epidural and intrathecal catheters
Opioids
Local anesthetic solution
Peripheral nerve blockade
Sympathetic blockade
Celiac plexus
Lumbar sympathetic
Surgical
Neuroablative procedures
Tumor debulking to reduce compression
Neurosurgical interventions
Physical Therapy
Transcutaneous electrical nerve stimulation
Acupuncture
Heat/cooling
Exercise
Anticancer Therapy
Radiation
Chemotherapy
Biologic therapy

Alternate novel methods for providing analgesia have been used in patients who do not have intravenous access. Nebulized opioids and transdermal delivery systems have been used in patients with intractable pain.[54,55] An adverse effect associated with long-term use of opioids can be tolerance and withdrawal. Careful rotation of opioids, along with the judicious use of other adjuvants, including *N*-methyl-D-aspartate–receptor antagonists, should be considered.

A child's view of death is very different from that of an adult. As a child grows older, there is a consistent progression of the conceptual aspect of death. The school-aged child finally understands the permanence of death. Home care may be very useful for the family to cope with the grief and sorrow. It also allows siblings to spend some time with a loved one. A home care coordinator should be available for the management of any adverse conditions. Knowing the family helps the coordinator understand the goals of the family. One of the basic tenets of hospice care is to enable patients to lead a fulfilled life, of the best quality, for whatever time they have remaining. Cooperation between the family and the caregiver should allow the child to die with as much dignity as possible. The combination of various techniques for the management of cancer pain will help to reduce pain and enhance the child's motivation to lead as normal a life as possible.

Summary

Chronic pain in children remains mostly an underreported phenomenon. For children with chronic pain, a multidisciplinary approach helps determine the course of action and prognosis of the particular patient. When pediatric pain is severe, most management techniques initially will include the use of opioids. Resistance to the use of opioids in children remains because of the fear of addiction or the occurrence of adverse effects, including respiratory depression. This also may pose an ethical dilemma to the nursing staff if they view the analgesic medication as a potential respiratory depressant, which may hasten the end of life.[56] The use of various methods, including physical therapy and the services of a child psychiatry/psychology department, can help children cope and overcome persistent pain. Chronic pain can be devastating to a child's morale and has to be recognized and treated just like any other chronic disease. The key to effective continuing care for these children is a multidisciplinary approach with a psychologist, physical therapist, and pain management specialist.

References

1. Thompson KL, Varni JW. A developmental cognitive-biobehavioral approach to pediatric pain assessment. *Pain.* 1986;25:283-296
2. Andrews K, Fitzgerald M. Biological barriers to paediatric pain management. *Clin J Pain.* 1997;13:138-143
3. McGrath PA. Pain in the pediatric patient: practical aspects of assessment. *Pediatr Ann.* 1995;24:126-133, 137-138
4. Merlijn VP, Hunfeld JA, van der Wouden JC, et al. Psychosocial factors associated with chronic pain in adolescents. *Pain.* 2003;101:33-43
5. Merlijn VP, Hunfeld JA, van der Wouden JC, Hazebroek-Kampschreur AA, Passchier J. Shortening a quality of life questionnaire for adolescents with chronic pain and its psychometric qualities. *Psychol Rep.* 2002;90:753-759
6. Blount RL, Schaen ER, Cohen LL. Commentary: current status and future directions in acute pediatric pain assessment and treatment. *J Pediatr Psychol.* 1999;24:150-152
7. Masek BJ, Russo DC, Varni JW. Behavioral approaches to the management of chronic pain in children. *Pediatr Clin North Am.* 1984;31:1113-1131
8. Keefe FJ, Bonk V. Psychosocial assessment of pain in patients having rheumatic diseases. *Rheum Dis Clin North Am.* 1999;25:81-103
9. Lewin DS, Dahl RE. Importance of sleep in the management of pediatric pain. *J Dev Behav Pediatr.* 1999;20:244-252
10. Hershey AD, Vockell AL, LeCates S, Kabbouche MA, Maynard MK. PedMIDAS: development of a questionnaire to assess disability of migraines in children. *Neurology.* 2001;57:2034-2039
11. Varni JW, Seid M, Smith KT, Knight T, Burwinkle T, Brown J, Szer IS. The PedsQL in pediatric rheumatology: reliability, validity, and responsiveness of the Pediatric Quality of Life Inventory Generic Core Scales and Rheumatology Module. *Arthritis Rheum.* 2002;46:714-725

12. Hunfeld JA, Perquin CW, Duivenvoorden HJ, et al. Chronic pain and its impact on quality of life in adolescents and their families. *J Pediatr Psychol.* 2001;26:145-153
13. Powers SW, Mitchell MJ, Byars KC, Bentti AL, LeCates SL, Hershey AD. A pilot study of one-session biofeedback training in pediatric headache. *Neurology.* 2001;56:133
14. McGrath PJ, Vair C. Psychological aspects of pain management of the burned child. *Child Health Care.* 1984;13:15-19
15. McGrath PJ, Johnson GG. Pain management in children. *Can J Anaesth.* 1988;35:107-110
16. Fanurik D, Zeltzer LK, Roberts MC, Blount RL. The relationship between children's coping styles and psychological interventions for cold pressor pain. *Pain.* 1993;53:213-222
17. Kuttner L. Managing pain in children. Changing treatment of headaches. *Can Fam Physician.* 1993;39:563-568
18. Zeltzer L, Bursch B, Walco G. Pain responsiveness and chronic pain: a psychobiological perspective. *J Dev Behav Pediatr.* 1997;18:413-422
19. Chen PP, Ma M, Chan S, Oh TE. Incident reporting in acute pain management. *Anaesthesia.* 1998;53:730-735
20. Sanders MR, Rebgetz M, Morrison M, et al. Cognitive-behavioral treatment of recurrent nonspecific abdominal pain in children: an analysis of generalization, maintenance, and side effects. *J Consult Clin Psychol.* 1989;57:294-300
21. Sanders MR, Shepherd RW, Cleghorn G, Woolford H. The treatment of recurrent abdominal pain in children: a controlled comparison of cognitive-behavioral family intervention and standard pediatric care. *J Consult Clin Psychol.* 1994;62:306-314
22. Wilder RT, Berde CB, Wolohan M, Vieyra MA, Masek BJ, Micheli LJ. Reflex sympathetic dystrophy in children. Clinical characteristics and follow-up of seventy patients. *J Bone Joint Surg Am.* 1992;74:910-919
23. Stanton-Hicks M. Reflex sympathetic dystrophy: a sympathetically mediated pain syndrome or not? *Curr Rev Pain.* 2000;4:268-275
24. Stanton-Hicks M. Complex regional pain syndrome (type I, RSD; type II, causalgia): controversies. *Clin J Pain.* 2000;16:S33-S40
25. Konen A. Measurement of nerve dysfunction in neuropathic pain. *Curr Rev Pain.* 2000;4:388-394
26. Arner S. Intravenous phentolamine test: diagnostic and prognostic use in reflex sympathetic dystrophy. *Pain.* 1991;46:17-22

27. Stanton-Hicks M, Baron R, Boas R, et al. Complex Regional Pain Syndromes: guidelines for therapy. *Clin J Pain.* 1998;14:155-166
28. Suresh S, Wheeler M, Patel A. Case series: IV regional anesthesia with ketorolac and lidocaine: is it effective for the management of complex regional pain syndrome 1 in children and adolescents? *Anesth Analg.* 2003;96:694-695
29. Brown CR. Pain management. Biofeedback and relaxation therapy. *Pract Periodontics Aesthet Dent.* 1997;9:1068
30. Kesler RW, Saulsbury FT, Miller LT, Rowlingson JC. Reflex sympathetic dystrophy in children: treatment with transcutaneous electric nerve stimulation. *Pediatr Ann.* 1988;82:728-732
31. Kemper KJ, Sarah R, Silver-Highfield E, Xiarhos E, Barnes L, Berde CB. On pins and needles? Pediatric pain patients' experience with acupunc ture. *Pediatr Ann.* 2000;105:941-947
32. Arner S, Killander E, Westerberg H. [Poor leadership behind poor pain relief. Medical audit of cancer-related pain treatment]. *Lakartidningen.* 1999;96:33-36
33. O'Neill WM. The cognitive and psychomotor effects of opioid drugs in cancer pain management. *Cancer Surv.* 1994;21:67-84
34. Richlin DM. Nonnarcotic analgesics and tricyclic antidepressants for the treatment of chronic nonmalignant pain. *Mt Sinai J Med.* 1991;58:221-228
35. Wheeler DS, Vaux KK, Tam DA. Use of gabapentin in the treatment of childhood reflex sympathetic dystrophy. *Pediatr Neurol.* 2000;22:220-221
36. Mellick GA, Mellick LB. Reflex sympathetic dystrophy treated with gabapentin. *Arch Phys Med Rehabil.* 1997;78:98-105
37. Paulson RR. Reflex sympathetic dystrophy in a teenaged girl. *Postgrad Med.* 1987;81:66-67
38. Connelly NR, Reuben S, Brull SJ. Intravenous regional anesthesia with ketorolac-lidocaine for the management of sympathetically-mediated pain. *Yale J Biol Med.* 1995;68:95-99
39. Varni JW. Behavioral medicine in hemophilia arthritic pain management: two case studies. *Arch Phys Med Rehabil.* 1981;62:183-187
40. Ashwal S, Tomasi L, Neumann M, Schneider S. Reflex sympathetic dystrophy syndrome in children. *Pediatr Neurol.* 1988;4:38-42
41. McGrath PJ, Beyer J, Cleeland C, et al. American Academy of Pediatrics Report of the Subcommittee on Assessment and Methodologic Issues in the Management of Pain in Childhood Cancer. *Pediatrics.* 1990;86:814-817

42. Brown RE Jr, Schmitz ML, Andelman P. The treatment of pain in children with cancer. *J Ark Med Soc.* 1993;90:316-318
43. Collins JJ, Grier HE, Kinney HC, Berde CB. Control of severe pain in children with terminal malignancy. *J Pediatr.* 1995;126:653-657
44. Collins JJ. Intractable pain in children with terminal cancer. *J Palliative Care.* 1996;12:29-34
45. McGrath PA. Development of the World Health Organization Guidelines on Cancer Pain Relief and Palliative Care in Children. *J Pain Symptom Manage.* 1996;12:87-92
46. Hollen PJ. Intervention booster: adding a decision-making module to risk reduction and other health care programs for adolescents. *J Pediatr Health Care.* 1998;12:247-255
47. Dunbar PJ, Buckley P, Gavrin JR, et al. Use of patient-controlled analgesia for pain control for children receiving bone marrow transplant. *J Pain Symptom Manage.* 1995;10:604-611
48. Chiang JS. New developments in cancer pain therapy. *Acta Anaesthesiol Sin.* 2000;38:31-36
49. Kasai H, Sasaki K, Tsujinaga H, Hoshino T. Pain management in advanced pediatric cancer patients—a proposal of the two-step analgesic ladder. *Masui.* 1995;44:885-889
50. Rosner H, Rubin L, Kestenbaum A. Gabapentin adjunctive therapy in neuropathic pain states. *Clin J Pain.* 1996;12:56-58
51. Montgomery GH, DuHamel KN, Redd WH. A meta-analysis of hypnotically induced analgesia: how effective is hypnosis? *Int J Clin Exp Hypn.* 2000;48:138-153
52. Rusy LM, Weisman SJ. Complementary therapies for acute pediatric pain management. *Pediatr Clin North Am.* 2000;47:589-599
53. Belgrade MJ. Control of pain in cancer patients. *Postgrad Med.* 1989;85:319-323, 326-329
54. Howe JL. Nebulized morphine for hospice patients. *Am J Hosp Palliat Care.* 1995;12:6
55. Collins JJ, Dunkel IJ, Gupta SK, et al. Transdermal fentanyl in children with cancer pain: feasibility, tolerability, and pharmacokinetic correlates. *J Pediatr.* 1999;134:319-323
56. Siever BA. Pain management and potentially life-shortening analgesia in the terminally ill child: the ethical implications for pediatric nurses. *J Pediatr Nurs.* 1994;9:307-312

Index

*Page numbers with *f* indicate figures; page numbers with *t* indicate tables.

A

Abdomen, blockade of, 165–167, 165*f*, 166*f*
Abdominal pain, 381, 392
  following traumatic injury, 401
Abdominal visceral injury, 401
Abrasions, 399
Abstinence syndrome, 44–45
Acetaminophen
  for burns, 404
  for chest pain, 392
  for headache pain, 389
  for mild to moderate pain, 324, 325, 326–327, 454
  for moderate to severe pain, 331–332
  for neonatal pain and surgery, 369–370, 371*t*
  for otitis media, 390, 391
Acetaminophen toxicity, 328
Acetylsalicylic acid for mild to moderate pain, 324, 325
Achilles tendon, 162
Acidosis, 99
Acid sensing ion channels (ASICs), 7, 8
Activities of daily living, impact of headaches on, 382
Acupuncture, 419, 427, 430–431
  for headache pain, 389
Acute cancer-related pain, 453–454
Acute medical illness, 323
Acute otitis externa, 390
Acute otitis media, 390
Acute pain, 231
  etiologies of, 323
  management of, 323–324
  neonatal
    acetaminophen for, 369–370
    assessment of, 359–360, 361*t*
    epidural analgesia for, 370–373, 371*t*, 372*f*
    opioid analgesics for, 366–369, 368*t*
  treatment of, when associated with medical illnesses, 381–411
    burns, 403–406
    chest pain, 392, 393*t*, 394–398
    headache pain, 382–389, 384*t*, 385*t*
    hemoglobinopathies, 406–411
    otitis media, 390–391
    traumatic injury, 398–403
Addiction, 293
Adenosine triphosphate (ATP) receptors (P2X3), 7, 8
Adjunctive techniques for circumcision, 365–366
Adrenergic agonists, 4
Agitation-Sedation Scale in assessing depth of sedation in pediatric intensive care unit, 237
Agonists, 42
Aldosterone, 63

Alfentanil
for moderate to severe pain, 338
in pediatric intensive care sedation, 266
Allium sativum for otitis media, 391
Allodynia, 443
α_2-adrenergic agonists
in opioid withdrawal, 313, 314
in pediatric intensive care unit sedation, 272–274
for procedure-related pain and anxiety, 206–207
Alprazolam, benzodiazepine withdrawal and, 296
Alternative medicine therapies, 419
American Academy of Pediatrics
on analgesia during circumcision, 364, 365
guidelines for preoperative evaluation/preparation, 186
American Society of Anesthesiologists (ASA) sedation classification system, 189, 189*t*, 190
Aminophylline in pediatric intensive care unit sedation, 240
Amitriptyline, for neuropathic pain, 405, 446
Analgesia. *See also* Epidural analgesia; Nurse-controlled analgesia; Patient-controlled analgesia (PCA); Spinal analgesia
adverse effects from, 323
for circumcision, 363–366
interpleural, 165–167, 165*f*, 166*f*, 170
ketamine in, 209–211
opioids in, 207–208
for painful medical procedures in the neonate, 361–363
plexus, 164
Analgesic effect, 42
Analgesic ladder, 323–324, 324*t*, 410, 454
Anemia, chronic hemolytic, 406
Anesthetic agents
barbiturates as, 211–212
nitrous oxide as, 214–215
propofol as, 213–214
Ankle block, 161–162, 161*f*
complications in, 162
Antagonists, 42–43
Anticonvulsants, 48
for neuropathic pain, 405, 446
Antidepressants for headache pain, 389
Antihistamines, 53, 109
Anxiolysis, 422
Apnea, 60, 68, 123
post-anesthetic, 95
Arthritis, 428
Aspiration, 103
negative, 103
Asthma
ketamine and, 248–249
migraines and, 387
AstraZeneca, 260, 261–262
Atherosclerotic coronary artery disease, 395–396
Atropine, 61
in pediatric intensive care unit sedation, 250
Auditory canal, 390
Aura, 387–388
Auralgan for otitis media, 391
Auriculotemporal nerve, 390
Axillary block to the brachial plexus, 147–149, 148*f*
complications of, 148–149
disadvantages of, 148
transarterial approach, 148–149
Axonal degeneration, 442

B

Bacteremia, 404
Barbiturates, 45, 63–65
  addiction and dependency, 298
  effects on cardiorespiratory function, 265
  in pediatric critical care unit sedation, 254
  in pediatric intensive care unit sedation, 263–265
  for procedure-related pain and anxiety, 211–212
  tolerance to, 314–315
Baxter Pharmaceuticals, 262
Behavioral measures. *See also* Cognitive-behavioral techniques in pain management
  for assessing pain in neonates, 359–360
  for chronic pain, 440
  for neuropathic pain, 445
Benzocaine, 79
Benzodiazepines, 45, 68–70, 217–218
  addiction and dependency, 296–297
  in pediatric intensive care unit sedation, 241, 242–247
  for procedure-related pain and anxiety, 204–206, 217–218
  tolerance and, 305
β-adrenergic antagonists
  for headache pain, 389
  in pediatric intensive care unit sedation, 241
Biofeedback
  for headache pain, 389
  for neuropathic pain, 444
  for sickle-cell pain, 410
  for terminal illness, 455
Biophysical techniques in pain management, 419, 425–426, 425*t*
  acupuncture as, 430–431
  cold therapy as, 428
  cutaneous stimulation as, 427
  heat therapy as, 428
  hydrotherapy as, 428
  massage as, 429
  nonnutritive sucking as, 426–427, 426*t*
  therapeutic exercise as, 429
  transcutaneous electrical nerve stimulation as, 430
Biopsychosocial perspective in assessing chronic pain, 437
Bispectral Index (BIS), 197–198
  in assessing depth of sedation in pediatric intensive care unit, 238
  documentation of tolerance with, 292–293, 306
Bleeding, following circumcision, 364
Bleeding dyscrasias, 333
Bloody diarrhea, 381
Body meridians, 431
Bone marrow aspirations, 424, 452
Bone marrow biopsy, 248
Bone marrow transplantation for sickle cell disease, 408
Bony infarctions, 407
Bovie pad, placement of, 133
Brachial plexus, 146
  anatomy of, 146–147
  axillary approach to, 147–149, 148*f*
  parascalene approach to, 149–150, 149*f*
Bradycardia, 47
Brain-derived neurotrophic factor (BDNF), 7

Brain tumor, 386, 449
Bretylium, 100
  for neuropathic pain, 448
Bupivacaine, 98–100, 102, 121
  in continuous brachial anesthesia, 164
  continuous infusion of, in neonates, 371–373
  in head and neck blockade, 174
  in ilioinguinal/iliohypogastric nerve block, 172
  in interpleural analgesia, 166
  in peripheral nerve blockade, 403
  via interpleural catheter, 167
Bupivacaine-induced cardiotoxicity, 100
Buprenorphine, analgesic effects of, 367
Burns, 324
  dressing changes for, 248
  pain related to, 403–406
Butorphanol (Stadol), 43, 49, 53, 107, 108
  for moderate to severe pain, 336
Butyrate in fetal hemoglobin production, 408
Butyrophenones in pediatric intensive care unit sedation, 270–272

C

Calcium channel blockers, 100
  for headache pain, 389
Calendula flores for otitis media, 391
Cancer pain, 344, 452–456
  treatment of, 323–324, 324*t*
Carbamazepine
  for benzodiazepine withdrawal, 314
  for neuropathic pain, 405, 447
  in terminal illness, 454
Carbon monoxide poisoning, 386
Cardiac catheterization, sedation during, 202
Cardiac causes of chest pain, 395–396
Cardiorespiratory function, effect of barbiturates on, 265
Cardiotoxicity, 98
  bupivacaine-induced, 100
Cardiovascular collapse, 99
Cathartic agents, 349
Caudal epidural block, 95, 110, 118–122
  comparison of, with spinal anesthesia, 122*t*
Ceiling effect, 333
Celecoxib (Celebrex)
  for moderate to severe pain, 335
  for neuropathic pain, 446
Cell-cycle kinetics, 12
Cellular injury, 428
Central afferent terminals, 9–10
Central line placement, 248
Central nervous system
  effects of ketamine on, 251
  effects of propofol on, 254
Central nervous system infection, 385
Central nervous system toxicity, 340
Cerebral cortex, 4, 5*f*
Cervical plexus, 146, 390
Checklists in assessing chronic pain, 437
CHEOPS (Children's Hospital of Eastern Ontario Pain Score), 351
Chest pain, 392, 394–398
  cardiac causes of, 395–396
  differential diagnosis of, 393*t*, 400–401
  functional, 396
  gastrointestinal etiologies of, 394
Chest tube removal, pain from, 397–398
Chest wall rigidity, 47–48, 267
Children's Comprehensive Pain Questionnaire, 437

Chiropractic manipulation, 419, 425
2-chloroprocaine, continuous infusion of, in neonates, 373
Chloral hydrate, 67–68
  in pediatric intensive care unit sedation, 272
  for procedure-related pain and anxiety, 203–204
  route of delivery for, 235
Cholecystitis, 407
Choline magnesium trisalicylate, platelet function and, 402
Choreoathetoid movements, withdrawal and, 303
Chronic hemolytic anemia, 406
Chronic pain
  assessment and evaluation of, 437–438
  multidisciplinary approach to, 437
  psychological methods in management of, 438–441
Chronic Pain Clinic, 450
Chronic pain syndromes, 403, 437
Chronic regional pain syndrome type I, 381
Circumcision, 123, 359, 361
  analgesia for, 363–366
Cleft lip repair, 175
Clonazepam for neuropathic pain, 447
Clonidine, 70, 107
  adverse effects from, 313
  in benzodiazepine withdrawal, 314
  in opioid withdrawal, 313–314
Closed head injury, 399–400
Cluster headaches, 386
Coagulopathy, 404
Coccyx, 119f
Codeine
  for mild to moderate pain, 328–329
  for otitis media, 390
  for sickle cell disease pain, 409
Cognitive-behavioral techniques in pain management, 420–424, 421*t*, 440
  distraction in, 421–422
  music therapy in, 422–423
  preparation in, 20–421
  relaxation and imagery in, 423–424
Cold therapy, 419, 425, 428
Collagen vascular diseases, 395
Colon puncture, 173
Comfort and consciousness monitoring, 196–198
COMFORT scale in assessing depth of sedation in pediatric intensive care unit, 237
Compartment syndrome, 403
Complementary therapies, 419
Complex regional pain syndrome (CRPS)-1, 440–441, 442–449
  management of, 445*f*, 447
Compression injuries, 442
Computed tomography (CT) in evaluating headaches, 382
Concurrent physical therapy, 447
Conduction blockade, 96
Conduction velocity, 428
Constipation, 394
Contingency management in chronic pain management, 440
Continuous brachial plexus anesthesia, 164
Continuous infusion for moderate to severe pain, 331
Continuous peripheral nerve catheters, 163–164
Controlled breathing, 423

Contusions, 399
Cookbook approach to sedation, 234, 274
Coping skills for neuropathic pain, 444
Coracobrachialis muscle, 148
Coronary artery disease
  atherosclerotic, 395–396
  ischemic, 395
Cortex, development of, 12–13
Corticosteroids
  effect of etomidate on, 63
  for sickle-cell pain, 410
Corticosterone, 63
Cortisol, 63
Costochondral instability, 394
Costochondritis, 392, 394
Crawford needles, 112
Crush injuries, 442
Cushing's triad, 384
Cutaneous nerve, 168
Cutaneous receptors and nerve terminals, 7–8
Cutaneous stimulation, 425, 427
Cyclooxygenase, inhibition of, 325
Cyclooxygenase type 1 (COX-1) for moderate to severe pain, 335
Cyclooxygenase type 2 (COX-2)
  for moderate to severe pain, 335
  for neuropathic pain, 446
  for traumatic pain, 402
Cyriax syndrome, 392
Cystic fibrosis, 396
Cytochrome P_{450} system, 244, 245

D

Dactylitis, 408
Day, William Henry, 382, 449
Debridements, 404
Deep peroneal nerve, 161–162
Deep sedation, 186
Demyelination injuries, 442
Dental problems, 386
Dependence
  opioids and, 294–296
  physical, 293
  psychological, 293
  treatment of, 308–315
Descending inhibitory controls, development of, 10–11
Desflurane in pediatric intensive care unit sedation, 239, 240
Desimipramine for neuropathic pain, 446
Dexmedetomidine (Precedex), 70–74
  in opioid withdrawal, 314
  in pediatric intensive care unit sedation, 273–274
Diamorphine (heroin), 105
  medical use of, 105, 107
Diaphragmatic hernia repair, 370
Diazepam, 68
  benzodiazepine withdrawal and, 296
  in pediatric intensive care unit sedation, 243
  for procedure-related pain and anxiety, 204
  tolerance and, 314
Diffuse noxious inhibitory controls (DNICs), 11
Digital block, 143, 162–163, 163*f*
Diphenhydramine, 53, 350
Direct sympathetic blockade, 448
Discharge procedure following procedures, 199*t*, 198–199
Dispositional tolerance, 292
Distal reconstructive surgery, 161

Distraction
in pain management, 422–423
in terminal illness, 455
Dolasetron, 349–350
Dorsal horn, 4
Dorsal penile nerve block for circumcision, 364, 365
Dorsal ramus, 170
Dorsal root ganglia, 8, 442
Dose titration, 303–304
DPT (Demerol, Phenergan, and Thorazine), 271–272
Dressing changes, pain associated with, 404, 405
Drug-addicted mothers, 294
Drug-drug interactions, 231
Drug incompatibilities, intravenous administration and, 235
Drug-rehabilitation centers, 312
Duodenal atresia, 367
Dysphoria, 340
Dysrhythmia, 395, 401

E

Ecchymosis, 175, 176
Eczema, migraines and, 387
ELA-Max, 80
Elective subspecialty evaluation, 381
Emergence phenomena, ketamine and, 58, 61, 210, 251
Emotional distress, 231, 419
Emotional input, 14
Empyema, 395
Endogenous analgesic systems, 15
Endogenous endorphins, 41
Endogenous opioids, 4
End-order failure, 231
Endorphins, 22
Endoscopic sinus surgery, 175
End-tidal carbon dioxide ($ETCO_2$), 196
Enflurane in pediatric intensive care unit sedation, 239, 240
Enkephalins, 43
Epidural abscess, 131
complications of, 132–133
Epidural analgesia, 95
anatomy, general considerations and dosing regimes, 110–118, 110*f*, 113*f*, 115*t*, 117*t*
needles for, 113
for neonatal pain and surgery, 370–373, 371*t*, 372*f*
for neuropathic pain, 449
for sickle-cell pain, 410
special considerations of caudal, 118–122
thoracic, 165
Epidural blockade, thoracic levels of, 133
Epidural hematoma, 131, 399
Epidural local anesthetic spread, 168
Epidural space, 95, 110, 131
Epinephrine
addition of, to peripheral regional blockade, 145
in digital block, 163
Equipment in preparing for sedation, 192, 193*t*, 194*t*
Ergotamine derivatives (dihydroergotamine), for headache pain, 389
Erythema, 65
Esophageal spasm, 394
Esophagitis, 394
Essays on Diseases in Children (Day), 382, 449

Ethyl chloride spray, 428
Ethylenediaminetetraacetic acid (EDTA), 262
Etomidate, 61–63
  in pediatric critical care unit sedation, 254
Eustachian tube, 390
  dysfunction of, 390
Eutectic mixture of local anesthetics (EMLA), 79–80, 219–220, 310
  for chest tube removal, 398
  for circumcision, 365
  for neonates, 362
Excitatory ion channels and receptors, 20–21
Excitatory neurotransmitters and receptor systems, 18–21
  excitatory ion channels and receptors, 20–21
  glutamate and its receptors, 18–19
  neurotrophins and their receptors, 18
  substance P and neurokinin receptors, 19–20
Extensor pollicis brevis tendon, 151
Extensor pollicis longus tendon, 151
Extracorporeal membrane oxygenation (ECMO), 244, 294
  sedation during, 264–265
Extracorporeal techniques, 99

F

Faces Pain Scale, 351
Familial Mediterranean fever, 396
Family, involvement of, in chronic pain management, 441
Fascia iliaca compartment block, 153–154
  complications with, 154
Femoral nerve, 151–152, 153, 157
Femoral nerve block, 143, 152–153, 152*f*, 157
Fentanyl, 44, 47, 104–105, 108, 350
  analgesic effects of, 367
  infusion rate of, 234
  for medical procedures in neonate, 361, 368*t*
  mode of operation for, 236
  for moderate to severe pain, 338
  in pediatric intensive care sedation, 264, 265, 266
  for procedure-related pain and anxiety, 207–208
  for sickle cell disease pain, 409
  starting infusion rates for, 368, 368*t*
  tolerance and, 305
  withdrawal and, 303, 308
Fetal hemoglobin, 407–408
Fibromyalgia, 394
Finger reimplantation, 147
Finnegan Score, components of, 295, 295*t*, 308–309
First-order neurons, 4
Flexor carpi radialis tendon, 150, 150*f*
Fluidotherapy, 428, 429
Flumazenil, 69
  in pediatric intensive care unit sedation, 247
  for procedure-related pain and anxiety, 217–218
Fluoride, nephrotoxicity and, 240
Focal neurologic deficits, 383
Forearm fracture, 147
Forehead reflectance sensors, 195

Foreign body removal, 161, 162
Frontal craniotomies, 174
Frontal ventriculoperitoneal shunts, 174
Functional chest pain, 396
Functional residual capacity, 60

G

GABA (γ-aminobutyric acid), 11, 22, 47, 204, 242, 253
Gabapentin
 for neuropathic pain, 405, 447
 in terminal illness, 454
Gastric distension, 394
Gastritis, 394
Gastroesophageal reflux, 394
Gastrointestinal etiologies of chest pain, 394
Gastrointestinal pain, 392
Gastroschisis, 123, 367
Gate control therapy, 430
Gate theory, 427
General anesthesia, 187
 administration of neuraxial blockade with, 95
 in combination with spinal analgesia, 128–129
Genitofemoral nerve, 153, 155
Glossopharyngeal nerve, 390
Glucuronidation, 68, 69
Glutamate and its receptors, 18–19
Glutathione peroxidase (GSH), 369
Glycopyrrolate, 61
 in pediatric intensive care unit sedation, 248, 250
Gomco clamp during circumcision, 366
G proteins, 42
Graft-versus-host disease, 350
Granisetron, 349–350
Greater auricular nerve, 176–177, 390
Greater auricular nerve block, 176–177
Greater occipital nerve block, 175
Greater trochanter, 158, 159
Guanethidine for neuropathic pain, 448
Guided imagery, 424

H

Hallucinations, ketamine and, 58, 61, 210, 251
Haloperidol in pediatric intensive care sedation, 270
Halothane in pediatric intensive care unit sedation, 239, 240
Headache diary, 388
Headaches, 381, 449–452. *See also* Migraines
 acute, 386
  recurrent, 386–387, 387
 in child with ventriculoperitoneal shunt, 450–452, 453*f*
 chronic
  nonprogressive, 387
  progressive, 387
 classification of, 386, 450, 451*t*
 differential diagnosis of, 383–385, 384*t*
 evaluating, 449, 450*t*
 organic causes of, 449
 pathogenesis of, 383
 primary, 386
 secondary, 386
 signs and symptoms suggestive of pathology in, 383, 385*t*
 tension, 386
 treatment of, 388–389

Headaches in Children (Friedman and Harms), 449
Head and neck blockade, 174–177, 174*f*, 175*f*, 176*f*, 177*f*
  complications of, 175
Head trauma, 386
Heat therapy, 419, 425, 428
Heel lance, 359, 361
  nonnutritive sucking during, 363
Heel stick, 427
Hematoma, 148
  epidural, 131, 399
  following circumcision, 364
  retroperitoneal, 157
  subdural, 399
Hemidiaphragmatic paralysis, 146, 150
Hemodialysis, 259
Hemoglobin S-β thalassemia, 407
Hemoglobinopathies, 396
  pain related to, 406–411
Hemoglobin SC disease, 407
Hepatic degradation, 96
Hepatic dysfunction, 248
Hepatic metabolism, 248
Hepatitis, 240
Hernia repair, diaphragmatic, 370
Heroin. *See* Diamorphine (heroin)
Herpes zoster, 396
Hirschsprung's disease, 128
Home care coordinator, 456
Hooking maneuver, 394
Horner syndrome, 150, 177
Hospice care, 24–25
Hydrocelectomy, 123, 172
Hydrocephalus, 385
Hydrocodone
  for mild to moderate pain, 328, 329
  for otitis media, 390
  for sickle cell disease pain, 409
Hydrolysis, 96
Hydromorphone, 44, 105, 108, 350
  for acute pain, 340
  mode of administration of, 344
  in pediatric intensive care sedation, 268
  for sickle cell disease pain, 409
Hydrotherapy, 425, 428
Hydroxyurea in fetal hemoglobin production, 408
Hydroxyzine, 53
Hyperalgesia, 24, 443
Hypercarbia, 47, 99
Hypericum perforatum for otitis media, 391
Hypertension, 385, 386, 388
Hypertriglyceridemia, 262
Hypnosis, 424
  for headache pain, 389
  in terminal illness, 455
Hypotension, 68, 133
Hypothalamus, development of, 14–15
Hypoventilation, 263
Hypovolemia, 133
Hypoxemia, 47
Hypoxia, 99

I

Ibuprofen
  for mild to moderate pain, 324, 327–328
  for moderate to severe pain, 331–332
  for otitis media, 390, 391
Iliohypogastric nerve, 155
Ilioinguinal/iliohypogastric nerve block, 172–173
  complications from, 173

Ilioinguinal nerve, 155
Imagery in pain management, 423–424
Imidazolines, 70
Indomethacin
for headache pain, 389
for moderate to severe pain, 332
Infants, non-pharmacologic pain management techniques for, 426, 426*t*
Infection, as risk in neuraxial anesthesia, 130
Inflammatory bowel disease, 381
Infraorbital block, 175
complications of, 176
Infraorbital foramen, 176
Infraorbital nerve, 175–176, 176*f*
Inguinal hernia repair, 172
Inguinal herniorrhaphy, 123
Inhalational anesthetic agents
addiction and dependency, 300–301
in pediatric intensive care unit sedation, 239–242
Inhibitory neurons, 42
Inhibitory neurotransmitters and receptor systems, 21–23
GABA and its receptors, 22
nitric oxide and its synthetases, 23
opioid peptides and their receptors, 21–22
Innate tolerance, 292
Inpatient records, 352
Insulin-like growth factor (IGF-1), 12
Intercostal nerve block, 143, 167–168, 167*f*, 170
for chest pain, 397–398
complications of, 168–169
patient positioning in, 169*f*
for slipping rib syndrome, 394
Intercostal nerves, 146, 167
Intercostal neuralgia, 396
Intercostal space, 167, 167*f*
Intercostobrachial nerve, 146, 148
Intermittent recording of respiratory rate, 196
Internal regulatory inputs, 15
International Headache Society, 450
Inter-observer reliability, 352
Interpleural analgesia, 165–167, 165*f*, 166*f*, 170
Interpleural catheter, complications from inserting, 166–167
Interscalene block, 149
Interscalene groove, 146
Intracranial hypertension, 233
Intracranial mass, 385, 386–387
Intracranial surgery, 333
Intralipid, 100
Intraneural injection, 144
signs of, 144
Intravenous administration, drug incompatibilities and, 235
Intravenous opioid therapy, for sickle cell disease pain, 409–410
Iontophoresis, 220
Ischemia, 442
Ischemic coronary artery disease, 395
Ischial tuberosity, 158, 159
Isoflurane
in pediatric intensive care unit sedation, 235, 239, 240, 241
route of delivery for, 235
withdrawal, 301–302, 308
Itching, opioid-induced, 52

J

Joint Commission on Accreditation of Healthcare Organizations (JCAHO)
  focus on pain assessment and treatment, 26
  standards for sedation monitoring, 187, 191, 192

K

Kangaroo care, 15
Kawasaki disease, 396
Ketamine, 58–61, 107
  addiction and dependency, 298–299
  anesthetic and analgesic properties of, 58–59
  bioavailability of, 59
  for burns, 405
  cardiovascular function of, 59
  effect on protective airway reflexes, 60–61
  effects on pulmonary vascular resistance, 60
  effects on respiratory mechanics, 59
  emergence phenomena from, 58, 61, 210, 251
  hallucinations and, 58, 61, 210, 251
  in pediatric critical care unit sedation, 254
  in pediatric intensive care unit sedation, 248–253
  for procedure-related pain and anxiety, 209–211
Ketorolac
  for moderate to severe pain, 332–334
  in regional blocks, 447, 449
Knockout drops, 67

L

Lacerations, 399
Laparotomy, 324
Lap belt injury, 401
Laryngospasm, 47
Learned tolerance, 292
Leukocytosis, 408
Levobupivacaine, 100, 102, 121
  in continuous brachial anesthesia, 164
  in digital block, 163
  in head and neck blockade, 174
  in ilioinguinal/iliohypogastric nerve block, 172
  in interpleural analgesia, 166
  in peripheral nerve blockade, 403
Lidocaine, 79, 96, 100, 102
  continuous infusion of, in neonates, 373
  in digital block, 163
  for neuropathic pain, 405
  in pediatric intensive care unit sedation, 241
  for procedure-related pain and anxiety, 221
  in regional blocks, 449
Ligamentum flavum, 95, 110, 118
Liposome-encapsulated lidocaine, 80
Local anesthetics, 74–79
  allergic reactions to, 103
  amides, 96, 97*t*
    bupivacaine, 76–77
    levobupivacaine, 78
    lidocaine, 75
    ropivacaine, 77–78
  classification of, 97*t*
  esters, 78–79, 96–97, 97*t*
  management of toxicity of, 100, 101*t*, 103

maximum recommended bolus doses of, 99*t*
maximum recommended continuous infusion doses of, 99*t*
in neuraxial blockade, 96–103
in pediatric intensive care unit sedation, 241
in peripheral regional blockade, 144–145, 145*t*
for procedure-related pain and anxiety, 218–221
rate of absorption from various administration sites, 98–99, 98*t*
uptake of, 97–98
Local erythema, 265
Lorazepam, 68
for burns, 405
in pediatric intensive care unit sedation, 236, 245–247
for procedure-related pain and anxiety, 204
tolerance and, 314
Lumbar plexus, 151, 154
Lumbar plexus block, 153, 155–157, 155*f*
complications with, 157
needle in, 155–156
nerve stimulator in, 155–156
Lumbar puncture, 424, 452–453
Lumbar spinal injury, 401
Lumbar sympathetic block for neuropathic pain, 449
LY274614, 307
Lytic cocktail, 215–216
for procedure-related pain and anxiety, 215–216

M

Magnesium, tolerance and, 307
Magnetic resonance imaging in evaluating headaches, 382
Malignant hyperthermia, 153, 241
Mallampati Classification, 189
Malnutrition, 231
Malrotation repair, 367
Massage, 419, 425, 429
Mastoidectomy, 176
Maternal conditioning, 16
Mechanical ventilation, sedation during, 232–233, 243, 252, 264, 265, 274
Medial malleolus, 161
Medical illnesses
acute, 323
treatment of acute pain associated with, 381–411
burns, 403–406
chest pain, 392, 393*t*, 394–398
headache pain, 382–389, 384*t*, 385*t*
hemoglobinopathies, 406–411
otitis media, 390–391
traumatic injury, 398–403
Meningitis, as risk in spinal anesthesia, 130–131
Meningomyelocele, 123
Meperidine (Demerol), 48, 50, 105, 107
for acute pain, 340–341
analgesic effects of, 367
in pediatric intensive care sedation, 268–269
for procedure-related pain and anxiety, 207
for sickle cell disease pain, 409
Mepivacaine, 96

Methadone (Dolobid)
for acute pain, 340
mode of administration of, 344
in pediatric intensive care sedation, 268
for sickle cell disease pain, 409
withdrawal and, 310–312
Methemoglobinemia, 80
risk of, in neonates, 362
Methohexital, 63–64
in pediatric critical care unit sedation, 254
in pediatric intensive care sedation, 263
for procedure-related pain and anxiety, 211–212
Methylprednisolone for sickle-cell pain, 410
Metoclopramide, 349
Mexiletine for neuropathic pain, 405
Michigan, University of, Sedation Scale, 197, 197*t*
Mickey Finns, 67
Midazolam
benzodiazepine withdrawal and, 297
for burns, 405
mode of operation for, 236
in pediatric critical care unit sedation, 254
in pediatric intensive care unit sedation, 243–245, 265
for procedure-related pain and anxiety, 204–206, 210
route of delivery for, 235
withdrawal and, 303
Migraines, 381, 383, 386–387. *See also* Headaches
associated conditions, 387
classification of, 387–388
gender and, 387
Mild to moderate pain
inpatient setting, 331–335
outpatient setting, 325–331
treatment of, 324
Milk of Magnesia, 349
Mindfulness mediation, 424–425
Minimum alveolar concentration (MAC), 300
Minute ventilation, 60
Mixed agonist/antagonists, 42
MK-801, 307
Moderate sedation, 186
Moderate to severe pain in inpatient setting, 336–350
Mogen clamp during circumcision, 364, 366
Monitoring during sedation, 192–199
comfort and consciousness, 196–198, 197*t*
post-procedure and discharge criteria, 198–199, 199*t*
record keeping, 199
Monotherapy, 247
Morphine, 43, 49, 105, 109, 111
analgesic effects of, 367
antinociceptive effects of, 307
half-life of, 43, 367
for medical procedures in neonate, 361, 368*t*
metabolism route, 43, 44
for mild to moderate pain, 329
mode of administration of, 344
for moderate to severe pain, 339, 339*t*
in pediatric intensive care unit sedation, 236, 267–268
for procedure-related pain and anxiety, 207
for sickle cell disease pain, 409
side effects associated with, 107

starting infusion rates for, 368, 368*t*
subcutaneous administration of, 345–346
Morphine-6-glucuronide (M6G), 43, 268–269, 339–340
Motion sickness, migraines and, 387
MS Contin, 312
Multidimensional assessment of chronic pain, 441
Multidisciplinary approach to chronic pain, 437, 448–449
Muscle atrophy, 429
Muscle spasm, 392
Musculocutaneous nerve block, 147, 148
Musculoskeletal pain syndromes, 394
Musculoskeletal trauma, control of pain related to, 400
Music therapy, 422–423
Myocardial contusion, 401
Myocardial depression, 99
Myocardial dysfunction, 133
Myocardial ischemia, 241, 395, 396, 401
Myocarditis, 395
Myoclonic movements, 56, 62, 239, 258
withdrawal and, 303

N

Nalbuphine (Nubain), 43, 53, 109
for moderate to severe pain, 336
Nalmefene for procedure-related pain and anxiety, 217
Nalmefine (Revex), 43, 45
Naloxone (Narcan), 43, 44–45, 53, 109
effects of, 51
overdoses of, 51–52
for procedure-related pain and anxiety, 216–217, 218
for respiratory depression, 347–348
Nasal reconstruction, 175
Nausea and vomiting
acupuncture for postoperative, 431
from opioids, 349
N-desmethyldiazepam, in pediatric intensive care sedation, 243
Neck blockade. *See* Head and neck blockade
Neck pain, 400
Necrotizing enterocolitis, 363
Negative aspiration, 103
Neonatal abstinence syndrome (NAS), 294–295
Neonatal Facial Coding System, 360
Neonatal Infant Pain Scale, 360, 361*t*
Neonatal intensive care unit (NICU), preterm and term neonates in, 359
Neonatal pain management, 24–26, 357–374
for acute pain and surgery, 366–373, 371*t*, 372*f*
assessment of acute pain in neonates, 359–360, 361*t*
for circumcision, 363–366
for painful medical procedures, 361–363
Neonates, assessment of acute pain in, 359–360, 361*t*
Nephrotoxicity, 404
Nerve block at the wrist, 150–151, 150*f*
Nerve growth factor (NGF), 7
Nerve of Arnold, 390
Neuraxial blockade, 95–134
administered with general anesthesia, 95
adverse effects of, 130–133
for burns, 404

for chest pain, 397–398
increased use of, 95
medications for, local anesthetic agents, 96–103
opioids for, 106*t*
potential contraindications to, 95, 96*t*
for sickle-cell pain, 410
technical complications of, 129*t*
for traumatic pain, 402–403
Neurogenesis, 7
Neurogranin, 12
Neurokinin receptors, 19–20
Neuroleptic malignant syndrome, 271
Neurologic imaging in evaluating headaches, 382, 388
Neuromuscular blocking agents, 143, 233
Neuronal depolarization, 96
Neuronal hyperpolarization, 242, 253
Neuropathic pain, 405, 429, 442, 443*t*
management of, 444–445, 444*t*
Neurotrophic factors, 7–8
Neurotrophins and their receptors, 18
Nifedipine for neuropathic pain, 447
Nitric oxide and its synthetases, 23
Nitrous oxide, 65–67
for procedure-related pain and anxiety, 214–215
N-methyl-D-aspartate (NMDA) receptors, 12, 18–19, 59, 107
in terminal illness, 456
tolerance and, 307
Nociceptive nerve factors, 8
Nociceptive nerve tracks, 10
Nociceptive neurotransmission, 42
Nociceptive pain, 442, 443*t*
Nociceptive receptors, 3
Nociceptive system, 3
Nociceptor-specific sodium channels, 7, 8
Nonnutritive sucking, 15, 362–363, 426–427, 426*t*
Nonopioid agents, 107
Non-pharmacologic techniques in pain management, 222, 419–432
biophysical techniques, 425–426, 425*t*
acupuncture, 430–431
cold therapy, 428
cutaneous stimulation, 427
heat therapy, 428
hydrotherapy, 428
massage, 429
nonnutritive sucking, 426–427, 426*t*
therapeutic exercise, 429
transcutaneous electrical nerve stimulation, 430
cognitive-behavioral techniques, 420–424, 421*t*
distraction, 421–422
music therapy, 422–423
preparation, 420–421
relaxation and imagery, 423–424
Nonsteroidal antiinflammatory drug (NSAID), 326*t*
adverse effects of, 334–335, 334*t*
for burns, 404
for chest pain, 392
for mild pain, 454
for mild to moderate pain, 324, 325, 382
for neuropathic pain, 446
platelet function and, 401–402
in terminal illness, 454
for traumatic injury pain, 400
Norketamine, 59
in pediatric intensive care unit sedation, 248
renal excretion of, 248

Normeperidine
for acute pain, 340
in pediatric intensive care unit sedation, 50, 269
for sickle cell disease pain, 409
Nortriptyline for neuropathic pain, 405, 446
NPO guidelines, 190–191, 190*t*
Nurse-controlled analgesia
for chest pain, 397
for traumatic pain, 402

O

Occipital pain, 175
Omphalocele, 367
Oncologic diseases, pain associated with, 381
Ondansetron, 349
Ongoing assessment of chronic pain, 440
Ongoing education, 352
Open-ended questions in assessing chronic pain, 437
Operative myringotomy, 391
Opioids, 104–109, 216–217
adverse effects of, 45, 46*t*, 47–53, 52*t*, 107–109, 108*t*, 109*t*, 326, 346–350, 346*t*
agent, mode, and route of administration, 338–343
age-related respiratory effects of, 367
antagonists, 44–45
for burns, 404
cardiorespiratory effects of, 3
cardiovascular effects of, 49–50
chemistry and metabolism, 43–44
for chest pain, 397
classification of, 337*t*
dependence and withdrawal, 294–296
gastrointestinal effects of, 52
genitourinary effect of, 52
hemodynamic effects, 49
itching induced by, 52
long-term use of, 456
methadone in withdrawal from, 310–312
for mild to moderate pain, outpatient setting, 325–331
for moderate to severe pain, inpatient setting, 331–335
in modulating cytokine production, 53
for neonatal pain and surgery, 366–369
neuraxial, 104
for neuropathic pain, 446
non-intravenous administration of, 343–346
in pediatric intensive care unit sedation, 265–270
pharmacokinetic characteristics of, 51–52, 52*t*
potency and half-life of, 337*t*
for procedure-related pain and anxiety, 207–208, 216–217
receptors, 21–22, 41–43, 42*t*
recommended dosing ranges for, 106*t*
in reducing intraocular pressure, 51
for severe pain, 382
short-term use of, 52–53
tolerance and, 304–305
for traumatic pain, 402
withdrawal from, 313–314
Opisthotonic posturing, 56, 258
Opium, tincture of, in opioid withdrawal, 312
Oral administration, 344
Oral methadone taper, 292
Orchidopexy, 123, 172

Orogustatory inputs, 15
Orthostatic hypotension, 447
Osmotic agents, 349
Otic drops for otitis media, 390–391
Otitis externa, acute, 390
Otitis media
  acute, 390
  pain associated with, 390–391
  recurrent, 391
  serous, 391
Otolaryngologic surgery, 333
Otoplasty, 176
Oxalozepines, 70
Oxazepam in pediatric intensive care sedation, 243
Oxycodone
  for mild to moderate pain, 328, 329, 382
  for otitis media, 390
  for sickle cell disease pain, 409
Oxycontin for mild to moderate pain, 329
Oxymorphone, 350

P

Pacifiers, sucrose, 362–363, 365
Pain. *See also* Acute pain
  anatomy of, 3–6, 5*f*, 6*f*
  decreased threshold to, 443
  intensity of, 421–422
  measurement of, 350–352
  multidimensional nature of, 438–439
  perception of, 3, 4, 6, 419, 422
  physiology of, 17
  reaction to, 323
  sleep and, 438
  during terminal stages of illness, 454–456, 455*t*
Pain Coping Questionnaire, 438
Pain system, development of, 7–9
Pain threshold, regulation of, 23–24
Palliative care, 24–25
Palmaris longus tendon, 150, 150*f*
Para-amino benzoic acid (PABA), 103
Para-amino phenol derivatives, 325
Parascalene approach to the brachial plexus, 149–150, 149*f*
  complications of, 150
Paravertebral nerve block, 170–172, 171*f*
  continuous, 170
  patient positioning, 171
Paravertebral space, 170, 171
Parecoxib
  for moderate to severe pain, 335
  for neuropathic pain, 446
Paregoric in opioid withdrawal, 312
Parenteral therapy for otitis media, 390–391
Patellar kick, 153, 156
Patient-controlled analgesia (PCA), 236
  for acute pain, 340, 341–343
  for burns, 406
  for chest pain, 397
  for moderate to severe pain, 331
  in terminal illness, 454
  for traumatic pain, 402
Patient-controlled anxiolysis, 236
Patient variables, pain and, 323
Pediatric gastroenterologist, evaluation by, 381
Pediatric intensive care unit (PICU)
  opioid tolerance and withdrawal in, 294
  patient care in, 231, 291
  pharmacodynamic tolerance in, 292–293
  variability in patient, 231–233

Pediatric intensive care unit sedation, 231–276
agents for, 233–235, 233*t*, 234*t*, 238–239
α_2-adrenergic agonists, 272–274
barbiturates, 263–265
benzodiazepines, 242–247
butyrophenones, 270–272
chloral hydrate, 272
inhalational anesthetic, 239–242
ketamine, 248–253
opioids, 265–270
phenothiazines, 270–272
propofol, 253–263
mode of administration options for, 235–236
preparation for, 231, 232*t*
route delivery options for, 235, 235*t*
tools for assessing depth of, 236–238
Pediatric neurologist, referral to, 381
Pediatric pain management, 24–26
PedMIDAS, 438
Pentazocine (Talwin) for moderate to severe pain, 336
Pentobarbital, 63
benzodiazepine withdrawal and, 297
in pediatric intensive care unit sedation, 236, 264
Pericardial effusion, 395, 401
Pericardial tamponade, 395
Pericarditis, 395
Peripheral nerve blockade
for sickle-cell pain, 410
for traumatic pain, 400, 402–403
Peripheral nerves, 8
injury to, 442
Peripheral nociceptors, 4
Peripheral pain mechanisms, 7–9
Peripheral regional blockade, 143–178
addition of epinephrine, 145
blockade of the thorax and abdomen
ilioinguinal/iliohypogastric nerve block, 172–173, 173*f*
intercostal nerve block, 167–168, 167*f*, 169*f*, 170
interpleural analgesia, 165–167, 165*f*, 166*f*,
paravertebral block, 170–172, 171*f*
for chest pain, 397–398
continuous peripheral nerve catheters, 163–164
digital block, 162–163, 163*f*
dosing guidelines in, 144–145, 145*t*, 156*t*
general techniques in, 143–145
head and nerve blockade, 174–177, 174*f*, 175*f*, 176*f*, 177*f*
lower extremity blockade, 151–152, 151*f*
ankle block, 161–162, 161*f*
fascia iliaca compartment block, 153–154, 154*f*
femoral nerve block, 152–153, 152*f*
lumbar plexus block, 155–157, 155*f*
sciatic nerve block, 157–160, 158*f*, 159*f*, 160*f*
needle insertion in, 143–144
nerve stimulator in, 143
reducing the risks of toxicity, 144–145
safety of, 143
success of, 144
upper extremity blockade
anatomy of brachial plexus, 146–147
axillary approach to brachial plexus, 147–149, 148*f*

nerve block at the wrist, 150–151, 150*f*
parascalene approach to the brachial plexus, 149–150, 149*f*
uses of, 143
Peripheral sensory receptors, 4
Peripheral vasodilation, 240
Permissive hypercapnia, 232
Peroneal nerve, 162
Personnel in preparing for sedation, 191–192
Pethidine for acute pain, 340
Phantom pain, 403
Pharmacodynamic tolerance, 292
Pharmacokinetic studies, 231
Phenacetin, 325
Phenobarbital
for benzodiazepine withdrawal, 314–315
in treating infants of drug-addicted mothers, 313
Phenothiazines, 45, 349
in pediatric intensive care unit sedation, 270–272
in treating infants of drug-addicted mothers, 313
Phenoxybenzamine for neuropathic pain, 447
Phentolamine
in diagnosing chronic pain, 443–444
for neuropathic pain, 448
Phenylethylamines, 70
Phenytoin, 100
for neuropathic pain, 447
Phonophobia, migraine headaches and, 388
Photophobia, migraine headaches and, 388
Phrenic nerve block, 177
Physical dependence, 293
Physical therapy, 425, 426, 428, 430
for neuropathic pain, 444, 448
Pleural effusion, 395, 400
Pleuritic pain, 332, 394–395
Pleuritis, 395
Plexus analgesia, 164
Pneumonia, 395
Pneumothorax, 168, 395, 400
risk of, 146
Polymodal nociceptors (PMNS), 7, 8
Popliteal fossa approach to the sciatic nerve, 159–160, 160*f*
Popliteal triangle, 160, 160*f*
Post-anesthetic apnea, 95
Post-dural puncture headache, 131–132
Postoperative nausea and vomiting, acupuncture for, 431
Postoperative pain, 323
Postoperative respiratory dysfunction, 123
Post-procedure monitoring and discharge criteria, 198–199, 199*t*
Prazosin for neuropathic pain, 447
Precordial catch syndrome, 394
Premature Infant Pain Profile, 360
Pre-sedation assessment, 187–191, 188*t*
Priapism, 410
Prilocaine, 79
Primary headaches, 386
Procedural sedation, 187
Procedure-related pain and anxiety, 185–222, 452
anesthetic agents
barbiturates, 211–212
nitrous oxide, 214–215
propofol, 213–214
combination of agents, lytic cocktail, 215–216

definitions in, 186–187
local and topical anesthetics, 218–221
monitoring during sedation, 192–196
choice of agent, 200, 201*t*, 202
comfort and consciousness monitoring, 196–198, 197*t*
post-procedure monitoring and discharge criteria, 198–199, 199*t*
record keeping, 199
non-pharmacologic methods, 222
opioid and benzodiazepine reversal agent, 216
benzodiazepine antagonists, 217–219
opioid antagonists, 216–217
preparation for sedation
equipment, 192
personnel, 191–192
pre-sedation assessment, 187–191, 188*t*, 189*t*, 190*t*
sedation for, 185, 185*t*
during cardiac catheterization, 202
sedatives
α-adrenergic agonists, 206–207
analgesic agents, 207–208
benzodiazepines, 204–206
chloral hydrate, 203–204
ketamine, 209–211
Progressive disability, 429
Prolonged QT syndrome, 446
Promethazine, 349
Propofol, 45, 54–58
addiction and dependency, 299–300
adverse effects with, 257*t*
for burns, 405
cardiovascular effects of, 55–56
initial formulation of, 58
neurologic effects of, 56
pain with administration of, 57–58
in pediatric critical care unit sedation, 254, 255–258
in pediatric intensive care unit sedation, 235, 253–263, 265
pharmacodynamic profile of, 54–55
physiologic effects of, 55
for procedure-related pain and anxiety, 213–214
as respiratory depressant, 56
route of delivery for, 235
Propofol infusion syndrome, 57, 258–260
Propranolol for benzodiazepine withdrawal, 314
Propylene glycol, 247
Prostaglandin synthesis inhibitors, 325, 325*t*, 326
for mild to moderate pain, 324
agent and route of administration, 326–331
outpatient setting, 325–331
for moderate to severe pain, inpatient setting, 331–335
Protective airway reflexes, effect of ketamine on, 250
Pruritus, 53, 103, 108, 340, 350
Pseudotumor, 385
Psoas muscle, 154
Psychological dependence, 293
Psychological methods in chronic pain management, 438–441, 448
Psychosocial stress, headaches and, 387
Pulmonary edema, 51–52
Pulmonary embolism, 395, 400
Pulmonary processes as cause of chest pain, 394
Pulmonary vascular resistance (PVR), 60, 233, 249
Pulse oximetry, 195

Q

Quantitative pain-rating scales, 437

R

Radial nerve block, 151
Radiopaque catheters, 371
Raj approach to the sciatic nerve, 158–149, 159*f*
Rami communicantes, 170
Ramsay score in assessing depth of sedation in pediatric intensive care unit, 237, 274
Reactive airway disease, 395
Record keeping, monitoring and, 199
Recurrent otitis media, 391
Recurring painful crises, 406
Reduced joint mobility, 429
Reflex sympathetic dystrophy, 381, 442
Reflex tachycardia, 240–241
Refractory status epilepticus, 258, 264
Regional (Bier) blocks, 447, 449
Rehabilitative approach to chronic pain management, 439
Relaxation
  for neuropathic pain, 444, 448
  in pain management, 423–424
Reliability, inter-observer, 352
Remifentanil, 44, 47
  for moderate to severe pain, 338
  in pediatric intensive care sedation, 266–267
  for procedure-related pain and anxiety, 208
  tolerance and, 305
Renal dysfunction, 259
Renal failure, 259, 347
Renal papillary necrosis, 325
Respiratory depression, 105, 346–347, 348
  from morphine, 367
  risk of, 43
Respiratory distress, 47
Respiratory rate, intermittent recording of, 196
Retroperitoneal hematoma, 157
Reverse inspiratory-expiratory ratio ventilation, 232
Reye syndrome, 325
Rhabdomyolysis, 259
Rhinoplasty, 175
RICE (rest, ice, compression, and elevation) regimen, 428
Rocuronium, 65
Rofecoxib (Vioxx)
  for moderate to severe pain, 335
  for neuropathic pain, 446
Ropivacaine, 100, 102, 121
  in continuous brachial anesthesia, 164
  in digital block, 163
  in head and neck blockade, 174
  in ilioinguinal/iliohypogastric nerve block, 173
  in interpleural analgesia, 166
  in peripheral nerve blockade, 403

S

Sacral cornua, 118, 119*f*
Sacral hiatus, 118
Sacral plexus, 151, 152
Sacrococcygeal membrane, 118
Sacrum, 119*f*
Salicylates, 326*t*
  for mild to moderate pain, 325
Saphenous nerve, 151–152, 157, 161
Scalp, innervation of, 174, 174*f*

Scalp excisions, 174
Scarpa's triangle, 153
School absence, headache pain as cause of, 382
Sciatic groove, 159
Sciatic nerve, 17, 152, 158, 159
Sciatic nerve block, 157–160
 popliteal fossa approach to, 159–160, 160*f*
 posterior approach to, 157–158, 158*f*
 Raj approach to, 158–159, 159*f*
Secondary headaches, 386
Second-order neurons, 4, 10
Sedation. *See also* Pediatric intensive care unit sedation
 during cardiac catheterization, 202
 deep, 186
 during mechanical ventilation, 232–233, 243, 252, 264, 265, 274
 moderate, 186
 monitoring during, 192–199
  comfort and consciousness, 196–198, 197*t*
  post-procedure, and discharge criteria, 198–199, 199*t*
  record keeping, 199
 pre-assessment, 187–191, 198*t*, 199*t*, 200*t*
 preparation for
  equipment, 192, 193*t*, 194*t*
  personnel, 191–192
 procedural, 187
 procedures requiring, in children, 185*t*
 route of delivery for, 200, 202
Sedatives and analgesics, 41–81
 α-adrenergic agonists, 206–207
 barbiturates, 63–65
 benzodiazepines, 68–70, 204–206
 chloral hydrate, 67–68, 203–204
 choosing agent, 200, 201*t*, 202
 dexmedetomidine, 70–74
 etomidate, 61–63
 ketamine, 58–61
 local anesthetics, 74–79
  amides, 96, 97*t*, 76–77
   bupivacaine, 76–77
   levobupivacaine, 78
   lidocaine, 75
   ropivacaine, 77–78
  esters, 78–79, 96–97, 97*t*
 nitrous oxide, 65–67
 opioids
  adverse effects of, 45, 46*t*, 47–50, 50–53, 52*t*
  antagonists, 44–45
  chemistry and metabolism, 43–44
  receptors, 41–43, 42*t*
 propofol, 54–58
 topical anesthesia, 79–80
Seizure disorders, 62, 258
Seldinger technique, 163–164
Self-hypnosis for sickle-cell pain, 410
Self-report pain scales, 351
Semimembranosus tendon, 159
Semitendinosus tendon, 159
Sensory neurons, 8, 18
Serotonin, 4
 headaches and level of, 383
Severe pain, treatment of, 324
Sevoflurane, 145
 in pediatric intensive care unit sedation, 239, 240
Sickle cell disease, 350, 396
 pain related to, 406–411
Sickle cell trait, 407

Sickle cell vaso-occlusive crisis, 324, 332, 381, 407, 408, 424, 428
Signal Extraction Technology, 195
Signaling proteins, 42
Sinus thrombosis, 385
Situational factors, influence on pain expression, 439–440
Skull fractures, 399
Sleep, pain and, 438
Slipping rib syndrome, 392, 394
Small-bowel puncture, 173
Social stigmata, migraine headaches and, 387
Sodium metabisulfite, 262
Sodium pentobarbital for procedure-related pain and anxiety, 212
Somatic pain, long-term effects of, 16–17
Somatosensory input, 14
Somnolence, 105
Spinal analgesia, 95, 123–129
  addition of epinephrine to spinal solution, 127
  in combination with general anesthesia, 128–129
  comparison with causal epidural anesthesia, 122*t*
  duration of, 127
  meningitis as risk in, 130–131
  success of, 126–127
  techniques of, 123–127
Spinal blockade, thoracic levels of, 133
Spinal cord compression, 452
Spinal cord injury, 400, 401
Spinal local anesthetic spread, 168
Spinal nerve tracks, 10
Spinal pain mechanisms, 9–11
Spinal projection neurons, 10
Spinothalamic afferents, 14
Splenic infarction, 407
Status epilepticus, 258
Stellate ganglion block for neuropathic pain, 449
Sternocleidomastoid muscle, 177
Steroids in terminal illness, 454
Stranger anxiety, 185
Stroke, 385
Subarachnoid block, 177
Subarachnoid space, 95
Subcutaneous administration, 344–345
Subcutaneous ring block for circumcision, 365
Subdural hematoma, 399
Substance P, 4, 19–20, 272
  headache pain and, 383
Sucrose pacifiers, 362–363, 365, 427
Sudden cardiac death, 395
Sufentanil
  for moderate to severe pain, 338
  in pediatric intensive care sedation, 47, 106–107, 266
  tolerance and, 305
Sumatriptan (Imitrex) for headache pain, 389
Superior triangle, 159
Supraorbital nerve, 174
Supraorbital notch, 174
Supraspinal pain mechanisms, 11–17
  development of the cortex, 12–13
  development of the hypothalamus, 14–15
  development of the thalamus, 14
  endogenous analgesic systems, 15
  long-term effects of somatic pain, 16–17
  long-term effects of visceral pain, 15–16

Supratrochlear block, 174
Supratrochlear nerve, 174
Sural nerve, 162
Surgery
  acetaminophen for neonatal, 369–370
  epidural analgesia for neonatal, 370–373, 371*t*, 372*f*
  opioid analgesics for neonatal, 366–369, 368*t*
Swaddling, 427
Sympathectomy, 172
Sympathetic blockade, 95, 448
Sympathetic chain, 170
Sympathetic hyperactivity, 442
Syndactyly repair, 147
Systemic bacteria, contaminated propofol and, 261

T

Tachycardia after meperidine administration, 50
Tactile allodynia, 443
Tamponade, 401
TCAs, in terminal illness, 454
Tension headaches, 386–387
Terminal illness, pain during, 454–456, 455*t*
Tetracaine, 79, 80
  adrenaline, and cocaine (TAC), 220
Texidor's twinge, 394
Thalamic neurons, 13
Thalamic processing, 4, 6
Thalamus, development of, 14
Therapeutic exercise, 429
Thermal injury, 428
Thiamylal, 63, 64
  in pediatric intensive care sedation, 263
Thiobarbiturates, 63–64
Thiopental, 63, 64
  in pediatric intensive care sedation, 263
  for procedure-related pain and anxiety, 212
Thoracic blockade, 133
Thoracic epidural analgesia, 165
Thoracic epidural space, 112
Thoracotomy, 324
Thorax, blockade of, 165–167, 165*f*, 166*f*
3-in-1 block, 153
Thrombophlebitis, 65, 265
Tibial nerve, 162
Tidal volume, 60
Tissue-damaging procedures, pain of, in neonates, 359
Tissue injury, long-term effects of early, 8–9
Toe amputation, 161
Tolerance, 291–293. See also Withdrawal
  barbiturates, 298
  benzodiazepines, 296–297, 305
  defined, 291–292
  dispositional, 292
  documentation with Bispectral Index, 292–293
  factors affecting the development of, 304–307
  innate, 292
  ketamine, 298–299
  learned, 292
  opioids, 294–296, 304–305
  pharmacodynamic, 292
  treatment of, 308–315
Tonic-clonic movements, 48
Topical anesthesia, 79–80
  for otitis media, 390–391
  for procedure-related pain and anxiety, 218–221

Toradol for moderate to severe pain, 332
Tourniquet, 447–448
Tramadol, for mild to moderate pain, 330–331
Transcutaneous electrical nerve stimulation (TENS), 427, 429, 430
  for headache pain, 389
  for neuropathic pain, 448, 445–446
Transection injuries, 442
Transient neurologic deficit, 132
Transverse abdominal contusion, 401
Trauma, 323
Traumatic injury, 442
  abdominal pain following, 401
  chest pain and, 392
  headaches associated with, 383
  pain related to acute, 398–403
Trichloroethanol, 67–68
  in pediatric intensive care unit sedation, 272
Tricyclic antidepressants, 68, 272
  for neuropathic pain, 405, 446
Trifluoroacetic acid, 240
Trigeminal nerve, 175, 390
Tumor, brain, 386, 449
Tumor involvement, 452
Tuohy needles, 112, 164, 171
Tylenol #2, for mild to moderate pain, 328
Tylenol #3, for mild to moderate pain, 328
Tylenol #4, for mild to moderate pain, 328
Tympanic membrane, 390

U

Ulcer disease, 394
Ulnar artery, 151
Ulnar nerve, 146–147
  limited anesthesia of, 146
Ulnar nerve block, 151
Universal reversal, 51
Unmyelinated C fibers, 7, 8
Upper airway assessment, 188
Urinary retention, 105
Urticaria, 103, 350

V

Valdecoxib (Bextra), for moderate to severe pain, 335
Vanilloid receptor (VR1), 7, 8
Varni-Thompson Pediatric Pain Questionnaire, 437
Vascular insufficiency, 95
Vascular puncture, 148, 168
Vasoconstrictors, 74
Venipuncture, 361, 427, 453
Venous puncture, 150
Ventricular dysrhythmias, 99
Ventriculoperitoneal shunt, headaches in child with, 450–452, 453*f*
Vervascum thapsus, for otitis media, 391
Vicoprofen, for mild to moderate pain, 329
Viral illnesses, 386
Visceral input, 14
Visceral pain, 407
  long-term effects of, 15–16
Visual guided imagery for neuropathic pain, 444
Vomiting. *See* Nausea and vomiting

W

Waldon/Varni Pediatric Pain Coping Inventory, 438
Windup phenomenon, 23
Withdrawal, 293. *See also* Tolerance

barbiturates, 298
benzodiazepines, 296–297
central nervous system manifestations of, 302
clinical signs and symptoms of, 293, 301–304
fentanyl and, 303, 308
gastrointestinal manifestations of, 302
inhalational anesthetic agents, 300–301
isoflurane, 301–302
ketamine, 298–299
opioids, 294–296
pentobarbital, 298
propofol, 299–300
risk factors for, 308
sympathic nervous system signs and symptoms, 302
World Health Organization, ladder for pain treatment, 323–324, 324*t*, 410, 454
Wound infection, contaminated propofol and, 261
Wrist, nerve block at, 150–151, 150*f*

Y

Yoga, 419